BULLETS

IN

EMERGENCY
MEDICINE

REVIEW AND REMINDERS IN PURSUIT
OF EVIDENCE-BASED DECISIONS

BEENA WYCLIFFE, MD
Department of Emergency Medicine
Paradise Valley Hospital
National City, CA

PETER ROSEN, MD
Department of Emergency Medicine
Beth Israel Deaconess Medical Center
Boston, MA

JONES AND BARTLETT PUBLISHERS
Sudbury, Massachusetts
BOSTON   TORONTO   LONDON   SINGAPORE

World Headquarters

Jones and Bartlett Publishers
40 Tall Pine Drive
Sudbury, MA 01776
978-443-5000
info@jbpub.com
www.jbpub.com

Jones and Bartlett Publishers
Canada
6339 Ormindale Way
Mississauga, Ontario L5V 1J2
CANADA

Jones and Bartlett Publishers
International
Barb House, Barb Mews
London W6 7PA
UK

Jones and Bartlett's books and products are available through most bookstores and online booksellers. To contact Jones and Bartlett Publishers directly, call 800-832-0034, fax 978-443-8000, or visit our website, www.jbpub.com.

Substantial discounts on bulk quantities of Jones and Bartlett's publications are available to corporations, professional associations, and other qualified organizations. For details and specific discount information, contact the special sales department at Jones and Bartlett via the above contact information or send an email to specialsales@jbpub.com.

Production Credits
Executive Publisher: Christopher Davis
Senior Acquisitions Editor: Nancy Anastasi Duffy
Production Editor: Rachel Rossi
Senior Editorial Assistant: Jessica Acox
Associate Marketing Manager: Ilana Goddess
Cover Design: Brian Moore
V.P. of Manufacturing and Inventory Control: Therese Connell
Composition: Shawn Girsberger
Cover Image: © Digital Vision/age Fotostock
Printing and Binding: Malloy, Inc.
Cover Printing: Malloy, Inc.

Library of Congress Cataloging-in-Publication Data
Wycliffe, Beena.
  Bullets in emergency medicine : review and reminders in pursuit of evidence-based decisions / by Beena Wycliffe and Peter Rosen.
    p. ; cm.
  Includes bibliographical references and index.
  ISBN-13: 978-0-7637-5416-7
  ISBN-10: 0-7637-5416-1
  1. Emergency medicine--Handbooks, manuals, etc. 2. Evidence-based medicine--Handbooks, manuals, etc. I. Rosen, Peter, 1935- II. Title.
  [DNLM: 1. Emergency Medicine--methods--Handbooks. 2. Emergencies--Handbooks. 3. Emergency Treatment--Handbooks. 4. Evidence-Based Medicine--Handbooks. WB 39 W997b 2009]
  RC86.8W93 2009
  616.02'5--dc22
                            2008018599

6048

Printed in the United States of America
12 11 10 09 08   10 9 8 7 6 5 4 3 2 1

Contents

Preface

The genesis of this book started during my emergency medicine residency while I was preparing for the yearly in-service examinations. I found it easier to review quickly once the ideas and concepts were organized and grouped together. In keeping with that experience, the concepts presented in this text are intended to be simple, terse, and focused. In addition to studying review books and practicing questions, you may use this book as a last-minute study preparation tool before taking the examinations

The book contains the following five sections:

I. Presenting Signs and Symptoms—A typical scenario is presented followed by the disease entity. The best way to get the most out of this section is to cover the right column with a sheet of paper and test yourself to determine how many of the answers you know.

II. Similar or Confusing Terms—These terms are often confused with one another. By grouping them together, they can easily be referred to while reading the rest of the book, or while preparing for the examinations.

III. Emergency Medicine Reminders—These reminders are presented in a form comparable to the sort of quick decision-making ideas that one runs through clinically when trying to solve the clinical puzzle. The concepts are short, and treatments are neither detailed nor accompanied by drug dosages. Images and electrocardiograms (EKGs) are provided throughout this section.

IV. Most Commons in Emergency Medicine—This section is most useful for the student, who needs to quickly learn some of the dialect and jargon of clinical emergency medicine.

V. Practice Questions—The book contains an examination consisting of 55 multiple-choice questions. Some of them have stimuli such as x-ray studies, or EKG tracings. The best way to use the questions is to take them as a test before reading anything in the book. Check the answers, but don't look at any explanations. Look up the subject categories in the text. Then retake the examination and read all the explanations. Each question has four possible answers. There is an explanation for each of the possible choices, right or wrong. Take the test again.

This book is not meant to be a finished product. New abbreviations, eponyms, and mnemonics are constantly being created, not to mention all the ones with which you, the readers, are familiar and use yourself that don't appear in this book. We hope you will feel free to submit your own favorites, or argue about our definitions.

We believe this book is a good way to review not only for in-service and board examinations, but also for recertification.

Good luck, and we hope you will find this material useful.

—Beena Wycliffe, MD

Acknowledgment

I am deeply honored to have the opportunity to coauthor this book with Dr. Peter Rosen (aka THE ROSEN), and will be forever grateful for all his hard work. About 2–3 years ago, I asked Dr. Rosen at a conference in San Diego if he'd kindly look at my manuscript. He thought it was good and gave me some ideas. Some time later when J&B Publishers accepted my manuscript for publication it became necessary to find a medical editor. This wasn't easy, but it was time-consuming. One day at work, sitting at my desk (between curing fibromyalgia) and staring at the bookshelf with Rosen's three volume textbooks staring back at me, I gathered enough courage and texted him. I was in shock (yeah, and awe) when I got a return text from Dr. Rosen. I am still unsure what surprised me more: the fact that he answered my text, or that he knew how to send text messages. This turned out to be a good shift after all, as he asked me to send a disc for review and soon thereafter graciously (not to be confused with regret-fully) accepted my request to edit and coauthor the manuscript as well.

For all those who are currently working on projects and are afraid that no one knows you exist, and even if you have never published anything before, I highly recommend that you attend the professional society con-ferences, and seek out people after their lectures (attendence is highly recommended because you are planning to ask intelligent questions to start the conversation). Give them a copy of your manuscript. Someone will eventually look.

In addition, I would also thank Dr. Ann Dietrich for her support and encouragement, especially during the early phase of this book.

Credits

Figures 3-7, 3-16, and 3-18: From *12-Lead ECG: The Art of Interpretation*, courtesy of Tomas B. Garcia, MD

Figure 3-27: Courtesy Andrew Spackman, MD

Figure 3-75: Courtesy Nathaniel D. Wycliffe, MD

Dedication

I would like to dedicate this book to my parents, who have taught me the value of education and hard work, and also to my sons Ryan and Sean, for their patience and understanding.

—Beena Wycliffe, MD

Foreword

I have noticed, as I age in medicine, that I forget abbreviations almost as rapidly as I forgot the Krebs cycle during medical school biochemistry. Moreover, I find that mnemonics don't help me, since I can never remember what they stand for. Finally, it has always bothered me that eponyms are used. They may gratify the egos of the people for whom they have been named, but other than to show a rare ability to retain trivial facts—that is the eponymic names—I can never remember what they stand for and what it is that I should be concerned about. It would probably help if there were a version of the game Trivial Pursuit that was based solely on these three forms of trivia. There must be a generational gap here as well, since all the residents and students with whom I work always understand the abbreviations and instantly acquire the mnemonics whether or not they are slightly salacious (Never Lower Tillie's Pants, Mother Might Come Home, for the wrist bones: Navicular, Lunate, Triquetral, Psisform, Multiangular, Multiangular, Capitate, Hamate.). Of course the anatomists never cooperate when they change the name of things like "navicular" to "scaphoid."

Apparently, fortunately, I am not the only one to suffer from this problem, and also fortunately, Dr. Beena Wycliffe conceived of the great idea to try to collect common things that we are all supposed to instantly recognize into a book of useful reminders.

There is an ugly and overused piece of jargon in medicine: "You must have a high index of suscipion." No one ever tells you what to suspect or how to recognize the thing that you are being admonished to look for. In the first edition of the textbook on Emergency Medicine that I edited, it appeared in almost every chapter. When I realized that we were telling the readers to suspect the entire body of knowledge contained in a 2000 page textbook, it became clear that we need to do something else to help people think of something. Therefore this book is an attempt to give you the clues of when to think of something, what to think of, and often in what way to respond.

It is of course true that you cannot make a diagnosis if you don't think of it, but hopefully, this book will help you recognize the clues that make a diagnosis jump into your mind.

One of the hidden benefits of the board certifying process is that almost nobody ever takes a board examination without some preparation. Knowledge comes from exposure, but it also comes from repetition. We hope this book of reminders will help you to bring back those pieces of knowledge that you haven't used for a while. We also hope that by serving to refresh your memories, these reminders will give you confidence to successfully approach your examinations. More importantly, if you spend a few minutes with the book before working your next tour of duty in the Emergency Department, it will help relieve the common anxiety that you are going to encounter something you don't know how to deal with effectively.

All good physicians never lose their fear of failure. We cannot hope to know everything. We cannot hope to remember everything. We don't wish to harm anyone. When used correctly, this book of reminders will allow one a sense of confidence that you can avoid the errors of ignorance, of inexorable forgetfulness that comes with aging, and the means to appropriately, and quickly start your evaluations.

The book will evolve over time, especially as readers suggest their own favorite abbreviations, mnemonics, and eponyms. Nevertheless, this is a good place to start.

For those of you who need to know trivia, I proffer my own favorite piece: The first conductor of the Detroit Symphony Orchestra was an internationally famous Polish pianist named Ossip Gabrilovitch. You can still obtain recordings of his performance of the Shumann quintette with the Flonzaly Quartette on a digitized reissue of an old phonograph record set. While this is worth listening to, the main reason for pursuing this, is that Maestro Gabrilovitch was Mark Twain's son-in-law; having married Susie Clemens.

Good reading, and good luck with your examinations, and your practices.

—*Peter Rosen, MD*
    Boston, Tucson, and Jackson Hole

Abbreviations

AAA—abdominal aortic aneurysm
AC—alternating current
AC—acromioclavicular
ACA—anterior cerebral artery
ACE—angiotensin-converting enzyme
ACL—anterior cruciate ligament
ACLS—advanced cardiac life support
ACS—acute coronary syndrome
ADH—antidiuretic hormone
AED—automated external defibrillator
Afib—atrial fibrillation
AGE—arterial gas embolism
AHA—American Heart Association
AI—aortic insufficiency
AICD—automatic implantable cardioverter–defibrillator
AIDS—acquired immunodeficiency syndrome
AIVR—accelerated idioventricular rhythm
AKA—alcoholic ketoacidosis
ALC—absolute lymphocyte count
ALS—amyotrophic lateral sclerosis
AMS—acute mountain sickness
AMS—altered mental status
ANUG—acute necrotizing ulcerative gingivitis
AP—anterior posterior
ARDS—acute respiratory distress syndrome
ARF—acute renal failure
ASO—antistreptolysin O
AST—aspartate aminotransferase
ATN—acute tubular necrosis
ATP—adenosine triphosphate
AV—atrioventricular
AVM—arteriovenous malformation

AVN—avascular necrosis
A/W—associated with

BCP—birth control pill
BFD—bilateral facet dislocation
BS—blood sugar
BVM—bag–mask ventilation

CAD—coronary artery disease
CAH—congenital adrenal hyperplasia
CAP—community-acquired pneumonia
CC—coracoclavicular
cGMP—cyclic GMP
CHF—congestive heart failure
CISD—critical incident stress debriefing
CLL—chronic lymphocytic leukemia
COPD—chronic obstructive pulmonary disease
CPR—cardiopulmonary resuscitation
CMV—cytomegalovirus
CN—cyanide
CNS—central nervous system
CO—carbon monoxide
COBRA—Consolidated Omnibus Budget Reconciliation Act
CPK—creatinine phosphokinase
CPP—cerebral perfusion pressure
CPR—cardiopulmonary resuscitation
CRAO—central retinal artery occlusion
CRP—C-reactive protein
CRVO—central retinal venous occlusion
CryoPPT—cryoprecipitate

CSF—cerebrospinal fluid
CVP—central venous pressure
CXR—chest x-ray

DAI—diffuse axonal injury
DC—direct current
DCS—decompression sickness
DI—diabetes insipidus
DIC—disseminated intravascular coagulation
DIP—distal interphalangeal
DKA—diabetic ketoacidosis
DM—diabetes mellitus
DPL—diagnostic peritoneal lavage
DTR—deep tendon reflex
DUB—dysfunctional uterine bleeding
DVT—deep vein thrombosis

EAST—elevated arm stress test
ECF—extracellular fluid
EES—erythromycin
EKC—epidemic keratoconjunctivitis
EM—erythema multiforme
EMS—emergency medical services
EMTALA—Emergency Medical Treatment and Active Labor Act
EOM—extraocular muscles
ESR—erythrocyte sedimentation rate
ETT—endotracheal tube

FAA—Federal Aviation Administration
FAST—focused assessment with sonography for trauma
FB—foreign body
FEMA—Federal Emergency Management Agency
FENa—fractional excretion of sodium

FFP—fresh frozen plasma

GABHS—group A beta-hemolytic *Streptococcus*
GB—gallbladder
GCS—Glasgow coma scale
GE—gastroesophageal (junction)
GHB—gamma hydroxybutyrate
GI—gastrointestinal
GSW—gun-shot wound

HACE—high altitude cerebral edema
HAPE—high altitude pulmonary edema
HBcAg—hepatitis B core antigen
HBsAg—hepatitis B surface antigen
HHNC—hyperosmolar hyperglycemic nonketotic coma
HIDA—hepatobiliary iminodiacetic acid
HIV—human immunodeficiency virus
HS—hydrogen sulfide
HSK—herpes simplex keratitis
HSV—herpes simplex virus
HSP—Henoch-Schönlein purpura
HTN—hypertension
HUS—hemolytic-uremic syndrome
HVS—hyperviscosity syndrome

IBS—irritable bowel syndrome
ICF—intracellular fluid
ICH—intracranial hemorrhage
ICP—intracranial pressure
ICS—intercostal space
ICU—intensive care unit
IgE—immunoglobulin E
IHSS—idiopathic hypertrophic subaortic stenosis
IJ—internal jugular

IOP—intraocular pressure
ITP—idiopathic thrombocytopenic purpura
IUP—intrauterine pregnancy
IVDA—intravenous drug abuse
IVF—intravenous fluid

JRA—juvenile rheumatoid arthritis
JVD—jugular venous distention

KI—potassium iodide

LAFH—left anterior fascicular hemiblock
LATS—long-acting thyroid stimulator
LAD—left-axis deviation
LD—lethal dose
LDH—lactate dehydrogenase
LEs—lower extremities
LES—lower esophageal sphincter
LGL—Lown-Ganong-Levine
LGV—lymphogranuloma venereum
LMN—lower motor neuron
LOC—loss of consciousness
LP—lumber puncture
LPFH—left posterior fascicular hemiblock
LV—left ventricle
LVH—left ventricular hypertrophy

MAOI—monoamine oxidase inhibitor
MAP—mean arterial pressure
MAT—multifocal atrial tachycardia
MCA—middle cerebral artery
MCL—medial collateral ligament
MCP—metacarpophalangeal (joint)
MDA—methylene deoxyamphetamine
MI—myocardial infarction
MR—mitral regurgitation
MS—multiple sclerosis

MSG—monosodium glutamate
MVC—motor vehicle collision
MVP—mitral valve prolapse

NAC—*N*-acetylcysteine
NaHCO₃—sodium bicarbonate

NDMD—National Disaster Medical System
NEC—necrotizing enterocolitis
NMS—neuroleptic malignant syndrome
NPV—negative predictive value
NS—normal saline
NSTEMI—non–ST-elevation myocardial infarction
NSVD—normal spontaneous vaginal delivery

OR—operating room
ORIF—open reduction-internal fixation
OTC—over the counter

PAC—premature atrial contraction
PAT—paroxysmal atrial tachycardia
PCA—posterior cerebral artery
PCI—percutaneous coronary intervention
PCL—posterior cruciate ligament
PCP—*Pneumocystis carinii* pneumonia
PCP—phencyclidine
PCWP—pulmonary capillary wedge pressure
PDA—patent ductus arteriosus
PEA—pulseless electrical activity
PEEP—positive end-expiratory pressure
PID—pelvic inflammatory disease
PIP—proximal interphalangeal
PMT—pacemaker-mediated tachycardia

POPS—pulmonary overpressurization syndrome

PPV— positive pressure value

PROM—premature rupture of membrane

PTU—propylthiouracil

PVC—premature ventricular complex

RAD—right-axis deviation

RAS—reticular-activating system

RBC—red blood cell

RCA—right coronary artery

RDS—respiratory distress syndrome

RHD—rheumatic heart disease

RF—rheumatic fever

RMSF—Rockey Mountain spotted fever

RSI—rapid-sequence intubation

RSV—respiratory syncytial virus

RTA—renal tubular acidosis

RUQ—right upper quadrant

RVH—right ventricular hypertrophy

SA—sinoatrial

SBO—small bowel obstruction

SCFE—slipped capital femoral epiphysis

SCIWORA—spinal cord injury without radiographic abnormality

SGOT—serum glutamic oxaloacetic transaminase (same as AST)

SIADH—symptoms of inappropriate antidiuretic hormone

SQ—subcutaneous

SVC—superior vena cava

SL—sublingual

SLE—systemic lupus erythematosus

SOB—shortness of breath

S/P—status post

SSSS—staphylococcal scalded skin syndrome

START—simple triage and rapid treatment

STEMI—ST-elevation myocardial infarction

SVT—supraventricular tachycardia

TBI—traumatic brain injury

TCA—tricyclic antidepressant

TEN—toxic epidermal necrolysis

TM—tympanic membrane

TOF—tetralogy of Fallot

TPA—tissue plasminogen activator

TMJ—temporomandibular joint

TSS—toxic shock syndrome

TT—thrombin time

TTP—thrombotic thrombocytopenic purpura

UFD— unilateral facet dislocation

UMN—upper motor neuron

UOP—urine output

URI—upper respiratory infection

US—ultrasound

VBI—vertebrobasilar insufficiency

Vfib—ventricular fibrillation

VP—ventriculoperitoneal

VSD—ventricular septal defect

V/Q—ventilation-perfusion

VZIG—varicella zoster immunoglobulin

WPW—Wolff-Parkinson-White

Presenting Signs and Symptoms

I

SIGNS AND SYMPTOMS	DIAGNOSIS (alphabetical order)
	A
An elderly man with hypertension and flank pain becomes hypotensive	Abdominal aortic aneurysm
An elderly patient with diabetes mellitus, bad burn, or multiple trauma presents with right upper quadrant abdominal pain, nausea and vomiting, and fever	Acalculous cholecystitis
Dark, velvety, and thickened skin in posterior neck and axillae	Acanthosis nigricans
Deafness, ataxia, ipsilateral facial weakness, and cerebellar signs	Acoustic neuroma
Painful eye starting in a darkened room and cloudy cornea	Acute angle closure glaucoma
Sickle cell patient with cough, chest pain, tachypnea, elevated white blood cell (WBC) count, and chest x-ray study infiltrate	Acute chest syndrome
Painful ulcerated gray tissue on gums	Acute necrotizing ulcerative gingivitis (ANUG)
Weakness, anorexia, dehydration, and hyperpigmentation	Adrenal insufficiency (primary or Addison's disease)
Weakness, anorexia, and dehydration but no hyperpigmentation	Adrenal insufficiency (secondary)
Intubated patient deteriorates after helicopter take-off	Air embolism

SIGNS AND SYMPTOMS	DIAGNOSIS (alphabetical order)
Anorexia, abdominal pain, jaundice, and tender hepatomegaly	Alcoholic hepatitis
Chronic alcoholic with recent history of heavy alcohol consumption and now with nausea and vomiting, abdominal pain, and acidosis	Alcoholic ketoacidosis
Foul taste and painful gum site following tooth extraction	Alveolar osteitis
An elderly patient with sudden unilateral painless loss of vision, which has resolved	Amaurosis fugax
Absent motor function, loss of pain and temperature sensation distal to lesion, and normal vibration and position sensation	Anterior cord syndrome
Brief upper respiratory infection (URI) followed by hypoxia and dyspnea, chest x-ray showing mediastinal widening (adenopathy)	Anthrax (inhalation)
Hypertensive patient with tearing severe chest pain radiating to back	Aortic dissection (acute)
Elderly patient with dyspnea, chest pain, syncope, and systolic murmur radiating to neck	Aortic stenosis
Atrial fibrillation and apathy in elderly	Apathetic thyrotoxicosis
Multiple painful lesions on labial and buccal mucosa	Aphthous stomatitis
Erythematous, pruritic, and scaly patches on dorsal areas, palms, and soles	Atopic dermatitis
Sickle cell patient with pain in hip and difficulty walking	Avascular necrosis of femoral head

SIGNS AND SYMPTOMS	DIAGNOSIS (alphabetical order)
	B
<3 years of age, croup-like then toxic, stridor, thick sputum, but no dysphagia	Bacterial tracheitis
Pain, edema, and erythema of glans penis and foreskin	Balanoposthitis
Battle's sign (mastoid bruising) or hemotympanum following trauma	Basilar skull fracture
Unilateral mouth drooping, facial smoothing, and unable to close eye or wrinkle forehead	Bell's palsy
An elderly woman develops vertigo with head turning with reproducible nystagmus	Benign positional vertigo
An 8-week-old otherwise healthy infant with worsening jaundice for 1 week and hepatomegaly	Biliary atresia
Painful bite, target lesion, spreading erythema, and abdominal cramps	Black widow spider bite
Sudden acute severe pain in chest or abdomen following forceful emesis	Boerhaave's syndrome (Esophageal perforation with mediastinitis)
Diplopia, blurred vision, photophobia, and descending paralysis	Botulism
Infant with constipation, hypotonia, poor feeding, and lethargy	(Infant) botulism
A 2-month-old infant with URI, fever, tachypnea, wheezing, and chest retractions	Bronchiolitis
Initially painless bite, later necrotic eschar, disseminated intravascular coagulation (DIC), and hemolysis	Brown recluse spider bite

SIGNS AND SYMPTOMS	DIAGNOSIS (alphabetical order)
Ipsilateral loss of motor function and vibratory sensation; and contralateral loss of pain and temperature sensation	Brown-Séquard syndrome
An adolescent girl with secondary amenorrhea, weight fluctuations, and loss of dental enamel	Bulimia
Flaccid bulla filled with purulent material	Bullous impetigo
Tense bullae with blistering benign course seen mostly in elderly	Bullous pemphigoid
C	
Fall from a height with landing on the heel	Calcaneal fracture and possible vertebral fractures
Bradycardia, hypotension, altered mental status (AMS), generalized weakness, and sinus arrest	Calcium channel blocker overdose
Multiple family members with headache and lightheadedness	Carbon monoxide poisoning
Motor and sensory loss in legs, bowel and bladder dysfunction, and saddle anesthesia	Cauda equina syndrome
Infraorbital or periorbital cellulitis with meningeal signs, sepsis, and coma	Cavernous sinus thrombosis
Quadriplegia with sacral sparing, and arms weaker than legs	Central cord syndrome
Sudden, painless monocular vision loss, and "cherry-red spot" on pale retina	Central retinal arterial occlusion (CRAO)
(Sudden or gradual) Variable painless, monocular vision loss (mild to severe), and "blood and thunder" fundus	Central retinal venous occlusion (CRVO)
Sudden inability to walk or stand, vertigo, headache, and nausea or vomiting	Cerebellar infarct

SIGNS AND SYMPTOMS	DIAGNOSIS (alphabetical order)
Reddened tender lump at the eyelid or the lid margin	Chalazion
Irregular painful genital ulcers with unilateral painful large inguinal nodes that may later rupture	Chancroid
"Dew drop on a rose petal" and lesions in different stages	Chicken pox (varicella)
Foot edema and erythema after chronic exposure to dry nonfreezing temperature	Chilblains
Injuries in a child at different stages of healing with inconsistent history	Child abuse
5-week-old afebrile infant with 1 week of mild cough, and conjunctivitis	Chlamydia pneumoniae
A middle-aged patient with right upper quadrant (RUQ) abdominal pain, fever, elevated bilirubin, and dilated common bile duct	Cholangitis
An overweight woman in her 40s with RUQ abdominal pain, nausea, and vomiting	Cholecystitis (acute)
24 hours after eating tuna— nausea, vomiting diarrhea, perioral paresthesia, and hot cold reversal	Ciguatoxin poisoning
A middle-aged man with recurrent unilateral orbital headache, lacrimation, and conjunctival injection	Cluster headache
Severe and constant pain over the leg compartment; palpation elicits pain	Compartment syndrome
After a physical battery—lower jaw pain, and jaw deviates to left	(Left) condylar angle fracture
Cauliflower-like, pink flesh-colored lesions on genitalia	Condylomata acuminatum

SIGNS AND SYMPTOMS	DIAGNOSIS (alphabetical order)
A 2-week-old lethargic infant with vomiting, hyponatremia, hypoglycemia, and hyperkalemia	Congenital adrenal hyperplasia
Dyspnea, orthopnea, chest pain, jugular venous distention (JVD), rales, and respiratory distress	Congestive heart failure (CHF)
1- to 2-day-old infant with bilateral conjunctivitis	(Chemical) conjunctivitis
1- to 2-week-old infant with bilateral conjunctivitis	(Chlamydial) conjunctivitis
3- to 5-day-old infant with bilateral conjunctivitis	(Gonococcal) conjunctivitis
A 1-year-old with diffuse abdominal pain, no bowel movement for 2 days, and no nausea or vomiting	Constipation
Severe eye pain, tearing, blurred vision, and foreign body sensation	Corneal abrasion
Perirectal abscess, fever, weight loss, and diarrhea	Crohn's disease
A 6-month-old infant with barky cough and stridor that worsens at night	Croup
Rapid weight gain, truncal obesity, striae, fatigue, and hypertension	Cushing's syndrome
Anxiety, hyperventilation, and symptoms of hypoxia, but not cyanotic	Cyanide toxicity
A renal transplantation patient presents with fever and chills	Cytomegalovirus (CMV)
	D
Swelling, warmth, pain and tenderness in extremity	Deep vein thrombosis
Polyuria, hypernatremia, dehydration, and no response to dehydration but to antidiuretic hormone (ADH)	Diabetes insipidus (central)

SIGNS AND SYMPTOMS	DIAGNOSIS (alphabetical order)
Polyuria, dehydration, but no response to either dehydration or ADH	Diabetes insipidus (nephrogenic)
Diabetic with hyperglycemia, volume depletion, and acidosis	Diabetic ketoacidosis
Paralysis of palatal muscles, ptosis, and descending paralysis	Diphtheria
Young adult with bilateral wrist or knee pain and lesions on digits	Disseminated gonorrhea
Patients with left lower quadrant (LLQ) abdominal pain, diarrhea or constipation, and fever	Diverticulitis
An elderly patient with massive painless rectal bleeding	Diverticulosis
A tearful housewife with contusions and multiple visits to healthcare provider	Domestic violence
E	
Curious toddler with lip corner burns, drooling, and bloodless	Electric cord burns
Chipped tooth after attack or fall, but no pain	Ellis I fracture
Chipped tooth with yellow dentin	Ellis II fracture
Chipped painful tooth and reddish blue coloration or blood on the fracture site	Ellis III fracture
Family members with bilateral eye pain, red, and blurred vision	Epidemic keratoconjunctivitis (EKC)
Gradual scrotal pain and swelling, fever, and urinary symptoms	Epididymitis
Significant blunt head trauma with loss of consciousness and lucid intervals	Epidural hematoma
Well-circumscribed fiery red lesions on face and extremities	Erysipelas
Slapped cheek, lace-like rash, fever, coryza, and malaise	Erythema infectiosum (Fifth disease)

SIGNS AND SYMPTOMS	DIAGNOSIS (alphabetical order)
Annular plaques, distinct borders with pale center, and nonpruritic	Erythema marginatum
F	
A wide-eyed, wary, malnourished infant gains weight after admitted to the hospital	Failure to thrive
Swollen, red, throbbing pain, and tense finger pad	Felon
Pelvic inflammatory disease (PID) and RUQ abdominal tenderness with jaundice	Fitz-Hugh-Curtis syndrome
Small pustules involving hair follicles	Folliculitis
Diabetic male with scrotal, rectal, or genitalia pain out of proportion	Fournier's gangrene
Tender, fluctuating, and deep nodule around hair follicle	Furuncle
G	
A partygoer after drug consumption was comatose and wakes up during intubation	Gamma-hydroxybutyrate (GHB)
Sensation that something is always stuck in the throat	Globus hystericus
A child after a upper respiratory infection (URI) has periorbital edema, tea-colored urine, and hypertension	Glomerulonephritis beta-hemolytic streptoccoal induced
Mediterranean male ate fava beans and now has dark urine and jaundice	Glucose-6-phosphate dehydrogenase (G6PD) deficiency
Bilateral leg weakness, progressive ascending paralysis, and no reflex in legs	Guillain-Barré syndrome

SIGNS AND SYMPTOMS	DIAGNOSIS (alphabetical order)
	H
An infant with excessive crying and a purple toe	**Hair tourniquet syndrome**
Fever, malaise, and lesions on soles, hands, palms, mouth, and diaper area	**Hand-foot-mouth disease (Coxsackievirus)**
A 6-month-old infant to 3-year-old child with symmetric painful swelling of hands and feet	**Hand-foot syndrome (Sickle cell)**
A 10-year-old with bloody diarrhea, vomiting, abdominal pain, low hemoglobin, and low platelets	**Hemolytic-uremic syndrome (HUS)**
A 6-year-old with a purpuric rash on buttock or abdomen, diffuse abdominal pain, and ankle pain	**Henoch-Schönlein's purpura (HSP)**
A 2-year-old daycare child with fever, vomiting, and RUQ abdominal pain	**Hepatitis A**
Microvesicles on soft palate, uvula, and tonsillar pillars	**Herpangina**
Grouped vesicles following pain in a unilateral dermatome	**Herpes zoster**
An elderly patient with severe unilateral eye pain and lesions at tip of nose	**Herpes zoster keratitis**
A 1-to-3-year-old with shallow painful ulcers on lips, tongue, and gums; and fever	**Herpetic gingivostomatitis**
A healthcare worker with painful distal periungual digit and vesicular lesions, but no pus	**Herpetic whitlow**
Chronic, purulent, and tender nodules coalesce in axillae and groin	**Hidradenitis suppurativa**
A mountain climber with ataxia, confusion, and coma	**High altitude cerebral edema (HACE)**

SIGNS AND SYMPTOMS	DIAGNOSIS (alphabetical order)
High altitude exposure, tachypnea, dyspnea with cough, and rales	High altitude pulmonary edema (HAPE)
A 2-day-old infant with vomiting and abdominal distention, but no meconium	Hirschsprung's disease
A 6-year-old with chronic constipation and no stool in rectal vault	Hirschsprung's disease
Young, monocular eye pain, redness, photophobia, and back pain	HLA-B27 syndrome
Young patient with fever, night sweats, and painless firm cervical nodes	Hodgkin lymphoma
A 3-day-old female infant with vaginal bleeding	Hormone withdrawal (mother's)
Ptosis, miosis, and anhydrosis	Horner's syndrome
A patient with history of lung cancer presents with AMS, weakness, increased thirst, polyuria, and decreased deep tendon reflexes	Hypercalcemic crisis
Diastolic blood pressure > 120 mm Hg. and asymptomatic	Hypertensive urgency
A 1-month-old infant in status epilepticus and given only water at home	Hyponatremia
Fatigue, puffy eyes, hair loss, cold intolerance, and weight gain	Hypothyroidism
	I
Patient presents after a viral infection with purpura, gum bleeding, and appears clinically well	Idiopathic thrombocytopenic purpura (ITP)

SIGNS AND SYMPTOMS	DIAGNOSIS (alphabetical order)
Limited active abduction of shoulder with pain on flexion and internal rotation	**Impingement syndrome**
A 2-week-old infant with AMS, acidosis, and vomiting	**Inborn errors of metabolism**
A 1-year-old with colicky abdominal pain, bilious vomiting, and palpable abdominal mass	**Intussusception**
Abdominal pain, bloating, altered bowel function, and stressed out	**Irritable bowel syndrome (IBS)**
An intravenous drug abuse (IVDA) patient with status seizures and not responding to usual anti-seizure medications	**Isoniazid (INH) toxicity**
	K
Painless and raised brown-black or purple nodules that do not blanch	**Kaposi's sarcoma**
A child with persistent fever, strawberry tongue, conjunctivitis, rash, and enlarged lymph nodes	**Kawasaki's disease**
	L
A 4- to 8-year-old boy with painless limp, knee pain, and abnormal gait	**Legg-Calvé-Perthes disease**
Blow to orbit, blurred vision, and vision 20/200 that corrects with pinhole	**Lens dislocation**
Fever, brawny induration of anterior neck, molar infection, and trismus	**Ludwig's angina**
Malaise, headache, and annular erythematous rash with central clearing	**Lyme disease**
Painless shallow genital ulcers with unilateral or bilateral tender matted inguinal nodes	**Lymphogranuloma venereum**

SIGNS AND SYMPTOMS	DIAGNOSIS (alphabetical order)
	M
Unexplained fever, headache, and palpable spleen in a patient with foreign travel	Malaria
Hyperthermia, profound myalgias, and body cramps after general anesthesia	Malignant hyperthermia
A diabetic patient with external ear cellulitis and fever	Malignant otitis externa
A 10-day-old ill infant with bilious vomiting and distended abdomen	Malrotation with midgut volvulus
After yawning, unable to close mouth, and jaw deviated to left	Mandibular dislocation (right)
Fever, cough, coryza, conjunctivitis (3 Cs), 5-day rash, and Koplik's spots (white ulcerations in the oral mucosa)	Measles
An 8-year-old with painless rectal bleeding and nontender abdomen	Meckel's diverticulum
A 20-year-old with headache, fever, rash, and nuchal rigidity	Meningitis
Fever, chills, hypotension, meningitis, and petechial lesions	Meningococcemia
An elderly patient with moderate to severe abdominal pain, minimal abdominal tenderness, and atrial fibrillation	Mesenteric ischemia
A 4-week-old with diarrhea, tachypnea, cyanosis, and O_2 saturation still low despite administration of O_2	Methemoglobinemia
Asymptomatic dome-shaped papules with central umbilication	Molluscum contagiosum
Fever, exudative pharyngitis, cervical and epitrochlear adenitis, splenomegaly, and rash	Mononucleosis

SIGNS AND SYMPTOMS	DIAGNOSIS (alphabetical order)
Swollen tender parotid glands that may be unilateral	Mumps
Mother causing symptoms in the child	Munchausen's syndrome by proxy
An 8-year-old with progressive cough, rales, and rhonchi	Mycoplasma pneumoniae
An elderly patient with thyroid disease, altered mental status, hypothermia, bradycardia, hyponatremia, and hypoglycemia	Myxedema coma

N

Painful, tender cellulitis-like skin, crepitation, toxic signs, and fever	Necrotizing fasciitis
A playful child, yet holding hand held in pronation with elbow flexion	Nursemaid's elbow

O

A 1-week-old infant with erythema around umbilical chord stump	Omphalitis
A 20- to 40-year-old with gradual, unilateral, and painful diminished vision presents with retro bulbar pain	Optic neuritis
A child with fever, periorbital swelling, proptosis, and painful extraocular movements	Orbital cellulitis
Orbital blow, diplopia, unable to look up, and infraorbital anesthesia	Orbital floor fracture
A confused farm worker who is drooling, diaphoretic, and bradycardiac	Organophosphate poisoning
A 13- to 14-year-old boy with gradual knee pain that worsens with activities	Osgood-Schlatter's disease

SIGNS AND SYMPTOMS	DIAGNOSIS (alphabetical order)
	P
A child with fever, trismus, who is toxic with muffled voice and stiff neck	Parapharyngeal abscess
Painful retracted foreskin and unable to bring forward to glans tip	Paraphimosis
Lower abdominal pain, cervical motion tenderness, and bilateral adnexal tenderness	Pelvic inflammatory disease (PID)
Flu-like symptoms, hypotension, and diastolic collapse of right ventricle on echocardiography	Pericardial tamponade
Sharp chest pain worsening with inspiration, dyspnea, and fever	Pericarditis
Fever, periorbital edema, and no proptosis or extraocular muscle involved	Periorbital cellulitis
An adolescent with a severe sore throat, fever, and drooling	Peritonsillar abscess
Upper respiratory infection (URI), whoop-like cough, and subconjunctival hemorrhage that improves	Pertussis
Episodic, throbbing headache, palpitation, and sweating	Pheochromocytoma
Difficulty retracting foreskin from urethra toward shaft or base of penis	Phimosis
Third-trimester pregnancy, severe abdominal pain, and vaginal bleeding	Placental abruption
Nonproductive cough, dyspnea, fever, and history of intravenous drug abuse (IVDA)	Pneumocystis carinii (PCP) pneumonia
Painful, erect, and edematous penis; and flaccid glans	Priapism
A 2-month-old formula-fed well infant with blood-streaked stool	Protein (diet) allergy

SIGNS AND SYMPTOMS	DIAGNOSIS (alphabetical order)
Anxiety, chest pain, dyspnea, hemoptysis, tachycardia, and tachypnea	Pulmonary embolism
A 2-week-old male infant with nonbilious projectile vomiting and appears hungry	Pyloric stenosis
R	
Herpes zoster, CN VII involvement, and vesicles on eardrum	Ramsay-Hunt syndrome
Sudden loss of unilateral vision, sense of curtain coming down, and floaters	Retinal detachment
Eye proptosis and subconjunctival hemorrhage following trauma	Retrobulbar hemorrhage
An infant with stridor but no cough	Retropharyngeal abscess
Inferior-wall myocardial infarction with hypotension	Right ventricular infarction
Fever, myalgia, headache, abdominal pain, and rash spreading from wrists to palms and soles	Rocky Mountain Spotted Fever (RMSF)
4–5 days abrupt fever, defervescence, and a 1- to 2-day rash (6 months to 2 years old)	Roseola
3 days of rash with large postauricular and post cervical lymph nodes	Rubella (German measles)
S	
Pruritic papular lesions in finger web spaces that worsen at night	Scabies
Sandpaper rash, fever, strawberry tongue, and pharyngitis	Scarlet fever
Fever, hip pain with swelling and erythema, and leg flexed/externally rotated	Septic hip arthritis

SIGNS AND SYMPTOMS	DIAGNOSIS (alphabetical order)
Infant with retinal hemorrhage	**Shaken baby syndrome**
A 5-year-old with bloody diarrhea, abdominal pain, fever, and seizure	**Shigellosis**
Elderly patient with pain and swelling in submandibular area	**Sialolithiasis**
A 14-year-old limping obese boy with groin, thigh, or knee pain	**Slipped capital femoral epiphysis (SCFE)**
Fever and flaccid blisters exfoliate in sheets. Oral mucosa spared	**Staphylococcal scalded skin syndrome (SSSS)**
Small pustule at the eyelash line	**Stye**
Severe (thunderclap) and sudden onset of headache. Occipitonuchal most common location	**Subarachnoid hemorrhage**
An elderly or alcoholic patient, with or without trauma, dilated right pupil, and left hemiplegia	**Subdural hematoma (right)**
Headache, shortness of breath, facial plethora, and feeling of fullness in head	**Superior vena cava (SVC) syndrome**
Painless, indurated, and solitary lesion on genitalia	**Syphilis (primary)**
Fever, malaise, chills, arthralgia, and diffuse papulosquamous rash	**Syphilis (secondary)**
	T
An elderly patient with temporal tenderness, myalgia, and unilateral vision loss	**Temporal arteritis**
Sudden, acute, and painful scrotal swelling with horizontal lie	**Testicular torsion**
Trismus, jaw rigidity, fever, and autonomic dysfunction	**Tetanus**
Hypopigmented scaly macules on back with Christmas-tree pattern	**Tinea versicolor**
Gradual scrotal pain in prepubertal boys and "blue-dot sign"	**Torsion appendix testis**

SIGNS AND SYMPTOMS	DIAGNOSIS (alphabetical order)
Fever, diffuse rash, hypotension, three or more organs involved, and desquamation	Toxic shock syndrome
Children 5- to 6-years-old, nontoxic, inability to walk, and pain in thigh and knee	Transient synovitis
Recent visit to Mexico with sudden-onset watery diarrhea and cramps	Traveler's diarrhea
Painful paresthesia and foot pale from prolonged wet/cold environment	Trench foot (immersion foot)
Fever, night sweats, chest x-ray study with right upper lobe cavitary lesion, and infiltrate	Tuberculosis
Sickle cell patient with fever, headache, diarrhea, rash, and bradycardia	Typhoid fever
U	
Weight loss, constipation, diarrhea with rectal bleeding, fever, and anemia	Ulcerative colitis
Severe pain, foreign body sensation, tearing, chemosis, and conjunctival erythema	Ultraviolet keratitis
Widely dilated fixed pupil with decorticate posture	Uncal herniation
Young girl with "cherry-like doughnut" mass at introitus and vaginal bleeding	Urethral prolapse
Flank pain radiating to the ipsilateral testicle or labia majora	Urolithiasis
Abdominal trauma, loss of the palpable uterine contour, and palpable fetal parts	Uterine rupture

SIGNS AND SYMPTOMS	DIAGNOSIS (alphabetical order)
	V
Sudden painless loss of vision and absent red reflex	**Vitreous hemorrhage**
Pain to proximal forearm with passive extension of fingers, along with swelling and numbness	**Volkmann's contracture**
A < 1-year-old infant with bilious vomiting, bloody stool with rigid abdomen, and shock	**Volvulus with malrotation**
Severe vaginal pruritus, "cottage-cheese" discharge, and external dysuria	**Vulvovaginal candidiasis**
	W
An alcoholic patient with confusion, ataxia, and nystagmus	**Wernicke's encephalopathy**
Ipsilateral loss of facial pain sensation and temperature, contralateral loss of same in body, and gait ataxia	**Wallenberg's syndrome**

TERM	DESCRIPTION
Abdominal aortic aneurysm (AAA)	An atheromatous destruction of all layers of the vessel wall; a true aneurysm (swelling of the vessel itself).
Dissecting aneurysm (aortic dissection)	A misnomer: not a true aneurysm but a crack in the intima with blood tracking between the intima and the media. It can reenter the lumen of the vessel or rupture the vessel with extra vessel hemorrhage. The major damage is due to the false passage between the intima and the media occluding flow through major vessel branches.
Traumatic dissecting aneurysm (traumatic aortic dissection)	Also a misnomer: a rupture in one or more layers of the vessel caused by external trauma.
Achalasia	Dilated esophagus and "beaked" lower esophagus segment.
Scleroderma	Rigid and aperistaltic esophagus.
Acidemia	Net imbalance of H^+ in blood. A patient with acidosis and alkalosis of equal magnitude will have normal pH, so has no acidemia or alkalemia but has acidosis and alkalosis.
Acidosis	Elevated H^+ in blood.
Acoustic neuroma	Vertigo, hearing loss, but no tinnitus.
Ménière's disease	Vertigo, hearing loss, and tinnitus.

TERM	DESCRIPTION
Activated thyrotoxicosis	Typical symptoms include tachycardia, fever, anxiety, and exophthalmus.
Apathetic thyrotoxicosis	Variant of hyperthyroidism. Elderly patient with depressed mental state and usually do not see goiter or exophthalmus. Presents with atrial fibrillation with congestive heart failure (CHF).
Acute necrotizing ulcerative gingivitis (ANUG)	Painful and bacteria invade normal tissue.
Gingivitis	Painless and gingiva inflamed in response to plaque but not invaded by bacteria.
Acute rheumatic fever	CHF from myocarditis, murmur due to inflammation of valve leaflets, and rash but no petechiae.
Bacterial endocarditis	CHF from valve destruction, murmur due to vegetation, and no rash but petechiae.
Alcoholic hepatitis	AST (aspartate aminotransferase) level >> ALT (alanine transaminase) level.
Viral hepatitis	Opposite from above. ALT >> AST.
Allergic conjunctivitis	Pruritus, cobblestoning of upper lid, and reddish conjunctiva.
Bacterial conjunctivitis	No lymphadenopathy and purulent discharge.
Epidemic keratoconjunctivitis (EKC)	Painful, highly contagious, and eyes very red.
Viral conjunctivitis	Contagious, periauricular lymphadenopathy, eyes red, and watery discharge.
Anal fissure	Skin tears (fissures) usually in the midline.
Fistula in ano	Tract between rectum and skin causing drainage.

TERM	DESCRIPTION
Anterior circulation strokes	Rarely loss of consciousness (LOC) with face and body neurologic findings on same side.
Posterior circulation strokes	LOC and crossed deficits (one side of face, opposite side of body).
Anticholinergic	Dry skin with no bowel sounds.
Sympathomimetic	Diaphoretic skin with positive bowel sounds present.
Aortic rupture	Esophagus shifted to right on chest x-ray study.
Innominate rupture	Esophagus shifted to left on chest x-ray study.
Arsenic	Shock, radiopaque, peripheral neuropathy, but no acute renal failure.
Mercury	Shock, radiopaque, peripheral neuropathy, and causes rapid acute renal failure.
Aspirin poisoning	Uncouples oxidative phosphorylation.
Cyanide, carbon monoxide, or hydrogen sulfide (CN, CO, or HS)	Inhibit electron transport chain.
Ascending cholangitis	Fever, chills, right upper quadrant (RUQ) pain, and jaundice. Surgical emergency.
Primary sclerosing cholangitis	RUQ pain, jaundice, and pruritus. Associated with Crohn's disease.
Air in biliary tree	In abdominal x-ray study see air-filled biliary tree. Due to surgery, perforation of gallbladder into intestine, ulcer into gallbladder, or infection of biliary tree.
Air in portal vein	In abdominal x-ray study see small black dots in liver. Loss of mucosal integrity of bowel wall signifies dead bowel.

TERM	DESCRIPTION
Amyotrophic lateral sclerosis, Eaton-Lambert, Multiple sclerosis, Polio	Only motor involvement
Guillain-Barré	Motor and sensory involvement.
Angulation	Refers to the distal direction of the distal bone fragment. Opposite of displacement.
Displacement	Refers to the direction of proximal portion of distal bone fragment.
Anterior cord syndrome	Forced hyperflexion. Complete paralysis and loss of pain and temperature below the lesion. Not transient. Requires surgery.
Central cord syndrome	Forced hyperextension with upper extremity motor weakness > lower extremity. Some loss of pain and temperature upper > lower. Better prognosis and transient.
Anterior hip dislocation	Presents with abduction and external rotation.
Posterior hip dislocation	Presents with adduction and internal rotation. Remember PID (**P**osterior—**i**nternal and a**d**duction)
Aortic dissection	β-Blocker first then α-blocker.
Pheochromocytoma	α-Blocker then β-blocker.
Thyroid storm	β-Blocker first then propylthiouracil (PTU).
Atropine	Reverses muscarinic and central nervous system (CNS) effects of anticholinesterase.
2-Pralidoxime (2-PAM)	Reverses nicotinic plus muscarinic and CNS effects.
Bennet's fracture	Oblique fracture into the joint space of the thumb metacarpal.
Rolando fracture	Comminuted intra-articular fracture of the thumb metacarpal.

TERM	DESCRIPTION
Beneficence	Doing good.
Nonmalfeasance	Do no harm.
Black widow spider	Painful muscle cramps. Less local reaction.
Brown recluse spider	Severe local reaction leading to tissue necrosis.
Blepharitis	Cellulitis of eyelid. Treat with baby shampoo and instruct to scrub eyelids.
Dacrocystitis	Swelling over lacrimal sac.
Boerhaave's syndrome	Full thickness tear of esophagus leading to mediastinitis. Presents with pain and sepsis.
Mallory-Weiss	Longitudinal partial thickness mucosal tear at the gastroesophageal (GE) junction. Presents with upper gastrointestinal bleeding.
Bisferiens pulse	Pulse that feels double peaked.
Pulsus alternans	Can palpate every other pulse.
Pulsus paradoxus	Decrease in peripheral pulse during inspiration.
Botulism	Ptosis, weakness, and descending paralysis. Has anticholinergic symptoms.
Diphtheria	Ptosis, palatal paralysis, dysphagia, diplopia, cardiac symptoms, and fever.
Botulism	Descending paralysis.
Guillain-Barré	Ascending paralysis.
Tetanus	Tetany and spasm.
Boutonniere deformity	Extension of distal interphalangeal (DIP) joint, flexion of proximal interphalangeal (PIP) joint.
Mallet	DIP joint partially flexed.
Swan neck	Flexion metacarpophalangeal (MCP) joint, extension PIP, flexion DIP.

TERM	DESCRIPTION
Brainstem lesion	Looks away from the lesion side.
Intracerebral lesion	Looks toward the lesion side.
Bright red blood	Carbon monoxide poisoning.
Chocolate brown blood	Methemoglobinemia.
Brudzinski's sign	When you flex patient's neck, the knee flexes.
Kernig's sign	With hip flexed, cannot extend the knee. This causes contraction of the hamstrings.
Bullous myringitis	Vesicles on tympanic membrane associated with mycoplasma.
Cholesteatoma	Keratin deposit on tympanic membrane.
Bullous pemphigoid	Tense bullae and benign course.
Pemphigus vulgaris	Small flaccid bullae and positive Nikolsky's sign (outer layers of the epidermis lift easily upon application of horizontal, tangential pressure).
Burst fracture	Stable, vertical compression, and vertebral body protrudes anterior and posterior.
Chance fracture	Seat belt injury of pedicles and vertebral body with fracture of posterior spinous process.
Wedge fracture	Stable, diminished height, and increased concavity of anterior border of vertebral body.
Caput succedaneum	Diffuse and poorly demarcated. Crosses suture line.
Cephalohematoma	Sharply demarcated and limited to a single bone.
Carbamate poisoning	Reversible and requires only atropine.
Organophosphate poisoning	Irreversible and requires 2-PAM and atropine.

TERM	DESCRIPTION
Carbuncle	Bunch of boils.
Furuncle	One boil.
Cecal volvulus	Found in young marathon runners. Requires surgery.
Sigmoid volvulus	Found in constipated and debilitated elderly. Requires sigmoidoscopy. Surgery for mucosal cyanosis or if volvulus fails to unwind.
Central cord	Weakness and worse in upper extremities.
Guillain-Barré	Weakness and worse in lower extremities, and hyporeflexia.
Central CN VII palsy	Can wrinkle forehead. Spares frontalis muscle.
Peripheral CN VII palsy (Bell's palsy)	Paralysis of whole side of face including forehead.
Central diabetes insipidus	Will not respond to water restriction but to antidiuretic hormone (ADH) administration.
Nephrogenic diabetes insipidus	No response to either water restriction or ADH.
Cerebral hypoxia (or increased CO_2)	Causes intracranial vasodilatation.
Pulmonary hypoxia	Causes pulmonary vasoconstriction.
Cervical (C-6) nerve lesion	Sensation of burning hands.
Ciguatera fish poisoning	Sensation of burning hands and feet.
Chancre	Primary stage of syphilis. Painless genital ulcer.
Chancroid (Haemophilus ducreyi)	Painful genital ulcer and painful inguinal lymph nodes.
Lymphogranuloma venereum (LGV)	Painless genital ulcer but painful inguinal nodes.
Chilblains (pernio)	Dry, cold, and nonfreezing injury.
Trench foot	Wet, cold, and nonfreezing injury.

TERM	DESCRIPTION
Cholinergic crisis	Pronounced bronchorrhea and generalized weakness from overtreatment with cholinesterase inhibitors. Edrophonium challenge test worsens symptoms.
Myasthenia crisis	Respiratory failure and muscle weakness from undertreatment for myasthenia gravis. Edrophonium challenge test improves symptoms.
Chopart's joints	Between hind-foot and mid-foot.
Lisfranc's	Between mid-foot and forefoot.
Ciguatera poisoning	Fish feast on dinoflagellates, then you eat the fish. No specific treatment.
Scombroid poisoning	Toxin from dark-meat fish. Histamine-like effect. Give antihistamine.
Claims-based malpractice insurance policy	Policy in effect when the claim is made.
Occurrence-based policy	Policy in effect when the incident occurred.
Classic heat stroke	Very old and young. Skin hot, dry, and red.
Exertional heat stroke	Young athletes. Sweating present.
Classic migraine	With aura.
Common migraine	No aura.
Colles fracture	Distal radius fracture with dorsal angulation from fall on outstretched hand.
Galeazzi's fracture	Distal radius fracture with dorsal angulation and dorsally displaced ulna.
Smith's fracture	Distal radius fracture with volar angulation from fall on flexed wrist.

TERM	DESCRIPTION
Compensated acidosis	pH close to normal. Elevated CO_2 would otherwise result in lower pH. Never fully corrects the pH.
Mixed respiratory and metabolic acidosis	pH relatively normal. pCO_2 and HCO_3 abnormal.
Complete cord lesion	Permanent deficit.
Spinal shock	Temporary with deficit < 24 hours. Shock is over when bulbocavernous reflex returns.
Complete spinal cord lesion	Total loss of sensory and motor below level of injury. Functional recovery remote if symptoms last > 24 hours.
Incomplete spinal cord lesion	Anterior, central cord, and Brown-Séquard syndrome. All have some neurologic functions retained. Better prognosis.
Concussion	Injury is functional.
Contusion	Injury is organic.
Condyloma acuminatum	Cauliflower-like pink to gray genital warts caused by human papilloma virus (HPV).
Condyloma latum	Fleshy, pearly gray, pale, and flat-top genital ulcers seen in syphilis (second stage).
Congenital adrenal hyperplasia	Male appearing, virilizing rather than feminizing.
Testicular feminization	Female appearing owing to end-organ insensitivity to androgens.
True hermaphroditism	Both testes and ovaries present.
Conjugated hyperbilirubinemia	Direct bilirubin level is elevated. Urine positive for urobilinogen.
Unconjugated hyperbilirubinemia	Indirect bilirubin is elevated. Urine negative for urobilinogen.

TERM	DESCRIPTION
Coronary artery disease	Most common cause of primary cardiac arrest in adults.
Respiratory arrest	Most common cause of cardiac arrest in children.
Cullen's sign	Bluish discoloration around umbilicus seen in hemorrhagic pancreatitis.
Grey-Turner's sign	Periumbilical and flank echymoses hemorrhagic pancreatitis.
Crohn's disease (regional enteritis)	"Skip lesions," may affect any areas from mouth to anus, and involves all layers of the bowel wall.
Ulcerative colitis	Includes mucosal and submucosal layer of rectum and colon.
Curling's ulcers	Stress ulcers (stomach) from burns.
Cushing's ulcers	Stress ulcers (stomach) from head trauma.
Cushing's disease	Caused by pituitary tumor and see increase in cortisol production.
Cushing reflex	Hypertension, bradycardia, and respiratory irregularity.
Cushing's syndrome	Caused by adrenal tumor; see elevation in cortisol production. Patient with obesity, short stature, striae, and hypertension.
Decerebrate	Both upper and lower extremity extension. Has worse prognosis than decorticate.
Decorticate	Upper extremity flexed, lower extremity extended, and turning to the center (core).
Delirium	Sudden onset, fluctuating course, confusion, disorientation, and visual hallucinations. Acute changes.
Dementia	Insidious onset, stable course, alert, and no hallucinations. Chronic changes.
Psychoses (psychiatric)	Sudden onset, alert, and auditory hallucinations. Alteration in thought.

TERM	DESCRIPTION
Dermatomyositis	Skin involvement. Associated with cancer.
Polymyositis	No skin involvement. No cancer.
Dialysis dementia	Related to elevated brain aluminum levels. Progressive fatal disorder with no response to dialysis.
Uremic encephalopathy	Related to elevated brain calcium levels. Responds to dialysis.
Dislocation	Complete joint separation.
Subluxation	Partial joint separation.
Duodenal atresia	Newborn within first 24 hours of life. Bilious vomiting.
Pyloric stenosis	Develops later at 2–3 weeks of age. Nonbilious vomiting.
Dysphagia	Something wrong with swallowing. True pathology.
Globus hystericus	Sensation that something is always stuck in the throat.
Dysphagia	Difficulty swallowing.
Odynophagia	Painful swallowing.
Early diaphragm repair	Do laparotomy.
Late diaphragm repair	Do thoracotomy due to adhesion.
Eaton-Lambert	Muscular weakness improves with activity.
Myasthenia gravis	Muscular weakness worsens with activity.
Ecchymosis/black eye	More prominent over bony ridges.
Raccoon's eye	Appears to originate from the sulcus about the globe.
Ectopic pregnancy	Pseudogestational sac on ultrasound.
Intrauterine pregnancy	Double decidual sac sign.

TERM	DESCRIPTION
Endometriosis	Endometrial tissue outside endometrial cavity. May cause pain during menses.
Endometritis	Infection of endometrium. May be localized to decidua and myometrium.
Erythema chronicum migrans	Lyme disease. Erythematous lesion with central clearing.
Erythema infectiosum	Fifth disease. "Slapped cheeks."
Erythema marginatum	Rheumatic fever.
Esophageal atresia	Polyhydramnios on maternal ultrasound.
Potter's facies	Oligohydramnios (associated with bilateral renal agenesis) on maternal ultrasound.
Esophageal coin	Transverse orientation. The esophagus is wider in the bilateral axis (horizontal) so the coin is seen en face in the posteroanterior (PA) view of x-rays. See Figure 3-31.
Tracheal coin	In anteroposterior (AP) orientation. The tracheal coin is seen en face on the lateral x-ray because the trachea is wider in the AP axis due to the absence of cartilage in the tracheal rings posterior.
Ethanol, ethylene glycol, and methanol	Anion gap and osmolar gap.
Isopropanol	No anion gap but ketosis and osmolar gap.
Ethanol withdrawal and sedative-hypnotic withdrawal	Seizure.
Opioid withdrawal	No seizure (except in neonatal opioid withdrawal).

TERM	DESCRIPTION
Eversion fracture	Dorsiflexion, transverse fracture of medial malleolus, and oblique fracture of distal fibula.
Inversion fracture	Plantar flexion, transverse fracture of distal fibula, and oblique fracture of distal tibia.
Extension teardrop	Forced abrupt extension pulls off anterior inferior corner of vertebral body. Unstable.
Flexion teardrop	Forced flexion. Anterior inferior portion displaces anteriorly. Unstable.
External hemorrhoid	Painful, distal to pectinate line, and skin covered.
Internal hemorrhoid	Painless, proximal to pectinate line, and mucosa covered.
Extraperitoneal bladder rupture	Contrast material in retroperitoneum, scrotum, and anterior abdominal wall.
Intraperitoneal bladder rupture	Contrast material surrounds loop of bowel and fills pericolic gutter.
Extravascular hemolysis	Rh factor incompatibility. Less severe.
Intravascular hemolysis	Blood types ABO incompatibility. More severe.
Exudate	Seen in infection and malignancy.
Transudate	Found in CHF. Pleural protein: serum protein ratio < 0.5, lactate dehydrogenase (LDH) < 200 mg/dl, and protein < 3 gms/l.
Forchheimer spots	Palatal petechiae. Rubella and mononucleosis.
Herpangina	Painful lesions on posterior pharynx.
Koplik's spots	Buccal mucosa. Measles.

TERM	DESCRIPTION
Functional psychosis	Gradual onset, auditory hallucinations, normal vitals, and oriented. This is a thought affective disorder.
Organic psychosis	Sudden onset, visual hallucinations, abnormal vitals, and disoriented. This is confusion.
Gastroschisis	Defect in abdominal wall with evisceration of abdominal structures without sac.
Omphalocele	Defect in abdominal ring. Protruding intestines in a sac.
Gout	Needle-shaped uric acid crystals and negatively birefringent crystals.
Pseudogout	Ca^{2+} pyrophosphate crystals, rhomboid shape, and positively birefringent crystals.
Greenstick fracture	Cortex disrupted on one side and intact on the other side.
Torus fracture	Cortex buckled but intact.
Hand foot and mouth syndrome	Shallow whitish ulcers on soft palate with rash on palms, hands, and feet.
Hand-and-foot syndrome	<2 years of age with sickle cell disease and swelling of one or all extremities.
Hematuria	Urine dipstick positive for blood and smear positive for red blood cells (RBCs).
Myoglobinuria	Urine dipstick positive for blood but smear negative for RBCs. This can be seen in carbon monoxide poisoning.
Hemolytic-uremic syndrome (HUS)	No neurologic symptoms.
Thrombotic thrombocytopenic purpura (TTP)	Positive neurologic symptoms.

TERM	DESCRIPTION
Hemorrhagic stroke	Rapid development of coma.
Hypertensive encephalopathy	Headache and lethargy progressing slowly.
Subarachnoid hemorrhage	Sudden onset of headache and vomiting.
Hereditary spherocytosis	Defect in RBC membrane. Causes hemolytic anemia.
Sickle cell anemia	Defect in hemoglobin, which is abnormal. Causes hemolytic anemia.
Herpangina	No gingival involvement.
Herpetic gingivostomatitis	Gingival involvement.
Herpes simplex	Does not follow dermatome.
Herpes zoster	Follows dermatome.
Hutchinson's sign	Herpes zoster lesion on tip of nose and eye. CN V involvement.
Ramsey-Hunt syndrome	Herpes zoster lesion on tympanic membrane and facial palsy. CN VII involvement.
Hypertensive encephalopathy	Onset gradual with global cerebral dysfunction. Decrease blood pressure (BP) by 20% within 1 hour.
Stroke	Onset acute with focal neurologic deficit. Treat BP only if $>220/120$ mm Hg. In hemorrhagic stroke, treat if >160–180 systolic.
Hypoxemia	Abnormally low arterial O_2 tension. Measured as $PaO_2 < 60$ mm Hg.
Hypoxia	Insufficient O_2 delivery to tissues. Measured in low SaO_2.
Incarcerated hernia	Irreducible hernia. Safe to reduce in children.
Strangulated hernia	Irreducible with vascular compromise. It does not occur in children, so reduction attempts of incarceration are safe in children.

TERM	DESCRIPTION
Ischemic colitis	No vessel occlusion and angiography usually normal.
Mesenteric ischemia	Large vessel occlusion.
Janeway lesions	Painless lesions on palms and soles.
Osler's nodes	Painful lesions on fingers and toes.
Jones fracture	Transverse fracture through the base of 5th metatarsal. Treat with a non–weight-bearing cast.
Pseudo-Jones fracture	Longitudinal avulsion fracture occurs at the base of the 5th metatarsal where peroneus brevis tendon attaches. Use a cast shoe.
Shaft fracture	Middle transverse fracture of 5th metatarsal. Use a walking cast or an orthopedic shoe.
Kawasaki's	At least 5 days of fever, papular rash, conjunctivitis, strawberry tongue, and desquamation.
Scarlet fever	1–2 days of high fever, sore throat, and sandpaper rash.
Keratitis	Inflammation of cornea, perilimbal flush, and circumferential redness of sclera.
Uveitis	Inflammation of iris and ciliary flush.
Korsakoff's psychosis	End result of untreated Wernicke's encephalopathy. A chronic brain syndrome that is irreversible.
Normal pressure hydrocephalus	Confusion, ataxia, and urinary incontinence.
Wernicke's encephalopathy	Confusion, ataxia, and nystagmus. Seen in alcoholics. May be precipitated by giving glucose without thiamine.
Kussmaul's breathing	Seen in diabetic ketoacidosis (DKA). Involuntary deep rapid respirations.
Kussmaul's sign	Distended neck veins with inspiration.

TERM	DESCRIPTION
Labyrinthitis	Vertigo and hearing loss.
Ménière's disease	Vertigo, tinnitus, and hearing loss present.
Vestibular neuronitis	Vertigo and no hearing loss.
Lown-Ganong-Levin (LGL) syndrome	No delta wave.
Wolff-Parkinson-White (WPW) syndrome	Delta wave present.
Macrocytic anemia	Folate and vitamin B_{12} deficiency. Seen in patients with chronic alcohol abuse and pernicious anemia.
Microcytic anemia	Seen in iron deficiency, thalassemia, and anemia of chronic disease.
Malingering	Voluntary. Motivation by external incentives. No painful procedures.
Munchausen's syndrome	Voluntary. Wants to be hospitalized. Undergoes painful procedures.
Mandibular fracture	Jaw deviates to the fracture side.
TMJ (temporomandibular joint) dislocation	Jaw deviates to the opposite side of dislocation.
Methemoglobinemia	No response to O_2. Treat with methylene blue.
Sulfhemoglobinemia	Responsive to O_2. Supportive treatment.
Missed fracture or dislocation	Most common malpractice claim.
Missed myocardial infarction (MI)	Highest percentage of malpractice dollar loss.
Myopathy	Proximal weakness greater than distal. Sensation and reflex are normal.
Peripheral neuropathy	Distal weakness greater than proximal. Decreased reflex.
Neuroblastoma	Displaces kidney downward.
Wilms tumor	Distorts renal image. Mass is inside the kidney.

TERM	DESCRIPTION
Nifedipine toxicity	Hypotension and bradycardia.
Verapamil toxicity	Hypotension and reflex tachycardia.
Normal pressure hydrocephalus	Dilated ventricles and normal intracranial pressure.
Pseudotumor cerebri	Slit-like ventricles with increased intracranial pressure.
O_2 saturation	A measure of the degree to which oxygen is bound to hemoglobin.
PaO_2	Partial pressure of gas in the blood. PaO_2 of 30, 40, 50, and 60 corresponds to SaO_2 of 60, 70, 80, and 90%, respectively.
Oculocephalic reflex (doll's eyes)	In normal person, when turn head, eyes do not turn.
Oculovestibular reflex (cold calorics)	When you irrigate ear with cold water, eyes turn to that side and quickly return to center (normal).
Optic neuritis	Inflammation of optic nerve, dilated pupil, and painful. Seen in multiple sclerosis.
Uveitis	Inflammation of iris and ciliary body, painful, and miosis. Seen in rheumatic fever and trauma.
Orbital cellulitis	A toxic-appearing child with painful extraocular movement.
Periorbital cellulitis	Eye movements not restricted, not painful, and the patient is nontoxic.
Orthopnea	Dyspnea induced by lying flat.
Platypnea	Dyspnea induced by upright position and relieved by recumbency.
Papilledema	Bilateral and associated intracranial pressure elevation.
Papillitis	Unilateral, painful inflammatory process, and loss of central vision early leading to total loss of vision. Seen in multiple sclerosis.

TERM	DESCRIPTION
Paraesophageal hernia	Gastroesophageal (GE) junction stays fixed while a portion of stomach herniates through a rent in the diaphragm.
Sliding hernia	A portion of the wall of the colon (usually sigmoid) forms part of the inguinal hernia sac.
Sliding hiatal hernia	GE junction and stomach fundus herniated.
Paraphimosis	Inability to reduce the proximal edematous foreskin distally over glans penis.
Phimosis	Inability to retract the foreskin toward the penile shaft base (away from the meatus).
Phlegmasia alba dolens	White and swollen leg with massive ileofemoral thrombosis. Artery okay.
Phlegmasia cerulea dolens	Blue discoloration. If continues, retrograde thrombosis of artery. Needs fasciotomy.
Photoallergic	Requires previous exposure. Stop drug causing reaction.
Phototoxic	First exposure to drug. Occurs from reaction with sunlight. Stop sunlight exposure.
Premature atrial contraction (PAC)	Non-compensatory pause, sinoatrial (SA) node resets. Next P wave ahead of scheduled time.
Premature ventricular contraction (PVC)	Compensatory pause. SA node does not reset. Next P wave at usual time.
Primary aldosterone insufficiency (Addison's)	Decreased aldosterone level and hyperpigmentation.
Secondary aldosterone insufficiency	Normal aldosterone level and no hyperpigmentation.

TERM	DESCRIPTION
Psychogenic polydipsia	Urine maximally diluted. Euvolemic hyponatremia.
SIADH (syndrome of inappropriate antidiuretic hormone)	Urine concentrated (osmolality increased). Euvolemic hyponatremia.
Roseola	Human herpes virus type 6; high fever then rash.
Rubella (German measles)	Togavirus. Rash starts in face then spreads to limbs. Posterior auricular lymphadenopathy.
Rubeola (measles)	Paramyxovirus. 3 C's (conjunctivitis, cough, and coryza) and Koplik's spots.
Sestamibi scan	Isotope deposit in infarcted tissue.
Thallium scan	Isotope deposit in normal tissue.
Sialoadenitis	Salivary gland inflammation.
Sialolithiasis	Salivary gland calculi.
Small bowel x-ray	See plicae circulares that traverse entire bowel width.
Large bowel x-ray	See haustral pattern that does not traverse entire bowel width.
Somatic pain	Sharp, knife-like, and focal pain that exacerbates with movement. Caused by irritation of abdominal musculature.
Visceral Pain	Dull and poorly localized pain. Caused by inflammation or distention of bowel.
Spondylolisthesis	Forward slippage of the superior vertebra over the inferior >25%.
Spondylolysis	Defect in pars interarticularis. Seen best in oblique view on x-rays.
ST depression	Angina or subendocardial myocardial infarction (MI).
ST elevation	Transmural MI

TERM	DESCRIPTION
Staphylococcal scalded skin syndrome (SSSS) and toxic epidermal necrolysis (TEN)	Have positive Nikolsky's sign (easy separation of outer layers of the skin with firm digit pressure, as seen in pemphigus vulgaris or other bullous diseases). SSSS has better prognosis than TEN.
Toxic shock syndrome (TSS)	Negative Nikolsky's sign.
SSSS	No oral mucosa involvement. Use antibiotics.
Stevens-Johnson syndrome	Mucous membrane involved. Use antibiotics.
TEN	Lips and oral mucosa involved. No antibiotics.
TSS	May involve oral mucosa and more than three organ systems. Caused by staphylococcal toxins, although most physicians treat with antibiotics.
Strawberry cervix	Seen in trichomoniasis.
Strawberry tongue	Found in Kawasaki's, scarlet fever, and TSS.
Strychnine poisoning	Blocks glycine receptors.
Tetanus	Prevents glycine release from presynaptic neurons.
Supraventricular tachycardia (SVT)	Preceding ectopic P wave with varying coupling interval. May respond to carotid massage.
Ventricular tachycardia (V Tach)	Atrioventricular dissociation, postectopic pause, fusion beat, concordance, and QRS > 0.14.
Tamponade	Jugular venous distention (JVD), hypotension, midline trachea, and equal breath sounds.
Tension pneumothorax	JVD, hypotension, tracheal deviation, and absent breath sounds one side.

TERM	DESCRIPTION
Technetium-99	Produces "hot spot."
Thallium-201	Produces "cold spot."
Temporomandibular joint (TMJ) spasm	Muscle spasm and jaw "clicking." Treat with nonsteroidal anti-inflammatory drugs (NSAID).
Trigeminal neuralgia (tic douloureux)	"Electric like" sensation. Demyelinization of trigeminal nerve.
Tetralogy of Fallot (TOF)	Both TOF and transposition cause cyanosis. In TOF see diminished pulmonary circulation on chest x-ray study.
Transposition of great vessels	Immediate newborn period. Narrow mediastinum on chest x-ray study.
Transfer dysphagia	Occurs early in the swallowing process, affecting both solids and liquids. Neuromuscular disease such as stroke and myasthenia gravis.
Transport dysphagia	Occurs later in the swallowing process. Progressive dysphagia first to solids then to liquids owing to mechanical problems. These include motility disorders, esophageal carcinoma, webs, strictures, achalasia, and esophageal spasm.
Valgus	Bent outward. The deformity produces an angulation away from the midline.
Varus	Bent inward. The deformity produces an angulation toward the midline.

Emergency Medicine Reminders

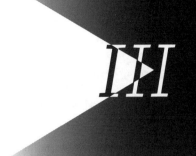

▶ALLERGY and IMMUNOLOGY

Allergic reaction (Table 3-1)—*All require antihistamine and steroids. H_2 blockers useful as well.*
- Minor—No hypotension or respiratory symptoms.
- Anaphylaxis:
    - Mild to moderate—No hypotension. *0.3 to 0.5 mL of 1:1000 epinephrine subcutaneous.* Repeat every 10 minutes up to 3 doses.
    - Severe—Hypotension and respiratory distress. *1.0 mL of 1:10,000 epinephrine intravenous (IV). Repeat every 5 minutes up to 5 mL maximum. Fluid resuscitation. May require intubation.*

Anaphylactoid reaction—No prior exposure. Seen in contrast dye reaction.

Angioedema:
- Drug-induced—angiotensin-converting enzyme (ACE) inhibitor. Not immunoglobulin E (IgE) mediated. *Treat with epinephrine, steroid, and antihistamine. Discontinue ACE inhibitor.*

Table 3-1: Types of Allergic Reaction

Types	Mechanisms of Action	Examples
I	IgE/IgG allergens bind to Ab on mast cells; releases vasoactive substances	Penicillin
II	IgG/IgM Ab reactions to cell surface Ag	Transfusion, hemolytic anemia, and idiopathic thrombocytopenic purpura (ITP)
III	Ag/Ab complex activates complement	Systemic lupus erythematosus (SLE), tetanus toxoid reactions, and serum sickness
IV	Cell mediated; no Ab involved	Positive skin tests (*Candida*, tuberculosis, etc.)

Ab, antibody; Ag, antigen; Ig, immunoglobulin.

- Hereditary angioedema—Autosomal dominant. C_1-esterase deficiency. *Treat with fresh frozen plasma (FFP).*

Chinese restaurant syndrome—From monosodium glutamate (MSG). Causes flushing, wheezing, nausea, vomiting, tightness of chest, and retro-orbital headache. *Treatment: supportive.*

Ciguatera fish poisoning—Ciguatoxin, heat-stable neurotoxin, and reversal hot–cold sensation. *Treatment: supportive.*

Erythema multiforme:
- Minor—Target lesions. Caused by drugs (penicillin or sulfa), herpes simplex, etc. Treatment: *Steroids and antihistamine.*
- Major (Stevens-Johnson syndrome)—Fatal form of erythema multiforme, mucus involvement, and multisystem failure.

Glucagon—Given in anaphylaxis if taking β-blocker (resistant to epinephrine). Also given in hypoglycemia if glucose cannot be administered.

Jarisch-Herxheimer reaction—Febrile reaction with rash after antibiotic treatment (penicillin) for syphilis.

Lidocaine—Allergy from the preservative (methylparaben). Use single-dose cardiac lidocaine.

Photoallergic reaction—Requires previous exposure. Skin appears like dermatitis. *Stop drug.*

Phototoxic reaction—First exposure. Drug plus adequate sunlight. (Like sunburn). *Stop sun exposure.*

Poison ivy vesicles—Linear lesions and no antigen, therefore, not contagious.
- Mild—*Topical steroids and oatmeal baths.*
- Face, genital, and larger area—*Systemic steroids for 10–14 days.*

Red man syndrome—Caused by histamine release when IV vancomycin is rapidly infused.

Scombroidosis—Spoiled fish. Headache, urticaria, itching, diarrhea, and "peppery taste." Antihistamine.

▶ BEHAVIORAL and PSYCHOLOGICAL

Agitation, delirium, fever, tachycardia, and hypertension—Alcohol withdrawal; phencyclidine (PCP), look for nystagmus; cocaine or crystal methamphetamine plus alcohol intoxications.

Akathisia—State of motor restlessness, physical need to move constantly. From acute neuroleptics side effect. *Treat with β-blockers or anticholinergics (benztropine).*

Anorexia nervosa—Body weight 15% below normal, fear of becoming fat, thinks "too fat," and absence of three consecutive menstrual cycles. Low electrolytes, osteoporosis.

Antabuse reaction—Flushing, headache, nausea, vomiting, and palpitation. Alcohol plus flagyl.

Antipsychotic agents:
- Low potency—Thorazine, mellaril, etc. Side effect is severe hypotension.
- High potency—Haldol, inapsine, etc. Fewer side effects.

Assault/battery—It is considered battery to draw blood for laboratory studies in an oriented patient who is refusing to have blood drawn. If the patient is not decisionally capacitated (deemed capable of making independent prudent decisions), studies need no consent.

Axis classification:
- Axis I—mental disorder
- Axis II—personality disorder
- Axis III—medical
- Axis IV—stressors

Barbiturate abuse—Noncardiac pulmonary edema, hypothermia, and clear vesicles and bullae with erythema base.

Bipolar disorder—Mania, grandiose ideas, pressured speech. Men equal to Women. Episodic.

Bulimia—Two episodes of binge eating per week for 3 months, laxative use, and overly concerned with body weight. See metabolic acidosis, parotid gland enlargement, and loss of dental enamel.

Chain of evidence—Samples collection as in a rape case clearly identifying all signatures.

Cocaine washout syndrome—Total depletion of catecholamines after cocaine binge use.

Conversion reaction—Following criteria: change or loss of physical functions, recent stress, unconsciously produces symptoms, and nonorganic etiology. Patient presents with subjective neurologic deficits (i.e., blindness) but not concerned. Physical examination is normal.

Delirium—Sudden onset, rapid deterioration, and clouded consciousness.

Delusions—Fixed false beliefs not amenable to argument.

Dementia—Insidious, alert, and no hallucination or delusion. Stable course.

Dysthymic disorder—More chronic and less severe form of depression. Women >> Men.

Dystonic reaction—Due to neuroleptics. *Give benadryl and cogentin.*

Factitious disorders—Intentionally produced. Two types:
- Munchausen's syndrome—Medical imposter who undergoes many tests and surgeries.
- Munchausen's syndrome by proxy—Parents produce abnormality in the child.

Grieving process steps—Denial, anger, bargaining, depression, and acceptance.

Hallucinations—False perceptions. In schizophrenia, auditory is the most common hallucination.

Hypochondriasis—Middle-aged woman with (+) review of systems. Has preoccupation with illness.

Hysterical conversion—Paralysis, numbness, and blindness. *La belle indifference. Referral.*

Involuntary psychiatric commitment—When patient is a threat to self or others. Initiated by any licensed MD.

Major depression—Dysphoric mood, distorted perception of self, and vegetative symptoms.

Manic (First) episode—Genetic. *Treatment with antipsychotic drugs. Hospitalization.*

Monoamine oxidase inhibitor (MAOI) and demerol—Do not use together. Dangerous combination.

Negligence in suit—Four components:
1. Duty of care
2. Breach of duty
3. Breach causes injury
4. Damages

Neuroleptic malignant syndrome (NMS)—Caused by neuroleptic drugs (haldol). Hyperthermia, muscle rigidity, altered mental status (AMS), autonomic instability, and tachycardia. *Treat with dantrolene. Intensive care unit (ICU) admission.*

Opiate withdrawal—Piloerection, lacrimation, yawning, rhinorrhea, nasal stuffiness, nausea, vomiting, and diarrhea. *Treat with antiemetics, antidiarrheal, and α-2 agonist (clonidine).*

Opioid intoxication—Triad: Central nervous system (CNS) depression, respiratory depression, and miosis. *Give naloxone.*

Optokinetic drum—Piece of paper with alternating black and white lines pulled laterally in front of patient's open eyes will produce nystagmus. Proves patient is not blind and is faking.

Personality disorders:
- Anti-social—Disregard for and violation of rights of others.
- Borderline—Impulsive, anger/depression, unstable, and self-mutilation.
- Histrionic—Drama-queen. Sexually seductive.
- Obsessive-compulsive—Orderliness, perfectionism, control, rigid, and stubborn.
- Passive-aggressive—Negativistic attitudes, dependent, and lacking in self-confidence.
- Schizoid—Loner, appears cold, and aloof.
- Schizotypal—Exhibition of odd behavior and social isolation.

Psychoses:
- Functional—Gradual, auditory hallucination, normal vital signs, alert, and intact cognition. Usually seen in patients < 40 years of age.
- Organic—Abrupt, visual hallucination, abnormal vital signs, and impaired mental status. Usually seen in patients > 40 years of age.

Somatoform disorders—Not deliberate. Secondary gain from "sick role."
- Conversion reaction—Tremors, seizures, paralysis, aphonia, blindness, and tunnel vision. *La belle indifference*—lack of appropriate concern regarding bodily dysfunction.
- Hypochondriasis—Preoccupation with potential serious illness. Goes doctor shopping.
- Somatization— < 30 years of age, pain in four different sites, two gastrointestinal symptoms, one sexual symptom, and one neurologic symptom. Not intentionally produced. A variety of medically unexplained symptoms. *Regular follow-up.*

Suicide risk—Women make more attempts. Men make more psychiatrically serious attempts, with a greater mortality from more medically serious methods.
- High risk—Male, alcoholic, single, divorced, widowed, separated, or unemployed. *Hospitalize.*
- Low risk— < 45 years of age, female, married, employed, no drug use, and normal personality.
- *First attempt. Discharge with stable, functional support system with specific follow-up.*

Tarasoff—"Duty to Warn" concept. Breach of confidentiality versus concern for safety. If the patient is a danger to others, the proposed victims must either be warned by the physician, or the patient must be placed on a mental health hold and admitted to an inpatient service.

Tardive dyskinesia—Writhing, grimacing, and tongue-twisting. Seen with chronic neuroleptic drug therapy.

Trigeminal neuralgia—Excruciating pain from the maxillary branch CN V. *Treat with carbamazepine.*

Vegetative symptoms—Depression. Disturbances in sleep, appetite, and sexual function.

Wernicke's encephalopathy—Ataxia, delirium, and ophthalmoplegia. Acute organic brain syndrome. *Give thiamine.*

▶ CARDIOVASCULAR

Accelerated idioventricular rhythm (AIVR)—*Do not suppress with lidocaine.*

Acute aortic insufficiency with endocarditis—Surgical emergency. *Valve replacement.*

Acute ischemic coronary syndrome (AICS)—Covers the following range:
- Non–ST-elevated myocardial infarction (NSTEMI)—No ST elevation but elevated cardiac enzymes. *No thrombolytics.*
- ST-elevated myocardial infarction (STEMI)—*Need reperfusion therapy. Thrombolytics or primary percutaneous coronary angioplasty (PCA).*
- Unstable angina (new onset or accelerating angina)—Normal cardiac enzymes.

Acute shortness of breath and normal chest x-ray study—Think pulmonary embolism.

Amyloidosis—Prone to digoxin toxicity due to amyloid fibril binding of digoxin.

Angina:
- Prinzmetal's angina—Occurs at rest; is associated with coronary spasm and ST elevation during attack.
- Stable—Lasts 5–15 minutes. Precipitated by exertion, cold, stress, and isometric exercise. Relieved by rest or sublingual nitroglycerine.
- Unstable—New or recent onset, increased frequency, more severe, on less exertion, and at rest.

Angiodysplasia—Associated with aortic stenosis.

Angiography (emergent)—Myocardial infarction (MI) with cardiogenic shock.

Aortic stenosis—Syncope in middle-aged patient with normal O_2 saturation, history of murmur, angina, and heart failure. Crescendo–decrescendo murmur at right second intercostal space (ICS). Left ventricular hypertrophy (LVH) on echocardiogram. *Do not treat with diuretics.*

Aortic transection or rupture—Severe deceleration injury with interscapular pain. Distal to left subclavian artery.

Atrial fibrillation—Irregularly, irregular rhythm. *Rate control.* (Figure 3-1)
- Stable—*Diltiazem, β-blocker, amiodarone, and digoxin.*
- Unstable—*Synchronized cardioversion 100 J.*

Atrial flutter—"Saw tooth," rate 250–300. Suspect in an unchanging ventricular rate of 150. (Figure 3-2)
- Treatment: *Rate control.*
  - Stable: *Diltiazem, β-blocker, and amiodarone.*
  - Unstable: *Synchronized cardioversion 50 J.*

Automatic implantable cardiovert-defibrillator (AICD)—Place magnet over it to deactivate. *Needs interrogation.*

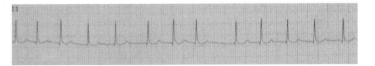

Figure 3-1: Atrial fibrillation

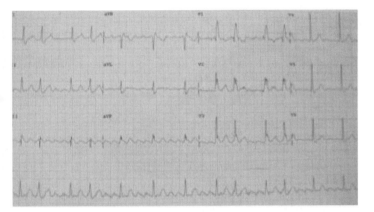

Figure 3-2: Atrial flutter

Axis deviation—Consider following differential:
- Left axis deviation (LAD)—Left ventricular hypertrophy (LVH), left anterior fascicular hemiblock (LAFH), and inferior wall MI.
- Right axis deviation (RAD)—Right ventricular hypertrophy (RVH), left posterior fascicular hemiblock (LPFH), and lateral wall MI.

Beck's triad (acute cardiac tamponade)—Elevated central venous pressure (CVP), hypotension, and muffled heart tones.

Bifascicular block and chest pain—*Needs transvenous pacemaker.*

Bigeminy—A premature ventricular contraction (PVC) alternating with sinus rhythm. (Figure 3-3)

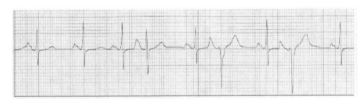

Figure 3-3: Bigeminy

Björk-Shiley prosthetic valve—Failure of the valve is associated with sudden pulmonary edema and loss of valve sounds.

Bradycardia—Heart rate < 60. Consider causes: node dysfunction, medications (calcium channel blocker, β-blocker, digoxin, and anti-arrhythmics), electrolyte abnormalities, hypoxia, and hypothermia. *Treat if symptomatic. Atropine, epinephrine, isoproterenol, calcium gluconate, and glucagon if indicated, and temporary transvenous pacemaker.* (Figure 3-4)

Brugada syndrome—Genetic cause. Mutation in cardiac Na channels. Right bundle-branch block (RBBB), ST elevation in V_1–V_3. Can cause sudden cardiac death. *Implantable cardioverter–defibrillator indicated.*

Cardiac arrest—Patients with ventricular fibrillation have greater survival from resuscitation than asystole or pulseless electrical activity.

Cardiac transplantation—Consider cytomegalovirus (CMV) in patients presenting with flu-like illness, fatigue, malaise, and nausea. *Use high dose of steroids if rejection present.* (Biopsy shows cytoplasmic inclusion bodies.)

Cardiogenic shock—When it occurs with an acute myocardial infarction (AMI), it means > 40% damage to the ventricular myocardium.

Cardiomyopathy:
- Dilated—Systolic pump failure with four- chamber enlargement.
- Hypertrophic—Asymmetric septum, septal Q waves, and sudden death.
- Restrictive cardiomyopathy—Diastolic pump failure. Low voltage QRS.

Cardioversion (synchronized)—For wide-complex tachycardia with hemodynamic instability. *For wide-complex tachycardia with stable vitals, use lidocaine, amiodarone, or procainamide first.*

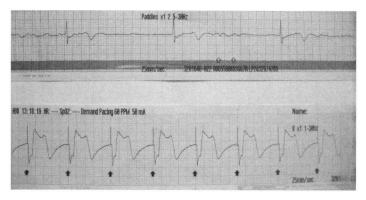

Figure 3-4: Bradycardia with external pacing

Chamber pressure equalization—Suspect pericardial tamponade or tension pneumothorax.

Chronic severe aortic regurgitation:

- Austin-Flint murmur—Soft diastolic rumble.
- Corrigan pulse—Quickly collapsing pulse after a sudden expansion (water-hammer pulse).
- De Musset's sign—Bobbing of head with the heart beat.
- Duroziez's sign—Bruit over the femoral arteries.
- Quincke's sign—Capillary pulsation of the nail bed.
- Water-hammer pulse—Visible, bounding peripheral pulses.

Congestive heart failure—See Table 3-2 and Figure 3-5.

Coronary artery disease—Important factors: left ventricular (LV) function and extent of coronary artery obstruction.

- Degree of LV function >> important than number of MIs.
- Number of vessels affected >> important than location.

Table 3-2: Congestive Heart Failure

Stages	Symptoms	Chest x-ray Findings	PAWP
I	Dyspnea	Cephalization	12–18
II	Dry cough	Interstitial Kerley B lines*	18–25
III	Pink, frothy sputum	Alveolar edema butterfly infiltrate	>25

PAWP, pulmonary artery wedge pressure.

*Interstitial Kerley B lines—horizontal lines at the edge of the pleural border seen on the posterior-anterior chest x-ray.

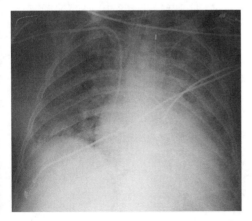

Figure 3-5: Pulmonary edema (Stage III)

Coxsackie virus—Associated with myocarditis.

Defibrillation—For witnessed ventricular fibrillation (before intubation).

Denervated heart—Atropine has no effect. Catecholamine effects increased due to upregulation.

Digitalis effect—Sagging ST ("hockey-stick"), short QT, and flat T. (Figure 3-6)

Digoxin—Contraindicated in Wolff-Parkinson-White (WPW) syndrome.

Digoxin toxicity—Atrial tachycardia and atrioventricular block. Flu-like symptoms, altered mental status, and visual disturbances (yellow–green halos). *Treat with Fab fragments. No calcium chloride if hyperkalemia. Atropine, phenytoin, magnesium, and lidocaine okay to use.*

Dressler's syndrome—Chest pain, fever, pleuropericarditis, and pleural effusion 2–6 weeks after MI. This is immunologic reaction. *Treat with nonsteroidal anti-inflammatory drugs (NSAIDs and steroids).*

Electrical alternans—Beat-to-beat variation in pericardial tamponade. Muffled heart sounds.

Endocarditis—Mitral > aortic > tricuspid > pulmonic valve.
- Cutaneous lesions:
  - Janeway lesions—Nontender plaques on palms and soles.
  - Osler nodes—Tender nodules on tips of fingers and toes.
  - Roth spots—Retinal hemorrhages with central clearing.
  - Splinter hemorrhages—On nail beds.
- Organisms:
  - Intravenous drug abuse (IVDA)—*Staphylococcus aureus.*
  - Mechanical valve—*Staph aureus* and *Staphylococcus epidermidis.*
  - Normal heart—Streptococcus viridans.

Fibrinolytics in acute myocardial infarction—Absolute contraindications: American Heart Association (AHA) guidelines:
- Active bleeding or bleeding diathesis (not including menses)
- Any prior intracranial hemorrhage
- Ischemic stroke within 3 months
- Known cerebral vascular lesion (i.e., arteriovenous malformation)
- Known malignant intracranial neoplasm (primary or secondary)
- Suspected aortic dissection

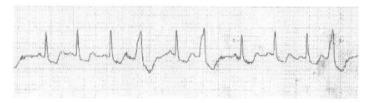

Figure 3-6: Digitalis effect

Globular heart—Dilated cardiomyopathy on chest x-ray study.
Heart block:
- *1st degree AV block*—PR interval > 0.20 seconds. *No treatment.*
- *2nd degree heart block*—Two types:
   - Mobitz Type I (Wenckebach—PR prolongs eventually no QRS complex.) *No treatment.* (Figure 3-7)
   - Mobitz Type II—Constant PR interval with preceding blocked P wave. Rhythm regular. Transvenous pacemaker.
- *3rd degree heart block*—Complete dissociation of atrial and ventricular activity. (Figure 3-8)

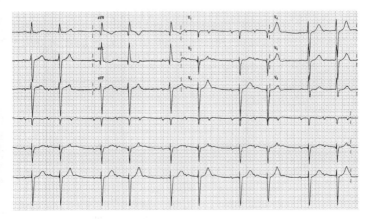

Figure 3-7: Wenckebach (Mobitz Type I)

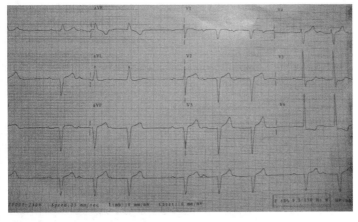

Figure 3-8: Complete heart block (3rd degree heart block)

— Treatment:
- Asymptomatic—Place transcutaneous pacemaker. If cannot capture, the patient needs a transvenous pacemaker.
- Symptomatic—Insert temporary transvenous pacemaker.

Heart failure:
- Diastolic dysfunction—Impaired relaxation of heart in diastole. Caused by: ischemia, hypertrophy, or amyloidosis.
- Systolic dysfunction—May be right or left sided. Impaired contractility. Caused by ischemia, high resistence, hypertension, dilated cardiomyopathy, etc.
  - *Left sided*—Dyspnea, orthopnea, tachycardia, and S_3 gallop.
  - *Right sided*—Peripheral edema, right upper quadrant (RUQ) abdominal pain, jugular venous distention (JVD), and enlarged liver.

Heart murmur:
- Diastolic murmur:
  - Aortic insufficiency—Diastolic decrescendo murmur at left sternal border.
  - Mitral stenosis—Diastolic rumble, loud S_1, and opening snap.
- Systolic murmur:
  - Aortic stenosis—Murmur radiating to neck. *Avoid nitrates or vasodilators.*
  - Mitral insufficiency—Loud holosystolic murmur at 5th intercostal space. Radiates to the left axilla.

High output cardiac failure—From thyrotoxicosis, anemia, arteriovenous fistula, or beriberi (thiamine vitamin B_1 deficiency).

Hypercalcemia—Shortened QT. In hypocalcemia: see prolonged QT.

Hyperkalemia—Prolonged PR → flattened P → tall T's → heart blocks → wide QRS (sine wave). (Figures 3-9–3-11)
- *Treat with calcium chloride, NaHCO3 , dextrose 50% in water (D50), IV insulin, kayexalate, and dialysis.*

Hypertrophy:
- Left ventricular hypertrophy (LVH)—S wave V_2 plus R wave of $V_5 > 35$ mm. (Figure 3-12)
- Right ventricular hypertrophy (RVH)—R wave $>$ S wave in V_1 and R wave decreases from V_1 to V_6.

Hypokalemia—Prominent U waves. Seen after T wave. *Oral or intravenous potassium replacement.* 20 mEq potassium increases level by approximately 0.25 mEq/L.

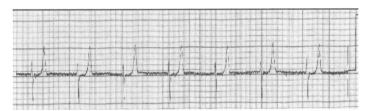

Figure 3-9: Hyperkalemia: peaked T waves

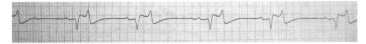

Figure 3-10: Hyperkalemia: (k + 7.4) with patient coding

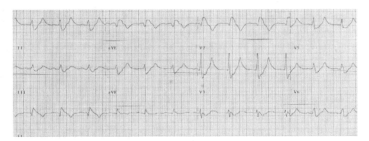

Figure 3-11: Hyperkalemia: sine waves

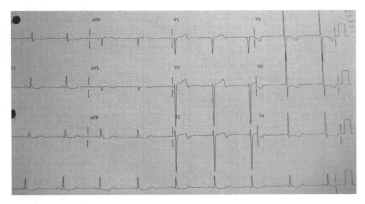

Figure 3-12: Left ventricular hypertrophy

Hypothermia with fibrillation—Need core temp >30°C (86°F) to
   defibrillate. See J (Osborne) wave: notched QRS down slope.
   (Figure 3-13)

Idiopathic hypertrophic subaortic stenosis (IHSS) murmur:
   • Increased with—Tachycardia, exercise, hypovolemia, valsalva
     maneuver, β-agonist, or nitrite.
   • Decreased with (by increased left ventricular filling)—Isometric
     handgrip, squatting, leg elevation, β-blocker, or α-agonist.

Idioventricular rhythm with thrombolytics—*DO NOT treat escape
   premature ventricular contractions or idioventricular rhythm with
   lidocaine. Will cause asystole!*

Infective endocarditis from intravenous drug abuse—*Staphylococcus
   aureus.* Tricuspid > aortic > mitral. Murmurs absent.

Initial EKG change—Seen only in 50% with acute myocardial infarction.

Ischemic heart disease and cardiomyopathy—Number 1 and 2
   reasons for heart failure. Number 3 is valvular heart disease.

Junctional rhythm—No P waves.

Kawasaki's and polyarteritis nodosa—Can cause an acute myocardial
   infarction.

Killip classifications of congestive heart failure (CHF)—See Table
   3-3.

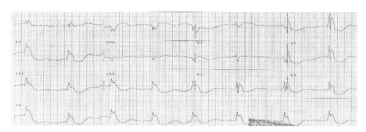

Figure 3-13: Hypothermia

Table 3-3: Killip Classifications of Congestive Heart Failure

Killip Class		Mortality
I	No LVH	5%
II	S₃ and rales	20%
III	Pulmonary edema	40%
IV	Cardiogenic shock	80%

LVH, left ventricular hypertrophy; S_3, third heart sound.

Kussmaul's sign—Quiet heart sounds, enlarged cardiomediastinal silhouette, tachycardia, and pulsus paradoxus. See in pericardial tamponade.

Liebman-Sachs—Vegetative growths on valves (noninfective endocarditis).

Lown-Ganong-Levine—James fibers, short PR, no delta wave, and normal QRS.

Marfan's syndrome—Cystic medial necrosis. One of the causes of aortic dissection.

Missed myocardial infarction (MI)—Cause of emergency department malpractice greatest monetary judgements.

Mitral valve prolapse—Mid-systolic click with late systolic murmur. Associated with amaurosis fugax.
- Infective endocarditis with mitral valve regurgitation—*Give antibiotics.*
- Valsalva—Brings murmur closer to S_1.
- Isometric grip—Brings murmur farther from S_1.

Multifocal atrial tachycardia—Variable P's (3) associated with chronic obstructive pulmonary disease (COPD), theophylline toxicity. *Treat with bronchodilator,magnesium, and verapamil. No β-blocker.*

Murmur:
- Idiopathic hypertrophic subaortic stenosis (IHSS) and mitral regurgitation—Increases with valsalva or standing.
- Other murmurs—Opposite to above (decrease with valsalva or standing).
- Left-sided murmurs—Loudest with expiration.
- Right-sided murmurs—Loudest with inspiration.

MI:
- *Anterior, lateral, or anterior–lateral MI*—See reciprocal changes in inferior leads.
- *Inferior MI*—See reciprocal changes in anterior or lateral leads.

MI and locations on electrocardiogram (EKG)—See Table 3-4

Table 3-4: Myocardial Infarction and Locations on EKG

Anteroseptal wall	V_1–V_2
Posterior wall (reciprocal)	V_1–V_2 (R/S ratio >1 in V_1 and V_2)
Anterior wall	V_3–V_4 (may → Mobitz type II or third-degree AV block)
Anterolateral wall	V_5–V_6
Inferior wall	II, III, aVF (may extend into first-degree AV block or Mobitz type I)
Lateral wall	I, aVL
Right ventricular	RV_4–RV_5

AV, atrioventricular

- Anteroseptal MI—ST elevation in anterior chest leads with reciprocal changes in inferior leads. (Figure 3-14)
- Inferior MI—ST elevation in II, III, aVF with reciprocal changes in anterior leads. Obtain right-sided V leads to look for ST elevation signifying a right ventricular infarction. (Figure 3-15)
- Posterior wall MI (acute)—ST depression in V_1 and V_2. Tall R in V_1. Often associated with inferior wall MI (II, III, aVF elevation). (Figure 3-16)

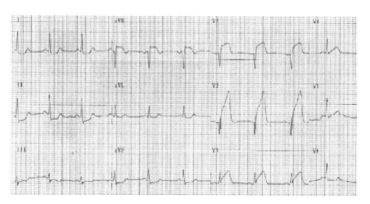

Figure 3-14: Anteroseptal MI

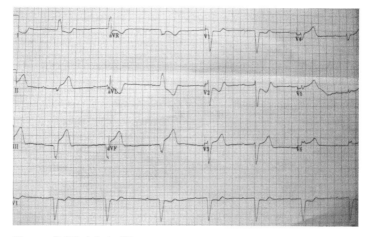

Figure 3-15: Inferior MI

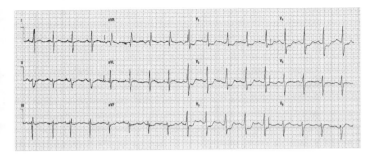

Figure 3-16: Posterior wall MI

MI treatment:
- Door to drug—30 minutes.
- Give oxygen (O_2), aspirin, nitrates, β-blocker (i.e., metoprolol), ace inhibitor (i.e., captopril) within 24 hours.
- Fibrinolytics (i.e., thromboplastin activator (TPA)—Indicated for acute MI meeting following criteria:
- Symptoms < 12 hours and one of the following:
  - ST elevation > 0.1 mV in at least two contiguous precordial leads or in at least two adjacent limb leads.
  - New left bundle-branch block (LBBB).
  - Anterior chest lead ST depression (posterior infarction).
  - PCA not available with patient meeting the EKG criteria for STEMI.
- Glycoprotein IIb/IIIa antagonists (ie, abciximab)—During PCA, MI, and acute coronary syndrome.
- Heparin—For percutaneous coronary angiography (PCA), and fibrinolytic therapy.
- PCA—Door to balloon time 90 minutes. Preferable to fibrinolytic therapy, but not universally available.

Myocarditis—Viral prodrome followed by dyspnea, tachycardia out of proportion, and CHF. *Do echocardiogram.*
- Viral—*Supportive. Immunosuppressive therapy—no value.*
- Rheumatic fever—*Antibiotics.*

Node blood supply:
- Atrioventricular (AV) node supply—90% right coronary artery (RCA)
- Sinoatrial (SA) node supply—55% RCA; 44% left circumflex coronary artery.

Pacemaker:
- Failure to pace—Absence of expected spikes. Most common cause: oversensing.
- Failure to sense—See spikes at wrong time.
- Failure to capture—See pacemaker spike but no QRS following the spike.
- Runaway pacemaker—Rate of 200–400. *Place a magnet over the pacemaker.*

Pacemaker-mediated tachycardia (PMT)—Only seen in dual chamber.

Papillary muscle rupture—Associated with inferior or posterior MI. See large V wave on pulmonary capillary wedge pressure (PCWP) monitor.

Paroxysmal atrial tachycardia—Associated with digitalis toxicity; 2:1 block.

Patient with hypotension, jugular venous distention (JVD), and clear lungs—Think right ventricular infarction secondary to inferior MI.

Pectus excavatum—Associated with pulmonary stenosis.

Pericardial effusion—See Figure 3-17.

Pericarditis—PR depression and upward concave diffuse ST elevation. Recent MI a few weeks prior, now fever, chest pain, and pleural effusion. *Aspirin in high dose. No aspirin for uremic pericarditis or with coexisting coagulopathy.* (Figure 3-18)

Pharmacology (limited list):
- Aspirin (ASA)—Decreases mortality by 20% when used in MI.
- β-blocker—14% reduction in mortality when used in MI.
- Digoxin—Enhances myocardial contractility.

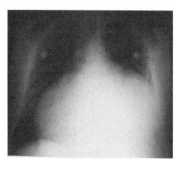 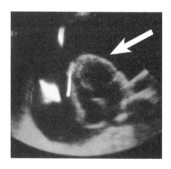

A   B

Figure 3-17: Pericardial effusion chest x-ray and echocardiogram (same patient)

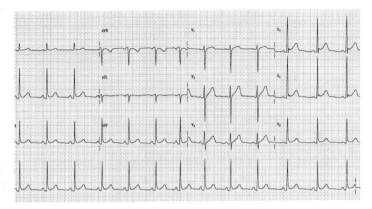

Figure 3-18: Pericarditis

- Dobutamine—Use for systolic blood pressure (SBP) >90 mm Hg.
- Dopamine—Use for SBP <90 mm Hg.
- Nitrate—Decreases preload and afterload.
- Nitroprusside—Through cyclic glucose monophosphate (cGMP) relaxes smooth muscle. Causes "coronary steal."
- Procainamide—For wide complex Wolff Parkington White (WPW) syndrome, not for torsades de pointes.

Phenothiazines—Mimics hypokalemia. Prolonged QT and prominent U wave.

Pheochromocytoma—Intermittent elevation in BP along with headache, flushing, and diarrhea.

Polymyositis and dermatomyositis—Associated with dysrhythmia and myocarditis.

Precordial catch syndrome—Short and sharp anterior chest pain resolves with respiration and rest.

Preexcitation syndrome (WPW)—*Avoid verapamil and digoxin.*

Prosthetic valves:
- Caged-ball (Starr-Edwards), Disk (Bjork-Shiley), Bileaflet (St. Jude's)—*Anticoagulation.*
- Porcine heterograph—*No anticoagulants needed* if the patient has a sinus rhythm.

Pseudo-infarction of Q waves—Hypertrophic cardiomyopathy.

Pulseless electrical activity (PEA)—40% to 50% with detectable waveform on arterial line. >80% wall-motion per ultrasound. Rhythm on monitor but no palpable pulse. *Cardiopulmonary resuscitation (CPR), endotracheal intubation, intravenous fluids, epinephrine, and atropine.* Consider causes. (Figure 3-19)

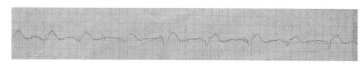

Figure 3-19: PEA (Patient coded and expired)

Pulsus alternans—Left ventricular (LV) dysfunction (alternating contractile force of LV).

Pulsus paradoxus—Drop of >10 mm Hg during inspiration, or the difference between the first onset of the first Korotkoff sound (blood pressure cuff audible beat) and its steady presence. Seen in tamponade, bronchial asthma, COPD, and superior vena cava (SVC) obstruction.

Q waves—Transmural MI.

QT prolongation—Caused by hyperphosphatemia, hypomagnesemia, and hypocalcemia.

Reperfusion dysrhythmias—Accelerated idioventricular rhythm (AIVR) appears during successful thrombolysis. *No treatment required.*

Rheumatic heart disease (RHD)—Jones criteria. Need 2 major or 1 major and 2 minor.
- Major—Carditis, arthritis, Sydenham's chorea, erythema marginatum, and subcutaneous nodules.
- Minor—Previous history of rheumatic fever or RHD, arthralgia, elevated erythrocyte sedimentation rate (ESR), prolonged PR, and fever.

Right coronary artery (RCA)—RCA supplies AV node 99%. Associated with inferior wall MI.

Right ventricular (RV) infarction—Elevated JVD, clear lungs (no LV failure), and onset of hypotension. *Give intravenous fluid.*

S_1 Q_3 T_3—Putative EKG pattern in pulmonary embolism, but not reliable. Usually see nonspecific ST-T changes. (Figure 3-20)

Septic thromboembolism of inferior jugular vein—From extension of peritonsillar abscess and indwelling catheter. *Treatment: surgical drainage of abscess, removal of thrombosed infected vein, and antibiotics.*

Statistics:
- 20% to 40% of acute MI patients have normal EKGs.
- <50% of acute MI patients have elevated creatine phosphokinase (CPK) on initial presentation.
- 50% of angina patients have normal-looking EKGs.

Supraventricular tachycardia (SVT)—Consider the following causes: coronary artery disease (CAP), congestive heart failure, chronic lung disease, pulmonary embolism, pneumonia, pericarditis, thyroid disorder, drugs, alcohol, caffeine, and stress. (Figure 3-21)

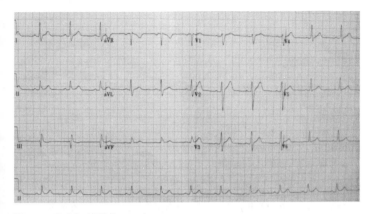

Figure 3-20: EKG for $s_1q_3t_3$

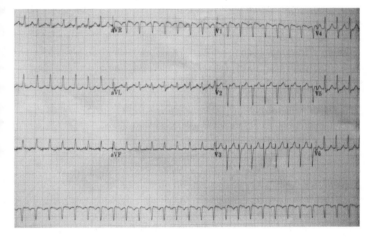

Figure 3-21: SVT

Survival from MI:

- 40% to 60% in witnessed ventricular fibrillation or tachycardia (V fib or V tach). *Prompt defibrillation and cardiopulmonary resuscitation (CPR).*
- <5% if not in V-fib or V-tach rhythm.
- 2% in PEA without rhythm.

SVT with digitalis toxicity—*Give magnesium, dilantin, digibind.* No calcium.

Syncope in the elderly patient—First test to order is EKG. High risk for age >55, congestive heart failure (CHF), and coronary artery disease (CAD).

Technetium-99 sestamibi—Deposited irreversibly in infarcted tissue showing up as hot spots on image.

Thallium-201—Hot spots → well perfused (normal myocardium). Cold spots → less perfused.

Thrombolytics—Converts plasminogen → plasmin. Lyses the fibrin content of clot.

Torsades de pointes—Rotating axis. *Treat with IV magnesium and overdrive pacing.* Caused by: Class I antidysrhythmics, tricyclic antidepressants (TCAs), organophosphates, antihistamines, and phenothiazine. (Figure 3-22)

Transcutaneous pacing—For Mobitz type II, 3rd-degree atrioventricular block unresponsive to atropine, early bradyasystole, bradycardia with hemodynamic compromise, and malignant escape rhythms unresponsive to treatment.

Transvenous pacing—See ST elevation when lead tip contacts ventricular wall.

Tricuspid incompetence—Signs of right heart failure, holosystolic murmur, and JVD. Located at the lower left sternal border. Found in intravenous drug abusers (IVDAs) with *Staphylococcus aureus* infection.

Tricyclic antidepressant (TCA) overdose—QRS and QT prolongation. *Charcoal, NaHCO3, IVF, and supportive treatment.*

Uremic pericarditis—Lateral chest x-ray study: lucent anterior pericardial stripe posterior to dark line of pericardial fat. *Definitive treatment: surgical pericardial window.*

Ventilatory Circulatory (VQ) scan—If normal, means negative pulmonary embolism. No further work-up and no anticoagulation needed.

Ventricular aneurysm—Patient with history of previous MI approximately 1 year ago, now presents with ST elevation on precordial leads and cardiomegaly on chest x-ray.

Ventricular fibrillation (V-fib)—See Figure 3-23.

Ventricular septal defect (VSD)—LVH, increased pulmonary vasculature, and systolic murmur.

Ventricular septal rupture—Patients with anterior wall MI present with chest pain, shortness of breath, new harsh systolic murmur along the left sternal border, and pulmonary edema.

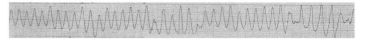

Figure 3-22: Torsades de pointes

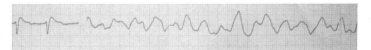

Figure 3-23: Ventricular fibrillation

Ventricular tachycardia (V-tach)—Atrioventricular dissociation, capture/ fusion beats, wide QRS, no RS wave in precordial leads, and ST-T wave concordance (ST elevation in the same direction as T wave). Wide beat supraventricular tachycardia can be hard to distinguish from V-tach. *Don't try!* Assume the tachycardia is ventricular; if the patient is unstable, cardiovert, and do not try to distinguish the two entities. (Figure 3-24)
- Clinically stable—*Lidocaine, procainamide, amiodarone, or β-blockers.*
- Pulseless—*Defibrillate at 200 J, 300 J, and 360 J.*
- Unstable—*Synchronized cardioversion with 100 J, 200 J, and 300 J. Amiodarone after cardioversion.*

Widened mediastinum on chest x-ray after motor vehicle crash (MVC)—Gold standard for diagnosis of aortic transaction is aortogram, computerized tomography (CT) angiogram, or esophageal echocardiogram. Institutional preferences and availability of these studies guides their choice.

Wolff Parkinson White (WPW) syndrome—Kent bundle, short PR, "delta wave" slurring upstroke of R wave, and wide or narrow QRS. (Figure 3-25)

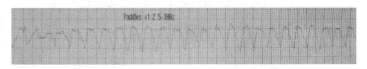

Figure 3-24: Ventricular tachycardia with wide QRS complex

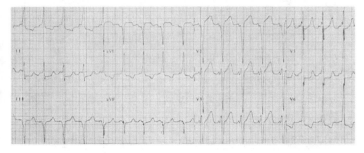

Figure 3-25: WPW

- Type A WPW—Right bundle-branch block (RBBB) pattern, deep S_1,V_1, RS, or RR′ in right precordium. See positive delta wave in V_1.
- Type B WPW—LBBB pattern, wide QRS, RR′ in left precordium. See negative delta wave in V_1.
- Narrow complex—Stable—*Adenosine, verapamil, β-blocker, digoxin, procainamide.*
- Wide complex—Stable—*Use procainamide;* **no verapamil.**

▶ VASCULAR

Abdominal aortic aneurysm (AAA) rupture—Classic triad: back, flank, or abdominal pain; pulsatile mass (palpable only 25% of the time); and shock. Syncope with new or chronic back or abdominal pain, hypotension, and hematuria. (Figure 3-26)

AAA repair history now presenting with gastrointestinal bleeding:
- Stable—*CT scan.*
- Unstable—*Immediate laparotomy.*

Afterload reduction—Use for all valvular disease except aortic stenosis.

Air embolism—*Place patient in Trendelenburg position, left side down.*

Aortic dissection—Tearing pain in chest. Pleuroapical cap, depressed left mainstem bronchus, pleural effusion, and wide mediastinum.
- Thoracic angiogram—Classic "gold-standard". Sensitivity 90%.
- Transesophageal echo—Preferred 1st imaging. Sensitivity 99%. (Figure 3-27)

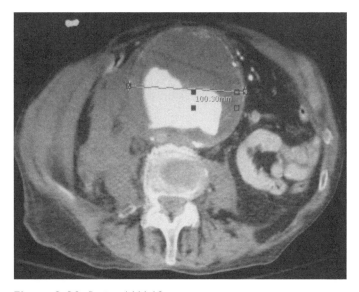

Figure 3-26: Ruptured AAA 10 cm

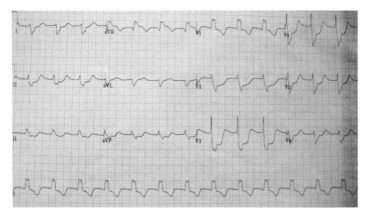

Figure 3-27: 76 y/o with sudden onset chest pain. DeBakey Type I aortic dissection.

- Classification:
    - DeBakey—I: Ascending and part of distal
        II: Ascending
        III: Descending
    - Stanford—A: Ascending (I and II); *Treatment: surgical*
        B: Descending (III); *Treatment: medical*

Aortic dissection versus MI:
- Aortic dissection—Chest pain and abnormal chest x-ray study. EKG usually normal or only nonspecific ST-T wave changes.
- MI—Chest pain, chest x-ray usually normal. EKG usually abnormal with ST elevations in contiguous leads. (Figure 3-28)

Aortoenteric fistula—Patient with aortic graft presents with GI bleed.

Aortography—Gold standard for identifying dissection. This is institutionally dependent. Can also be reliably diagnosed with transesophageal echocardiogram, or with CT angiography (CTA).

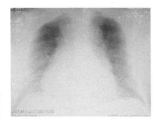
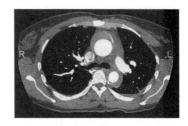

a   b

Figure 3-28: (a) Chest x-ray with widened mediastinum. (b) Aortic dissection.

Carotid artery bruit—~70% stenosis.

Carotid sinus hypersensitivity—Occurs with head turning.

Chest pain and neurological symptoms—Look for an aortic dissection.

Clotted external hemodialysis shunt—*Consult vascular surgeon.*

Compartment syndrome—6 P's: pain, paresthesia, paralysis, pallor, palpable tenderness, and pulselessness. Compartment pressure >30 mm Hg → *emergent fasciotomy.*

Computerized tomography (CT) scan—Gold standard for AAA in stable patients.

Contrast venography—Gold standard for ruling out deep venous thrombosis (DVT). Usually doplar studies are done to evaluate for DVT.

Digoxin—Causes constriction of mesenteric circulation → nonocclusive mesenteric infarction.

DVT—Most reliable sign: unilateral pain, swelling, and edema. Least reliable sign: Homan's sign.

Effort thrombosis—See in young people. Subclavian and axillary DVT. 15% chance of pulmonary embolus (PE).

Elderly patients—Apparent renal colic is AAA until proven otherwise. May present with hematuria.

Fat embolism—Do not use heparin. *Use high-dose steroids.*

Hypertensive emergency—Elevated blood pressure with evidence of end-organ damage. *Immediate lowering of 20% to 25% mean arterial pressure (MAP) in 1 hour.*
- Aortic dissection—Lower blood pressure with *labetalol.*
- Eclampsia—Lower blood pressure with *MgSO4, hydralazine, labetalol.*
- Hypertensive encephalopathy—Lower blood pressure with *nitroprusside.*
- Pheochromocytoma—Lower blood pressure with *both α- and β-blockers.*
- Pulmonary edema—*Use morphine, nitroglycerine, and lasix.*

Hypertensive urgency—Elevation of BP with diastolic >120 mm Hg. Potentially harmful but no symptoms. *Reduce BP in 24 hours using oral agents.*

Infraclavicular subclavian route—Central line with highest complication rate. Complications are lowered if the insertion is made using the aid of ultrasound probe.

Leriche's syndrome—Bilateral claudication causing bilateral hip or thigh pain and impotence.

Mesenteric infarction—Nausea and vomiting, anorexia, severe abdominal pain with normal physical examination, with or without bloody stool, metabolic acidosis, and leukocytosis. Thumb-printing (irregular thickening of bowel wall) and pneumatosis intestinalis (air within the wall of small bowel). *Mesenteric angiography.*

Mesenteric ischemia—Marked leukocytosis, elevated serum phosphate, and metabolic acidosis.
  • Arterial thrombosis—Progressive arteriosclerosis and unexpected weight loss.
  • Venous thrombosis—Risk factors: hypercoagulable states, antithromboplastin III (ATIII) deficiency, atrial fibrillation, congestive heart failure, myocardial infarction, and cancer.
Phlegmasia alba dolens (white)—Ileofemoral vein thrombosis with swollen leg and doughy white skin. From arterial spasm.
Phlegmasia cerulea dolens (blue)—Ileofemoral vein thrombosis with leg tensely swollen and cyanotic. May have blisters.
Protein C deficiency—*Do not use coumadin.*
Pulsus paradoxus—Not present in constrictive pericarditis.
Subclavian steal syndrome—Caused by upper extremity exercise. Blood shunted from vertebrobasilar system to supply ipsilateral subclavian. Abnormal narrowing of subclavian proximal to vertebrobasilar artery.
Thoracic outlet syndrome—Mimics ulnar nerve complaints (C8, T_1). *Conservative treatment, but if persistent problems, may require surgical release of the anterior scalene muscle.*
Vasovagal syncope—Bradycardia, hypotension, and pallor. (In contrast, see tachycardia, hypotension, and diaphoresis in anaphylaxis.) *Intravenous fluids.*
Virchow's triad—Venous stasis, hypercoagulability, and endothelial damage.

▶ DERMATOLOGY

Acanthosis nigricans—Brown to black velvety hyperpigmentation of the neck, axilla, or groin. Most common cause is insulin resistance. Other causes are obesity, malignancy (gastric cancer), and polycystic ovary syndrome.
Atopic dermatitis—Chronic pruritic eczema. Involve cheeks, legs, and antecubital fossa.
Basal cell carcinoma—Pearly rolled border with central ulceration.
Bullous pemphigoid—Tense bullae. Negative Nikolsky's sign. Benign course.
Chicken pox—Lesions in different stages. "Dew drops on a rose petal" starts on trunk and spreads to face. Includes mouth, spares palms and soles. Contagious before clinically evident and until all lesions are crusted. Crusting appears in 2 days. Acyclovir not helpful after crusting.
  • Adults run more complicated course—If immunosuppressed, febrile, has chest pain, or confused, *check for pneumonia and encephalitis, and admit for IV acyclovir therapy.*

- Pregnant with herpes zoster or chicken pox exposure—*Check titer: If negative, give varicella zoster immunoglobulin (VZIG) within 96 hours.* Peripartum varicella: May see disseminated herpes zoster in newborn.

"Coining"—Coin rubbing imprints on skin. Common practice in many Asian cultures. Do not confuse with child-abuse bruises.

Contact dermatitis—Two types: allergic and irritant. *Treatment: antihistamines and steroids.*

Dermatomyositis—Associated with skin findings and malignancy (6–55%).

Diaper dermatitis (candida)—Moist, beefy-red plaques, and marked edges with satellite lesions.

Disseminated gonorrhea—Young, women > men, fever, bilateral wrist or knee pain, and red papules on digits with a necrotic center. Cultures > positive from blood, genitalia, and pharynx than from joints.

Ehlers-Danlos—Easy bruising, loose joints, and hyperextensible skin.

Elongating pretibial tract-like skin lesion—Cutaneous larva migrans.

Erysipelas—"St Anthony's fire." Bright red, raised, and well-demarcated border. Group A streptococci. *Admit for IV penicillin.*

Erythema infectiosum (fifth disease)—Caused by parvovirus B19. "Slapped cheek." Fiery red erythema rash which fades to reticulated or lacy pattern. Hydrops fetalis if exposed during pregnancy. *Symptomatic treatment.*

Erythema multiform—Associated with herpes simplex. See target lesions.

Erythema nodosum—Painful, violet red nodule at dermis–adipose tissue junction. Most commonly seen on pretibial area.Causes: *yersinia*, tuberculosis, sarcoid, ulcerative colitis, Crohn's, pregnancy, streptococci, chlamydia, and BCP (birth control pills).

Erythroderma (generalized)—Pathognomonic for Hodgkin's disease.

Exfoliative dermatitis—Scaly, flaky, and erythematous rash that feels warm to touch. *Needs admission for diagnostic work-up, antihistamine, and topical steroids.*

Forchheimer's sign—Pinpoint petechiae on soft palate associated with German measles.

Gonococcal dermatitis—Tender lesions with gray necrotic or hemorrhagic center.

Henoch- Schönlein Purpura (HSP) triad—Symmetric palpable purpura on extensors, joint pain, and abdominal colic.

Herald patch—Pityriases rosea. Solitary round erythematous scaly plaque. Seen 5–10 days prior to generalized rash.

Herpangina—Coxsackievirus. Painful vesicles on posterior pharynx (not on buccal mucosa, tongue, or gingiva). Acute high fever and sore throat. *Treatment: hydration and viscous lidocaine.*

Herpes simplex—Painful grouped vesicles on erythematous base. Nondermatomal. Treatment does not prevent recurrence but decreases shedding and symptom duration and increases healing.
- Transmission: A person with chicken pox may give herpes zoster to susceptible individual. Opposite less common.

Herpes simplex with eye involvement—*Do not use steroid (worsens).*

Herpes zoster—Reactivation of varicella zoster virus. Thoracic: most common dermatome. Pain or paresthesia of dermatome followed by clusters of vesicles. Oral antiviral for immunocompetent and IV acyclovir for immunocompromised patients. Immediate ophthalmology consult for eye involvement. Nonimmune contacts can develop chicken pox. (Figure 3-29)

Herpes zoster with eye involvement—*Use topical steroid.*

Herpetic stomatitis—Child with fever, decreased oral intake, oral lesions only on lips, and painful lymphadenopathy. Caused by herpes simplex virus type 1 (HSV-1).

Herpetic whitlow—Herpes simplex I or II and involves only one finger.

Hydradenitis suppurativa—Occlusion of apocrine gland in groin, axillae, and vulva. Pitted, hypertrophic, or bridging scar.

Impetigo—Treat with either oral or topical antibiotics.
- Bullous—Staphylococcal aureus. Flaccid thin-walled bullae with purulent material, which ruptures forming "coin" lesions. Involves face and trunk.
- Nonbullous (classic):
  - Staphylococcus aureas—Mild erythema and superficial.
  - Group A beta-hemolytic streptococci (GABHS)—Vesicles with erythematous margins and honey-colored crusts. Acute post-streptococcal glomerulonephritis could occur, but not rheumatic fever.

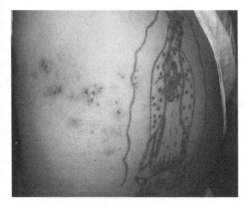

Figure 3-29: Thoracic herpes zoster lesions with tattoo

Kaposi's—Second most common manifestation of AIDS (after *Pneumocystis carinii* pneumonia). Painless, raised violaceous unblanching papules and nodules.

Koplik's spots—Measles. Bright red spots with bluish white center. Found on buccal mucosa.

Leptospirosis—Spirochete. From skin contact with urine of infected animal. Biphasic disease which begins with flu-like symptoms followed by asymptomatic period. The second phase is characterized by jaundice, renal failure, and meningitis.

Lyme disease—*Borrelia burgdorferi. Ixodes* ticks. Erythema chronicum migrans rash, which has central clearing. Spares palms and soles. Three stages: rash, neurologic/cardiac, and arthritis.

Macular rash—See Table 3-5.

Malignant melanoma—Sun-exposed areas. Metastases common.

Measles (Rubeola)—Begins on face and spreads to trunk. Koplik's spots on day 3–5. Three C's: coryza, conjunctivitis, and cough. *Treatment: supportive.*

Meningococcemia—Rash on palms and soles, fever, headache, and myalgias. Poor prognosis if petechiae, hypotension, and no meningismus.

Molluscum contagiosum—Firm, gray, and translucent dome-shaped umbilicated papules in sexually active patients.

Mononucleosis—Fever, pharyngitis, hepatasplenomegaly, and lymphadenopathy. One of very few diseases that causes enlargement of epitrochlear nodes. (Hodgkin's disease can also do so.)
  • Epstein-Barr virus (EBV)—Etiologic agent in 90% of acute cases. *If treated with ampicillin, because the throat looks like strep throat, 100% of patients will develop an erythematous rash that resembles a drug reaction.*

Mucormycosis—Rhinocerebral infection affects immunocompromised hosts.

Nikolsky's sign—Positive in toxic epidermal necrolysis (TEN), staphylococcal scalded skin syndrome (SSSS), and pemphigus vulgaris. Negative in bullous pemphigoid.

Table 3-5: Macular Rash

Meningococcemia	>100 skin lesions; petechial or maculopapular
Erythema marginatum	Begins as a macula that extends outward with central clearing
Secondary syphilis	Macular, pink, nontender
Rocky Mountain spotted fever	Macular erythematous rash begins on wrist and spreads to ankles, palms, and torso

Paronychia—Swelling and tenderness of nail fold. *Treatment: incision and drainage.*

Pediculosis capitis (head lice)—*Treat with lindane, pyrethrin, or permethrin.*

Pemphigus vulgaris—Adults. Involves skin and mucous membrane. Autoimmune. Bullous (flaccid), positive Nikolsky's sign, and positive Tzanck test. Mortality 10% to 15%.

Petechial rash and bleeding gums—Think idiopathic thrombocytopenic purpura (ITP).

Pityriasis rosea—"Herald patch" (single oval pink patch 3–6 cm in diameter with scaly border) seen most commonly on trunk. A week after the patch appears, there are pruritic papules with a "Christmas-tree" pattern.

Poison ivy or poison oak—With severe (bullae) give *oral steroids.*

Polymyositis—No skin involvement. Not associated with cancer.

Potassium iodide (KI)—For erythema nodosum.

Pseudomonas—Hot tub folliculitis.

Psoriasis—Erythematous plaques with white/silver scales. Involves elbows, knees, scalp, palms, and soles.

Pyogenic granuloma—Bright red shiny papule initially, and then a dull red to purple lesion.

Rocky Mountain spotted fever (RMSF)—2–12 incubating days, headache, fever, and myalgias followed by rash on the wrists, palms, and ankles. Uncommon in the Rocky Mountain region.

Roseola infantum—3–4 days of high fever. Maculopapular rash spreads from trunk to neck after defervescence.

Rubella (german measles)—1–5 days of fever, rash in face (blush), and suboccipital and posterior auricular lymphadenopathy.

Scabies—Itchy rash that worsens at night. Excoriated papular lesion in interdigital web spaces.

Scarlet fever—Caused by GABHS. Fever, strawberry tongue, and sandpaper rash.

Scleroderma—Follicular pattern skin depigmentation.

Seborrheic dermatitis—White and yellow scales with erythema. Involves scalp, eyebrows, and ears.

Secondary syphilis—Maculopapular rash with intraoral lesions.

Small pox—Incubation period: 12 days. All lesions are in same stage of eruption (unlike chicken pox).

Spider angioma—Erythematous vascular lesion. Seen in liver disease and pregnancy.

Staphylococcal scalded skin syndrome (SSSS)—<6 years of age. It follows an upper respiratory infection (URI) or purulent conjunctivitis. Flaccid bullae and skin desquamation. Perioral but no oral mucosal involvement. Pigment remains. Positive Nikolsky's sign. *Admit to burn unit.*

Stevens-Johnson syndrome—Remember M's: mycoplasma, malignancy, medications, mucous membrane, and multisystem involvement. Severe form of erythema multiforme. Bullous mucocutaneous lesions.

Squamous cell cancer—Rapid growth, central ulcer, and indurated raised border.

Syphilis—Spirochete treponema pallidum.
  - Primary: Painless chancre.
  - Secondary: Rash (palm or soles) or condylomata lata (infectious).
  - Tertiary: Cardiac and neurologic symptoms delayed.

Target lesions—Erythema multiforme (EM). Three zones color: central dark, pale next, and erythema on the periphery. Involves palms and soles.

Toxic epidermal necrolysis (TEN)—Adults with flu-like prodrome. Positive Nikolsky's sign. Involve drug reactions. Staphylococcus aureus is most common etiology. Mucous membrane affected. *Treat like burns. Admit, no antibiotics, and steroids controversial.* 25– 30% mortality. Involves >30% body surface area. Most severe form of EM. Severity scale: TEN >> Stevens-Johnson >> EM.

Toxic shock syndrome (TSS)—Fever, hypotension, rash, and at least three organs involved.

Varicella—"Dew drops on a rose petal."

Varicella zoster immunoglobulin (VZIG)—Give within 72 hours to susceptible immunocompromised or pregnant patients exposed to herpes zoster.

Waterhouse-Friderichsen syndrome—Shock, petechiae, and adrenal infarction. Meningococcemia.

Wound closure:
  - Primary closure—Closed before granulation tissue forms, 5–7 days.
  - Delayed primary closure—Closed before granulation tissue forms, but in 24–48 hours after initial wound occurs when there is a question of contamination.
  - Secondary closure—Closed after granulation tissue forms.
  - Tertiary closure—Healing by secondary intention. Allowed to granulate and epithelialize without formal closure.

Xanthelasma palpebrarum—Soft yellowish lesions around eye. Associated with familial hyperlipidemia.

▶ EMERGENCY MEDICAL SERVICE (EMS)/ ADMINISTRATION

"3rd service" model of EMS system—Police, fire services, and EMS. Three distinct entities.

Aeromedical:
- Primary response—Patient transport to receiving facility.
- Secondary response—Interfacility transport. From emergency department (ED) to another hospital.
- Tertiary response—Inpatient transfer to another hospital for definitive care.
- In rural areas, it converts a Basic Life Support (BLS) system to an Advanced Life Support (ALS) system.

Commercial flights—Contraindications: pregnancy >36 weeks, immobility, contagious disease, and severe anemia.

Critical incident stress debriefing (CISD)—Established in 1983. Should take place within 72 hours of disaster.

Disaster plans—Single disaster plan with subsections to cover specific requirement for particular type.

Disaster response:
- Level I—Provided by resources within the affected community.
- Level II—Mutual aid among adjacent communities or regions. Hours to days.
- Level III—Involvement by state or federal authorities. 48–72 hours.

Disaster response phase:
- 1st phase—Activation: initial response made and command center set up.
- 2nd phase—Implementation: search and rescue, triage, and patient management.
- 3rd phase—Recovery: orderly withdrawal from the scene, recheck for missed victim, and return to normal.

EMS classifications—80% volunteers. Requires 100 hours minimum instruction.
- Responder—BLS, spinal immobilization, splint, hemorrhage control, childbirth, and automated external defibrillator (AED).
- Emergency Medical Technician Basic (EMT-B)—Minimum required to staff BLS ambulance. Defibrillate.
- EMT-Intermediate (EMT-I)—IV, defibrillate, and adjunctive airway procedures.
- EMT-Paramedic (EMT-P) —Defibrillate, definitive airway, pacing, and needle cricothyrotomy.
- (These classifications are somewhat different in various locales. Permitted activities varies considerably from state to state. Become familiar with your own state and region.)

EMS Dispatch—Safely prioritize calls that need prompt or maximal response.

EMS Provider—Takes advice from on-line MD, which overrides orders from on-scene MD.

EMS resuscitation—Can honor valid written Do Not Resuscitate (DNR) orders. Resuscitate if there is any doubt regarding the DNR status.

External disaster—Event in the community leads to a sudden influx of patients for ED care.

Federal Aviation Authority (FAA)—Defibrillators not required. Dextrose, benadryl, nitroglycerine, einephrine, and oropharyngeal airway are required.

Federal Emergency Management Agency (FEMA)—The primary federal agency for emergency preparedness and response.

Hazardous materials—Decontaminated outside before coming inside the ED.

Helicopter ambulances—Cost $1000 to $2000. Flying prohibited if visibility <1 mile.

Incident commander—Management responsibility usually nonmedical.

Internal disaster—An event that disrupts the daily routine hospital functions, for example, labor dispute, power failure, etc.

Involuntary holds—Initiated by prehospital providers, physicians, safety officers, and family.

Mass gathering—>1000 people at one site.

Medical disaster—An event that overwhelms response capabilities.

Medical record essentials—EMS care, time, means of arrival, procedures, diagnosis, results, and orders.

Minors:
- Emancipated—Under 18 years, lives separately from parents, is independent, and self-supporting.
- With emergency (life or limb threat)—No consent needed for treatment. Make attempts to notify.
- Without emergency—Consent by special caretakers, adult relatives, foster parent, and judge.

National Medical Disaster System (NMDS)—Medical response, evacuation, and precommitted beds.

Off-line medical control—Prospective and retrospective patient care review.

On-line medical control—Critique and communication with paramedic after patient arrival. Overrides orders given by on-scene physician.

On-scene observation—Most effective way to assess quality of care.

Simple Triage and Rapid Treatment (START)—Respiration, perfusion, and mental status.

Triage:
- Categories—Walking wounded, critically ill, ill but can wait, and deceased.

- *Colors*:
    - Red—Critical priority, that is, shock, hypoxia, etc.
    - Yellow—Serious but can wait 45–60 minutes.
    - Green—Less serious and can wait hours to days.
    - Black—Dead.
- In a true disaster situation, care given to red patients, may cause yellows to deteriorate to red and die. Disaster triage is more like battlefield triage, where the less ill receive priority in order to be returned to combat status. Red needs recognition, but depending on numbers of victims, and availability of evacuation vehicles, may have to wait until all the yellows have been removed. Greens tend to remove themselves and clog up every nearby ED.

Unresponsive patient in out-of hospital setting:
- Adults—If there is only one responder, call the EMS system first before starting cardiopulmonary resuscitation (CPR). If multiple responders, start CPR while calling 911. Same process in infants and children.

▶ ENDOCRINE

Acanthosis nigricans—Cutaneous marker for endocrine disorder with insulin resistance.

Addison's disease—Adrenal cortex destruction causes the primary adrenal insufficiency. Small heart from low volume.

Adrenal crisis—Weak, confused, postural hypotension, fever, anorexia, nausea, vomiting, and abdominal pain. Hyponatremia is more common than hyperkalemia, but both can occur together.

Adrenal insufficiency:
- Primary—Decreased aldosterone increases the renin–angiotensin axis.
- Secondary—Normal aldosterone:
    - Acute adrenal insufficiency—Iatrogenic adrenal suppression (prolonged use).
    - Chronic adrenal insufficiency—Idiopathic atrophy adrenal cortex.

Alcoholic ketoacidosis (AKA)—Alcoholic with nausea, vomiting, and abdominal pain presents 2–3 days after binge drinking. Tachycardia, blood glucose <300 mg/dL, and ± urine ketones. *Often potassium and magnesium depleted as well as glycogen depleted.*

Aldosterone deficiency—Small heart size and low cardiac output. Dehydration with hyponatremia and hyperkalemia.

Apathetic thyrotoxicosis—Seen in elderly patients who present with atrial fibrillation with congestive heart failure (CHF).

Conn's syndrome (primary aldosteronism)—From overproduction of adrenal hormone.

Cortisol deficiency—Lethargy, anorexia, nausea, and vomiting. Hypoglycemia with fasting and inability to withstand minor shock.

Delayed deep tendon reflexes—Hypothyroidism.

Dexamethasone phosphate—*Treatment for unconfirmed diagnosis of adrenal insufficiency.*

Diabetes insipidus—Severe hypernatremia if the patient has no free water source; cannot excrete the sodium load of normal saline.

Diabetic ketoacidosis (DKA)—H_2O deficit 70–80 mL/kg and Na deficit 8–10 mEq/L. Usually history of diabetes mellitus (DM). Blood glucose <600 mg dL, Kussmaul breathing, ketoacidosis, and develops over short period.

Early morning hyperglycemia:
- Dawn phenomenon—Abrupt increase in fasting glucose not preceded by hypoglycemia. Normal circadian rhythm.
- Somogyi phenomenon—Hyperglycemic rebound from transient hypoglycemia.

Hydrocortisone hemisuccinate—Treatment for known adrenal failure.

Hyperosmolar hyperglycemic nonketotic coma (HHNC)—Usually no prior history of DM, blood glucose >800 mg/dL, no ketosis or acidosis, and develops over long period. If seizure, dilantin is contraindicated. It impairs endogenous insulin release.

Hyperpigmentation—Separates primary adrenal insufficiency (hyperpigmentation) from secondary adrenal insufficiency (no hyperpigmentation).

Hyponatremia—See Table 3-6.

Hypothyroidism:
- Primary—Thyroid stimulating hormone (TSH) level is increased.
- Secondary—TSH level normal or decreased.

Iodide—Blocks release of stored thyroid hormone. *Give 1 hour after propylthiouracil (PTU).*

Keyser-Fleisher ring—Wilson's disease. Copper deposits.

Table 3-6: Hyponatremia

Types	Common Causes	Urine Sodium	Treatment
Hypovolemic	Diuretics or vomiting	>20 mEq/L	Give NS IVF
Euvolemic	SIADH	>30 mEq/L	Restrict water
Hypervolemic	Cirrhosis or CHF	<10 mEq/L	Restrict water

CHF, congestive heart failure; IVF, intravenous fluid; NS, normal saline; SIADH, syndrome of inappropriate antidiuretic hormone.

Myxedema—Hypothermia, weight gain, constipation, and confusion to coma. *Treat with immediate IV thyroxine.*

Propranolol—Blocks peripheral effects of thyroid storm.

Propylthiouracil (PTU)—Blocks synthesis of new thyroid hormone only.

Salicylate—Contraindicated in thyroid storm fever. It increases free thyroxine (T_3) and triiodothyronine (T_4).

Stress hormone—Glucagon, cortisol, and somatostatin.

Syndrome of inappropriate antidiuretic hormone (SIADH) versus psychogenic polydipsia—In psychogenic polydipsia, urine maximally diluted (voids often and large quantities).

Thyroid storm—Fever, increased deep tendon reflexes, exophthalmus, conjunctivitis, corneal ulcer, weight loss, and confusion. Scenario: An elderly patient with fever, diarrhea, diaphoresis, tachycardia, and mental status change.

▶ ENVIRONMENTAL

▶ BIOTERRORISM

Agents:
- Chemical warfare:
  - Cyanides—Hydrogen cyanide and cyanogen chloride.
  - Nerve agents—Sarin, soman, and tabun.
  - Vesicants—Sulfur, mustard, and pulmonary agents (phosgene, chlorine).
- Biologic agents:
  - No person to person transmission—Inhaled anthrax, botulism, and tularemia.
  - Person to person transmission—Plague, smallpox, and Ebola.

Anthrax—*Bacillus anthracis.* "Bamboo or boxcar shaped" rods. *Postexposure. Oral ciprofloxacin for 60 days.*
- Cutaneous—Painless, pruritic, then vesicular eruption turning to a black eschar. Oral *ciprofloxacin for 60 days.*
- Inhalation—"Flu"/dyspnea followed by abrupt respiratory failure. Widened mediastinum, hilar nodes, and bloody pleural effusions. IV *ciprofloxacin for 60 days.*
- Prophylaxis—If exposed, give oral ciprofloxacin for 60 days and institute immunization.

Botulism—*Clostridium botulinum.* Descending flaccid paralysis. 4 D's: diplopia, dysarthria, dysphonia, and dysphagia. No fever.

Ebola—Three types. *All require contact and respiratory isolation.*

- Ebola virus (RNA filovirus)—Red eyes, maculopapular rash, and fever to shock. *ICU supportive care.*
- Lhasa fever (RNA arenavirus): Fever, pharyngitis; abdominal pain and edema; pleural and pericardial effusion. If AST > 150 IU/L, has worse prognosis.
- Marburg virus (RNA filovirus): Findings similar to those for Ebola. *ICU supportive care.*

Plague—*Yersinia pestis.* Sudden onset of fever, chills, headache, and myalgia. Rash due to disseminated intravascular coagulopathy (DIC) or necrosis of extremities ("black death"). Aspirate has a closed "safety pin" shape. *Treatment: streptomycin or gentamicin. Respiratory droplet isolation. Postexposure: ciprofloxacin, doxycycline, or chloramphenicol.*

- Bubonic—Painful lymph nodes in groin, axillae, and neck.
- Pneumonic—Cough, chest pain, hemoptysis and subsequent respiratory failure, and shock. Chest x-ray study: patchy, cavities, and consolidation.

Smallpox—Variola (DNA virus). Vaccinia (related virus) used in the vaccine. Vaccinia immunoglobulin (VIG) is used for serious vaccine reactions. *Contact and respiratory isolation. Vaccination 3–4 days after exposure offers protection.*

- Febrile prodrome—1–4 days before rash, temperature > 38.3 °C, (101°F), and one of the following: prostration, headache, backache, chills, vomiting, or abdominal pain.
- Lesions—Firm and round vesicles or pustules. May have umbilication or confluence. All lesions in same stage of development. Face first, then palms, soles, arms, and trunk.

Tularemia—Francisella tularensis.

- Pneumonic—Fever, cough, chest tightness, pleural effusions like tuberculosis, and skin rash. Laboratory personnel at risk. *Streptomycin, gentamicin, or ciprofloxacin. Postexposure: doxycycline.*
- Others—Ulcer, ulceroglandular, typhoidal, and meningeal.

> ▶ *BITES AND STINGS*

Black widow spider—Orange-red hourglass shaped coloration on abdomen. Neurotoxin. Digoxin like ST depressions on the EKG, and a board like abdomen. *Antivenin: use in patients younger than 16 years, older than 65, pregnant, or unstable.*

Brown recluse spider—Found in closets and attics. Causes DIC and renal failure. May not cause pain initially. "Bull's eye lesion" with necrosis and eschar.

Copperhead—No antivenin.

Coral snake bite—*Give antivenin, even before any symptoms develop.*
Crotalids—Pit vipers (rattlesnake, water moccasin, and copperhead).
Elapid—Coral snake and cobras. *Treat with antivenin.*
Honeybee—*Scrape to remove stinger.*
Pit viper—Immediate burning pain.
Pregnant with raccoon bite—*Human diploid cell vaccine and rabies immunoglobulin.*
Rattlesnake:
- Grades
  - Dry bite—No envenomation. Puncture wounds. No systemic effects. *No antivenin.*
  - Grade I—Mild envenomation. Swelling, pain, or ecchymosis confined to the local bite area. No systemic effects. No coagulation abnormalities. *No antivenin.*
  - Grade II—Moderate envenomation. Swelling, pain, or ecchymosis beyond the bite area. Nausea, vomiting, paresthesia, and mild hypotension. Mild coagulopathy. *Antivenin: 5–10 vials.*
  - Grade III—Severe envenomation. Swelling, pain, or ecchymosis beyond the extremity involved. Hypotension, shock, or altered mental status. Marked coagulopathy. *Antivenin: 15–20 vials.*
- Two types of antivenin—the conventional horse serum, which has a high incidence of anaphylaxis and serum sickness, and a newer human (similar to digibind) antiserum. It has a higher cost, but fewer side effects. Consult Poison Control Center for the recommended antivenin in your area.

Snakes:
- Elapid—Coral snakes and cobra. Causes neurotoxic symptoms.
- Crotalid—Pit viper: slit-like pupil and diamond head (rattlesnake, copperhead, cottonmouth). All venoms are hemolytic toxins.

Sting ray—Heat labile. *Immerse in hot water (decreases potency), x-ray for foreign bodies and débride.*
Toad toxicity—Similar to digoxin toxicity. *Treat with Digibind.*

▸ **BURNS**

Burns:
- First Degree—Superficial (sunburn).
- Second Degree—Blister.
- Third Degree—Skin charred, pearly white, and insensitive.
- Fourth Degree—Necrosis of tissues below the epidermis.

Major burn—*See Tables 3-7 and 3-8.*

Table 3-7: **Burn Center Criteria for Admission**

Age	Burn Thickness
<10 years of age	>3% full thickness >10% partial thickness Second-/third-degree burn >10% BSA
10–50 years of age	>5% full thickness >15% partial thickness Second-/third-degree burn >20% BSA
>50 years of age	>3% full thickness >10% partial thickness Second-/third-degree burn >10% BSA
Any age	Second-/third-degree burn to face, hands, feet, genitalia, perineum, or major joints Third-degree burn >5% with associated trauma, electrical, lightening, chemical, or inhalation injuries

BSA, body surface area.

Table 3-8: Rule of Nines

Adults	Body Surface Areas	Children
9%	Head and neck	18%
18%	Back	18%
18%	Front	18%
9% each	Upper extremity	9% each
18% each	Lower extremity	13.5% each
1%	External genitalia	1%

▶ CARBON MONOXIDE (CO)

CO—Crosses placenta, false high O_2 saturation with CO presence
- T½ life:
  - 6 hours—*Room air*
  - 1½ hours—*100% O_2*
  - 30 minutes—*Hyperbaric O_2*

CO poisoning—Red retinal veins and pale cyanotic skin (not cherry red).

Paint remover—Has methylene chloride that is metabolized to CO in the liver.

▶ DROWNING AND DYSBARISM

10% drowning—"Dry drowning" means without aspiration.
- Ascent:
  - Decompression sickness (DCS)—From ascending too quickly. Dissolved nitrogen bubbles reenters tissues and blood vessels. Risk factors: advanced age, obesity, post dive air travel, exertion, and cold dive.
    - *Type I DCS*—"skin bends," cutaneous; "the bends," musculoskeletal.
    - *Type II DCS*—"the chokes"—pulmonary, acute paraplegia, spinal cord; "the staggers"—cerebellar.
    - *Pulmonary overpressurization syndrome (POPS):* Acute gas embolism (AGE)—Sudden loss of consciousness on surfacing. Symptoms occur within 10 minutes. Most severe form of POPS. Others: pneumothorax and subcutaneous emphysema. Retinal gas bubbles on retinoscopy and Liebermeister's sign (a blue or pale tongue secondary to lingual artery emboli) are pathognomonic of AGE but rare.

Aspiration:
- Dry drowning—10–15%.
- Fresh water—Red blood cell (RBC) hemolysis, hypervolemia, and surfactant wash-out.
- Salt-water—Acute tubular necrosis is the major complication. Hypovolemia. Fresh water drowning is more common than salt water drowning.

Descent—All "squeezes."
- External ear squeeze—tympanic membrane (TM) bulging outward. Blockage due to plugs or cerumen.
- Middle ear squeeze—TM bulging **inward**, "ear squeeze."
- Inner ear barotrauma—Hemorrhage or rupture of the inner ear round window.
- Triad—Tinnitus, profound vertigo, and deafness.
- Nitrogen narcosis—Depths >70 feet. Euphoria, confusion, and disorientation. Known as "rapture of the deep."
- Perilymph fistula—Triad of deafness, vertigo, and tinnitus.
- "Sinus squeeze"—Sensation of fullness and pressure in the affected sinuses.

Drowning—Suffocation from submersion.

Fresh-water drowning—More common than salt-water drowning.

Hypoxemia—Can be caused from as little as 2.2 mL/kg fresh or salt water.

Near drowning—Recovery from drowning.

Recompression therapy—Indicated for DCS I and DCS II and AGE.

Secondary drowning—Acute respiratory distress syndrome (ARDS) and death.

▶ *ELECTRICITY*

Asystole—Caused by direct current (DC); also by high-voltage alternating current (AC).

Kissing burn pattern—Arc burns in flexor creases.

Labial artery hemorrhage—Delayed bleeding from bites on electrical cord.

Lightning strikes—Cause greater respiratory than cardiac depression. Therefore, victims will survive if given early vigorous artificial respiration.

Ventricular fibrillation—Caused by low-voltage AC.

▶ *HIGH ALTITUDE*

Acute Mountain sickness (AMS)—Headache, nausea, and weakness. *Treatment: Prochlorperazine and diamox.* Can prevent with diamox.

High altitude pulmonary edema (HAPE)—Noncardiogenic. Cough, shortness of breath, headache, and rales. *Treat with bed rest, O_2, and descent.*

High altitude cardiac edema (HACE)—Confusion, ataxia, and retinal hemorrhage leading to coma. *Treat with O_2, descent, and dexamethasone.*

▶ *HYPERTHERMIA*

Heat cramps—Benign muscle cramp. Excessive sodium loss replaced by water. *Rest and IVFs. Most commonly caused by intense exercise in heat, but can also be caused by hypokalemia in elderly patients on potassium wasting diuretics.*

Heat exhaustion—Volume depletion, fatigue, headache, nausea, vomiting, tachycardia, and hypotension. *Treat with IVFs.*

Heat loss:
  - Conduction—Transfer of heat through direct physical contact.
  - Convection (sweat evaporation)—Major mechanism for heat dissipation.
  - Evaporation—Conversion of liquid to gas phase.
  - Radiation—Heat transfer by electromagnetic waves.

Heat stroke—Hyperpyrexia and neurological symptoms (sudden loss of consciousness and bizarre behavior). *Rapid cooling.*

Heat syncope—Temporary loss of consciousness. Self-limited.
Heat tetany—Tingling and spasms in the extremities with hyperventilation.

▶ HYPOTHERMIA

Core temperature afterdrop—On rewarming, cold blood from periphery causes further cooling.
Freezing—Dry or wet.
  - Frostnip—Pale and numb skin with loss of discomfort and cold sensation. Reversible.
  - Frostbite—*Rapid rewarming in 42°C circulating water.*
Hypothermia—Sinus bradycardia with atrial fibrillation. J (Osborne) wave. Slow ventricular response most commonly seen. Sinus bradycardia → atrial fibrillation → ventricular fibrillation → asystole.
  - Mild: 32°–35°C. *Treatment: Passive external rewarming. Warmed humidified oxygen.*
  - Moderate: 30°–32°C. *Treatment: Active external rewarming. Heating blankets and lavage.*
  - Severe: < 30°C. *Treatment: Active core rewarming. Warm IVF, lavage, and warm humidified O₂.*
Non-freezing:
  - Dry (chilblains or pernio)—Erythema, pruritus, and burning.
  - Wet (trench or immersion foot)—Exposure in wet environment. Painful paresthesia.

▶ LIGHTNING

High voltage—> 1000 volts.
Keraunoparalysis—Transient and temporary. Cold pulseless leg secondary to lightning injury.
Lichtenberg figure—Superficial fern pattern from lightning.
Lightning—Asystole, > 50% tympanic membrane perforation, 50% fetal demise, cataracts, and lower extremity paralysis.
Reverse triage—Even with multiple victims, you cannot pronounce someone dead until you have supplied artificial respiration. In this situation, your attention must be given first to the apparent dead. Cardiac function returns before respiratory function, so many lightning-strike victims will survive with artificial respiration.

▶ MARINE

Jellyfish sting—Local irritation. *Treatment: Apply salt water (not fresh), vinegar, or isopropyl alcohol.*

Marine envenomation
- Spines—(sting-ray, catfish, and stone fish). *Treatment: Soak in hot water.*
- Nematocysts/sponges—*Treatment: Vinegar or salt water (not fresh water).*

Sea bather's eruption—Pruritic dermatitis in areas previously covered by bathing suit. By jellyfish *Linuche unguiculata.*

Swimmer's itch—Exposed areas. Flatworm schistosomes.

Venomous marine animal—*Treatment: Antihistamine, steroid cream, and topical anesthetics.*

▶ *PLANTS*

Dieffenbachia species (dumbcane, dumb plant)—Inability to talk. Plant contains calcium oxalate crystals.

Jimsonweed—Atropine-like symptoms (anticholinergic).

Mushroom—Although mild mushroom poisoning does occur, it is often impossible to know whether the patient has a fatal ingestion if the mushrooms are unidentified. The earlier that the symptoms appear after ingestion, the more likely it is a mild poisoning.
- Amanita—95%. GI effects: These progress from a quiet phase to hepatic necrosis and renal failure.
- Gyromitra—Hemolytic anemia and seizure.
- "Inky cap"—Disulfiram-like reaction when taken with alcohol.
- Muscarinic—SLUDGE (salivation, lacrimation, urination, defecation, GI symptoms, and emesis).
- Mushroom poisoning

Water hemlock—Neurotoxin causes seizure.

▶ *RADIATION*

More than 1 rad—Harmful to infants.

Acute radiation exposure—Highest rate of cell growth most sensitive (GI > CNS).

Absolute lymphocyte count (ALC)—Best indication of radiation exposure is ALC at 48 hours.
- $1200/mm^3$ good prognosis
- $300–1200/mm^3$ fair prognosis
- $<300/mm^3$ poor prognosis

LD 50 (Lethal dose 50%)—300 rad.

Rays—Alpha, epidermis only; beta, depth of 8 mm.; gamma, deeply.

Units and coversions:
- 1 gray (Gy) = 100 rad
- 1 sievert (Sv) = 100 rem
- 1 Gy = 1 Sv

Table 3-9: Symptoms of radiation exposure

Symptoms	Radiation
Within 2 hours	>400 rems
Diarrhea	>400 rems
Erythema	>300 rems
After 2 hours	<200 rems
No symptoms 6 hours later	<50 rems

▶ FLUID/ELECTROLYTE

ABGs (arterial blood gases):
- Winters' equation: $PCO_2 = [1.5 (HCO_3)] + 8 \pm 2$. Use it to predict PCO_2 when you know HCO_3.
- Primary respiratory alkalosis also present if ABG $PCO_2 <$ calculated PCO_2.
- Primary respiratory acidosis also present if ABG PCO_2 much greater than the calculated PCO_2.

Acetone—It is a ketone, but not a ketoacid; therefore, no acidosis is seen after ingestion.

Acidosis—This increases the ionized calcium function, but there is no change in total calcium.

Alcoholic ketoacidosis (AKA) versus diabetic ketoacidosis (DKA) versus hyperosmolar hyperglycemic nonketotic coma (HHNC)—All may present with nausea, vomiting, and abdominal pain. (Table 3-10)

Alkalosis—See hyperkalemia and hypocalcemia. Decreases ionized calcium function.

AKA—Chronic ETOH (ethanol alcohol) abuser who has an acute cessation from drinking.

Table 3-10: AKA versus DKA versus HHNC

Types	BS range	Symptoms
AKA	<300	Binge drinking with abrupt cessation. Ketones present
DKA	>300	Ketones present
HHNC	>800–1000	No ketones

AKA, alcoholic ketoacidosis; BS, blood sugar; DKA, diabetic ketoacidosis; HHNC, hyperosmolar hyperglycemic nonketotic coma.

Anion Gap—$Na-(HCO_3 + Cl)$ = normal ~10.
- Increases in MUDPILES: Methanol; uremia; diabetes; paraldehyde, phenformin, and propylene; iron and isoniazid; lactic acid; ethanol and ethylene glycol; salicylate, starvation, and solvents.
- Decreases in hypoalbuminemia, hyperviscosity (multiple myeloma), hyperlipidemia, and bromide.

Central pontine myelinolysis—Starts with confusion and progresses to cranial nerve deficits and quadriparesis. This is caused by overly rapid correction of hyponatremia.

Chronic renal failure with missed dialysis in cardiac arrest—Most common etiology is hyperkalemia.

Chvostek's sign—Facial nerve tapping causes ipsilateral facial muscles twitch.

Digoxin toxicity—Enhanced by hypercalcemia, hypokalemia, and hypomagnesemia.

DKA—Young or old with nausea, vomiting, Kussmaul's respirations, and acidosis.

DKA with normal potassium—*As the patient has fluids and glucose restored, the potassium level will fall. An initial normal potassium probably represents a true body hypokalemia. Add potassium as the patient recovers.*

Electrolytes:
- Calcium (Ca):
  - Hypercalcemia—Scenario: Elderly patient with history of lung cancer, confusion, and high calcium level. Etiology: Primary hyperparathyroidism, malignancy, Addison's disease, hyperthyroidism, lithium toxicity, thiazide use, tuberculosis, sarcoidosis, immobilization, and milk-alkali syndrome. Short QT interval.
- Magnesium (Mg):
  - Hypermagnesemia—This is often iatrogenic, seen in patients being treated for eclampsia. The deep tendon reflexes (DTRs) disappear followed by respiratory depression. *Treatment: Calcium gluconate. If not symptomatic, give IVF and diuretics. If renal failure is present, the patient needs dialysis.*
  - Hypomagnesemia (common in alcoholics)—Symptoms similar to hypocalcemia. The patient often also has hypokalemia.
- Phosphate (PO_4):
  - Hyperphosphatemia—Commonly accompanies hypocalcemia.

- Potassium (K):
  - Hyperkalemia—>5.5 mEq/L. Patient with a renal disease history or missed dialysis. The EKG shows high peaked T waves that with worsening hyperkalemia evolve into a sine wave. Acidosis causes the cells to leak potassium. Also seen with cell lysis, Addison's disease, potassium-sparing diuretics, and ACE inhibitors.
  - Hypokalemia—<3.5 mEq/L. From decreased intake, renal excretion, and gastrointestinal loss. Because the serum potassium is a poor reflection of the total body potassium, it is difficult to impossible to correct hypokalemia quickly. Follow the urinary pH; when it becomes neutral to basic, potassium losses have been replaced, and paradoxic acid excretion by the kidney, in an attempt to conserve potassium loss, ceases.
- Sodium (Na):
  - Hypernatremia—>150 mEq/L. Water deficit (in liters) 0.6 × wt in kg (1 – actual Na/desired Na). Each liter of deficit raises the serum sodium by 3–5 mEq. Correct 10–15 mEq/day.
    - *Hypervolemic*—From excess salt intake. *Treatment: Correct the cause.*
    - *Euvolemic*—Diabetes insipidus. Dilute urine in the face of concentrated serum.
      Central—Responds to ADH but not to dehydration. *Treatment: Give vasopressin (DDAVP).*
      Nephrogenic—No response to ADH or dehydration.
    - *Hypovolemic*—From reduced intake, or GI or renal losses. *Treatment: Give normal saline IVF.*
  - Hyponatremia—<135 mEq/L. Goes along with hypochloremia. If the patient has seizures, treat with hypertonic saline.
    - *Hypertonic*—Plasma osmolarity >295mOsm/L. See Hyperglycemia.
    - *Isotonic (pseudo)*—Plasma osmolarity 275–295mOsm/L. See Hyperlipidemia.
    - *Hypotonic*—Plasma osmolarity <275 mOsm/L.
      Hypervolemic—Edematous state. *Treatment: Restrict fluids.*
      Urinary sodium >20 mmol/L—From renal failure (unable to excrete free water).
      Urinary sodium <20 mmol/L—From CHF, cirrhosis, or nephrotic syndrome.

Euvolemic—*Treatment: Restrict fluids.*

Syndrome of inappropriate antidiuretic hormone secretion (SIADH)—Urine sodium >30 mmol/L. Urine concentrated.

Psychogenic polydipsia—Urine maximally diluted.

Hypovolemic—Urine sodium >20 mEq/L. GI, renal, and skin losses. Appears dehydrated. *Treatment: Give normal saline IV.*

High anion gap—MUDPILES.

High osmolar gap and normal anion gap— Isopropyl alcohol, glycerol, mannitol, and acetone.

Isopropanol alcohol—Osmolar gap but no anion gap.

Ketoacidosis—0.1 change in pH with 0.6 mEq/L change in potassium concentration in opposite direction.

Lactic acidosis:
- Type A—Associated with tissue hypoxia; sepsis frequent.
- Type B—Metabolic disease, drug, chemicals, toxins, and inborn errors of metabolism.

Metabolic acidosis:
- High anion gap—MUDPILES.
- Normal anion gap:
    - Low bicarbonate (HCO_3)—Pancreatic fistula, renal tubular acidosis (RTA), or diarrhea. Low potassium. *Treatment: Give HCO_3.*
    - High chloride (Cl)—From too much saline infusion or total parenteral nutrition (TPN). Normal potassium. *Treatment: Diuresis.*
- Low anion gap—Multiple myeloma (increases calcium), starvation (decreases albumin), or poison (halogens: iodides, bromides, etc.).

Metabolic acidosis and hypokalemia—RTA (except type IV), postobstructive diuresis, diuretics except potassium sparing; and Cushing's syndrome.

Metabolic alkalosis:
- Saline (chloride) responsive—Urine chloride <10 mmol/L. From vomiting, suction, or diarrhea. *Treatment: Give saline IV.*
- Saline (chloride) resistant—Urine chloride >10 mmol/L from mineralocorticoid excess. *Treatment: Give potassium.*

Methanol, ethanol, and ethylene glycol—Increased anion gap and increased osmolar gap.

Nitroprusside test—Tests for acetoacetate, not β-hydroxybutyrate. (β-hydroxybutyrate → acetoacetate with treatment). Early in therapy, the test is false negative, because it does not measure the high ketone that is present. Ask if your laboratory is able to perform β-hydroxybutyrate measurement.

Opioids—Causes hypoventilation and respiratory acidosis.

Osmolar gap—Difference between the calculated and measured osmolality of >10 mOsm/L.

Pseudohyponatremia—Caused by hyperglycemia, hyperlipidemia, or hyperproteinemia.

Psychogenic polydipsia—Patient with hyponatremia, a decreased serum osmolality, but the urine is maximally diluted (producing a lower urine sodium).

Rapid fluid administration—Single most important initial step in the treatment of diabetic ketoacidosis.

Rhabdomyolysis—See hypokalemia more commonly (63%) than hyperkalemia (40%).

Salicylism—Causes hyperventilation that produces a respiratory alkalosis. The metabolic acidosis is also present from the salicylic acid, thus produces a mixed acidosis and alkalosis.

Serum osmolarity= 2 Na + glucose/18 + BUN/2.7. Normal is 280–295 mOsm/L.

Sodium decreases by 1.6 mEq/kg—For each increase of 100 mg/dL glucose.

Syndrome of inappropriate antidiuretic hormone (SIADH)—Urine sodium >20 mmol/L, urine osmolality >150 mOsm/L, decreased blood urea nitrogen (BUN), and decreased serum osmolarity,

Trousseau's sign—Blood pressure cuff to upper arm maintaining pressure above systolic for 3 minutes produces carpopedal spasm.

Remember that for all metabolic diseases, they develop slowly, the patient looks sicker than what is complained about, and they cannot be corrected rapidly.

▶ GASTROINTESTINAL

▶ ESOPHAGUS

90%—Once an object passes the gastroesophageal junction, the probability of eventual passage through the gastrointestinal tract is high. (Figure 3-30)

Achalasia—Failure of lower esophageal sphincter to relax with absent peristalsis in the body of the esophagus. Dysphagia with solid or liquid, odynophagia, and

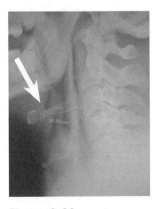

Figure 3-30:
Chicken bone in esophagus

valsalva to pass food. Bird's beak (distal) and dilated esophagus with air–fluid level on chest x-ray.

Aluminum cans pull tabs—Difficult to detect on plain films.

Boerhaave's syndrome—Sudden, forceful vomiting, chest pain radiates to back, full-thickness tear on distal left posterolateral esophageal wall, and a Hamman's crunch (a clicking rub heard posteriorly with respiration). *Chest x-ray—Use gastrografin preferentially over barium to prevent mediastinal soilage.*

Cafe coronary—Partially chewed meat lodged in upper esophagus causing cyanosis and death. Often seen with ill-fitted dentures, alcohol consumption, and too-rapid eating.

Caustic ingestion:
- Acids—Coagulation necrosis.
- Alkali—Liquefaction necrosis.

Coins—Transverse position in esophagus (anteroposterior position in trachea). (Figure 3-31)

Curling ulcer (stress)—Commonly located in body and fundus of stomach.

Distal esophageal food impaction—*Treatment: IV glucagon, sublingual nitroglycerine, and nifedipine. Manual removal per endoscopy if necessary.*

Dysphagia:
- Transfer dysphagia (oropharyngeal)—Difficulty initiating a swallow.
- Transport dysphagia (esopharyngeal)—Difficulty occurs after the swallowing process has started.

Esophagus veins—Inferior thyroid (cervical), azygous (thoracic), coronary, and short veins.

Gastrografin swallow—Diagnose esophageal trauma.

Globus hystericus—Sensation of foreign body in the throat.

Glucagon—Used in esophageal foreign body impaction (middle to distal third where there is more smooth than striated muscle; glucagon will not relax striated muscle, so upper third foreign body must be removed manually).

Intestinal obstruction—Most common parasite is *Ascaris lumbricoides.*

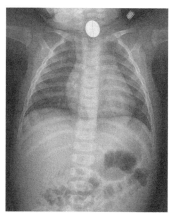

Figure 3-31: Swallowed coin

Lower esophageal dysphagia—Patient complains of a "sticking sensation." Rule out carcinoma.

Mallory-Weiss tear—Partial-thickness, longitudinal tear at the right posterolateral gastroesophageal junction with retching, dysphagia, and odynophagia. Upper GI bleed. Majority stop bleeding spontaneously. Common in bulimia. Look for posterior erosion of teeth from induced vomiting with gastric acid effect upon the teeth.

Mononucleosis-like—With Monospot negative and atypical lymphocytes. Suspect cytomegalovirus (CMV).

Nasotracheal intubation—Not precluded by known esophageal varices; neither is nasogastric intubation.

Nontraumatic chylothorax—Esophageal cancer.

Plummer-Vinson syndrome—Esophageal webs with iron deficiency anemia and cancer.

Schatzki's ring—Diaphragm-like stricture near gastroesophageal junction.

Zenker's diverticulum—Pharyngoesophageal pouch.

▶ GALLBLADDER, LIVER, PANCREAS, AND SPLEEN

Acalculous cholecystitis—5% to 14% cases. Elderly, postoperative, or post trauma patient.

Asterixis—Alternating flexion and extension of wrist when held in extension. Known as liver flap, and seen in hepatic failure.

Calcified gallbladder wall—Porcelain gallbladder.

Carcinoid syndrome—Vomiting, diarrhea, and hypotension, induced by the endocrine tumor that can implant anywhere in the gastrointestinal tract. Seen only if hepatic metastases are present.

Charcot's triad in ascending cholangitis—High fever with shaking chills, right upper quadrant (RUQ) abdominal pain, and jaundice. *Requires biliary tract decompression.*

Chronic hepatitis—50% of hepatitis C patients develop chronic hepatitis.

Chronic hepatitis carrier— + HBsAg, + HBcAg, and + anti-HB core.

Colon cut-off sign—Dilated bowel loop over pancreas. Seen in acute pancreatitis.

Courvoisier's sign—Nontender palpable gallbladder and jaundice associated with pancreatic cancer.

Cullen's sign—Periumbilical ecchymosis in acute hemorrhagic pancreatitis.

Entamoeba histolytica—Bloody diarrhea with chronic liver abscesses.

Gallbladder—Normal wall <3 mm thick.

Gallbladder cancer—Ampulla of Vater >> survival than biliary tree cancer. Early symptoms lead to early diagnosis.

Gas in gallbladder wall in x-ray—Emphysematous cholecystitis. Seen in diabetics. *Treatment: Emergent surgery.*

Grey-Turner sign—Flank ecchymoses in acute hemorrhagic pancreatitis.
Hemobilia—Bleeding into biliary tree, but presents as an upper GI bleed.
Most cases are of iatrogencic or traumatic origin.
Hemochromatosis—Increased iron deposited in liver tissue. Associated
with diabetes, hepatomegaly, and melanin deposit on skin. Skin has
metal-gray hue.
Hepatic encephalopathy—Precipitated by azotemia, GI bleeding,
hypotension, infection, and high-protein diet. Patient in coma with
asterixis (wrist flap) *Treatment: Lactulose, neomycin, thiamine, and
magnesium.*
Hepatitis—Incubation period:
  • Hepatitis A—½ to 2 months. RNA virus. Fecal-oral, subclinical
    anicteric, and no carrier state (no chronic hepatitis A).
  • Hepatitis B—2 to 6 months. DNA virus.
Hepatitis Serology:
  • HBeAg—High infectivity.
  • HBsAg—Carrier or active hepatitis. Appears in serum before
    hepatic enzymes increase.
  • HBsAb—IgM—early infection. IgG-protective. Present if had
    previous infection or vaccination.
  • HBcAb—Core antibody increases in window period.
Hepatitis distinction between infection and alcohol consumption:
  • Alcoholic—AST: ALT ratio >> 2. Viral—AST: ALT ratio << 1.
Hepatobiliary iminodiacetic acide (HIDA) Scan—More sensitive and
specific than ultrasound study. Used to diagnose acute cholecystitis.
Less readily available than ultrasound; cannot be done at the bedside,
and difficult to perform on a sick patient.
Hepatorenal syndrome—Acute renal failure in cirrhotic patient with
prior normal kidney function. *Treatment: Admit.*
Hypercalcemia—Causes pancreatitis, then pancreatitis causes
hypocalcemia.
Kala-azar—*Leishmania donovani*. Hepatomegaly, and splenomegaly.
Pancreatic pseudocyst—Pain, fever, and palpable mass.
Nonepithelialized wall-enclosing fluid.
Pancreatitis (acute)—Caused by gallstones > alcoholism.
Porcelain gallbladder—Nontender palpable gallbladder in RUQ
abdomen. Associated with pancreatic cancer.
Primary sclerosing cholangitis—RUQ pain, jaundice, and pruritus.
Ranson's criteria—Used to prognosticate pancreatitis:
  • On admission:
      —**A**ge : >55 years
      —**W**BC: >16,000/uL
      —**G**lucose: >200 mg/dL

- —**A**ST: >250 IU/L
- —LDH : >350 IU/L
- 48 hours after admission—Remember numbers 4, 5, and 6:
  - —**4's**: Base deficit>4 mEq/L. Calcium<8 mg/dL
  - —**5's**: BUN >5 mg/dL. Hct<10%
  - —**6's**: Fluid sequestration>6L. PO_2<60 mm Hg
- Mortality:
  - — <3 criteria: predicted mortality 1%
  - —3–4 criteria : predicted mortality 15%
  - —5–6 criteria: predicted mortality 40%
  - —>7 criteria: predicted mortality 100%

Rigler's triad—Gallstone ileus. Pneumobilia, dilated small bowel, and ectopic calcified gallstone. Seen in small bowel obstruction caused by gallstone rupture into the intestine; usually obstructs at the ileocecal valve.

Sclerosing cholangitis—Associated with inflammatory bowel disease.

Sentinel loop—Small bowel air seen over pancreas in acute pancreatitis.

Spontaneous bacterial peritonitis—Fever, abdominal pain, and tenderness. Ascitic fluid neutrophils >250 cells. Most common organisms are members of Enterobacteriaceae. uL and ascitic protein<gldL. *Treatment: Third- and fourth-generation penicillin or cephalosporin. Hospitalize.*

Spontaneous splenic rupture—History of mononucleosis, presents with left shoulder pain (Kehr's sign) and dizziness.

Wilson's disease—Cirrhosis of liver caused by excessive copper retention.

▶ STOMACH

Duodenal ulcer—More common than gastric ulcers. Burning between meals. Helicobacter pylori infection often accompanies.

Emergency endoscopy—Diagnostic procedure of choice for patients with significant GI bleed if they can be stabilized. If they cannot be stabilized, they need exploratory surgery.

Gastric outlet obstruction—Reflux, early satiety, weight loss, abdominal pain, and vomiting.

Gastric ulcer—Burning immediately after eating.

Gastric volvulus—Borchardt's triad: Sudden severe epigastric pain, distention, vomiting, and inability to pass nasogastric tube. Abdominal x-ray: large gas-filled bowel loop in abdomen or chest. *Treatment: emergency surgery.*

Gastritis—Burning pain worsens with eating.

Ulcer perforation—Sudden onset of severe epigastric pain. Chest x-ray often shows free air.

▶ SMALL AND LARGE BOWEL

Acute appendicitis:
- Symptoms—anorexia > nausea vomiting.
- Signs—Right lower quadrant (RLQ) abdominal tenderness > rebound > rectal tenderness > cervical motion tenderness.
  - *Obturator sign*—RLQ pain with internal rotation and flexed right thigh.
  - *Psoas sign*—RLQ pain with thigh extension lying on left side.
  - *Rovsing's sign*—RLQ pain with left lower quadrant (LLQ) palpation.

Adynamic ileus—No actual blockage or disturbance in gut motility. Seen after abdominal surgery.

Angiodysplasia—Most common in cecum and ascending colon.

Antibiotics—For treatment of conditions caused by *Campylobacter*. Not used for *Salmonella*. It will prolong the course.

Aortoenteric fistula—Patient with history of abdominal aortic aneurysm (AAA) repair, and now with upper GI bleeding.

Appendicitis—Outer diameter on ultrasound >6 mm.

Appendicitis in pregnancy—Incidence not increased, but perforation increases due to delay in the diagnosis caused by the obfuscation of the pregnancy.

Bacillus cereus:
- Staph-like—Only vomiting. From eating fried rice.
- Clostridium-like—Only diarrhea. Meats and vegetables.

Borborygmus—Visible peristalsis in small bowel obstruction.

Bowel ischemia—Postprandial abdominal pain. Elevated lactate dehydrogenase (LDH), and elevated lactic acid.

Bowel strangulation—Most common in small bowel secondary to vascular compromise.

Bright red blood per rectum (or maroon)—Upper GI source 14% of the time.

Campylobacter—Backpacker with WBCs and blood in stool. *Treatment: Antibiotics.*

Cecal volvulus—Younger patients. X-ray: dilated loop above pelvis. *Treatment: Surgery.*

Cholelithiasis and cholecystitis—See Figure 3-32.

Chronic appendicitis and right lower quadrant abdominal pain—Suspect Crohn's disease.

Ciguatera poisoning—Hot/cold reversal, perioral paresthesia, sensation of loose teeth, and lasts months. Gambierdiscus toxicus. Large fish, grouper, and snapper barracuda. *Treatment: Supportive care.*

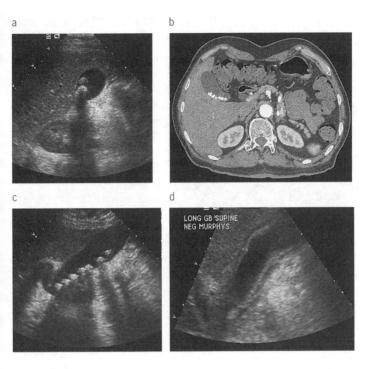

a   b

c   d

LONG GB SUPINE
NEG MURPHYS

Figure 3-32: (a-c) Gallstones: Ultrasound and CT scan (d) Thickened GB wall

Clams and paralytic shellfish poisoning—Saxitoxin. *Treatment: Supportive care.*

Closed loop obstruction—Volvulus, herniation of bowel loop into omentum/mesentery. Bowel segment that is blocked proximally and distally.

Coffee-bean sign—Distended, air-filled, and U-shaped bowel loops separated by edematous bowel wall. Seen in x-ray with small bowel obstruction.

Crohn's disease—All layers, mouth to anus, skip lesions, perianal fistulas, transmural, and ileum always involved. Most common complication: obstruction.

Diaphragmatic hernia—See Figures 3-33 and 3-34.

Diarrhea (causes and symptoms):
- Aeromonas hydrophilia—Rice water stools lasting >2 weeks but less volume.
- Bacillus cereus—Emetic syndrome: fried rice, meat, or vegetables. Diarrheal syndromes.

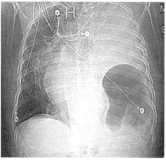

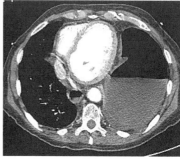

Figure 3-33 (above): Left diaphragmatic hernia. Chest x-ray and chest CT scan

Figure 3-34 (left): Left diaphragmatic hernia after repair. Left chest tube

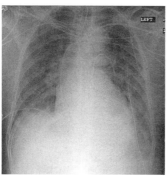

- Bloody diarrhea at camp—*Campylobacter.*
- Clostridium perfringens—Poultry or other meat.
- Cryptosporidium—Protozoa, chronic diarrhea in AIDS.
- Enterotoxin—*Vibrio cholera*, enterotoxigenic *Escherichia coli, Clostridium difficile, Clostridium perfringens, Bacillus cereus*, and *Staphylococcus aureus.*
- Enterovirus—No diarrhea.
- Giardia—Backpackers with abdominal pain, bloating, and frothy, foul smelling stool. *Treatment: Flagyl. Test contacts and treat if positive.*
- Norwalk virus—Nausea, vomiting, diarrhea, and abdominal cramps. No respiratory symptoms.
- Rotavirus—<1 year of age, fever, vomiting, and diarrhea. Diarrhea lasts 3 to 10 days. May have upper respiratory symptoms or pneumonia.
- Vibrio cholera—Rice water stools. From contaminated shellfish.

Diarrhea (types):
- Invasive—*Campylobacter, Giardia, Escherichia coli, Salmonella, Shigella*, amebiasis, *Vibrio parahaemolyticus*, and *Yersinia.*

- Toxigenic (noninvasive) —Staphylococcal toxin, *Clostridium perfringens*, Scrombroid, ciguatera. *Bacillus cereus, Escherichia coli,* and *Aeromonas*.

Diarrhea in AIDS:
- Campylobacter—Proctocolitis.
- Isospora and cryptosporidium—Chronic watery diarrhea.
- Salmonella—Bacteremia.

Diverticulitis—LLQ abdominal pain. Rectal bleeding uncommon. *No colonoscopy in acute phase due to risk of perforation.*

Emesis:
- Surgical cause—Pain followed by emesis.
- Medical cause—Emesis followed by pain.

Free air under diaphragm—See Figure 3-35.

Gallstone ileus—Gallstone eroding through gallbladder wall into a loop of small bowel until distal ileum where it causes mechanical obstruction.

Gastroenteritis and seizure in children—Think shigella.

Hematemesis and hypotension—Massive gastrointestinal bleeding. *Treatment: Give saline boluses and transfuse cross-matched blood.*

Hemolytic-uremic syndrome (HUS)—Bloody diarrhea associated with undercooked hamburger (Escherichia coli). History of invasive enteritis treated with bactrim.

Hemorrhoids—Internal, painless; external, painful. *Treatment: Incise external if thrombosed. Do not incise thrombosed prolapsed internal hemorrhoid.*

Hernia (types):
- Hesselbach's—Femoral and indirect same side.
- Littre's—Incarcerated Meckel's diverticulum within an inguinal hernia.
- Pantaloon—Direct and indirect same side.
- Richter's—Antimesenteric border herniates in the hernia sac.
- Sliding—Portion of hernia sac composed of organ (i.e., cecum, ovary). Only one wall.

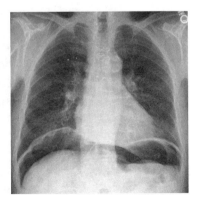

Figure 3-35 (left): Free air under diaphragm

Hernia—Incarcerated: irreducible. Strangulated: vascular compromise. (Figure 3-36)

Hiatal hernia—In chest x-ray see retrocardiac air–fluid level.

Internal hemorrhoids—Painless bright red rectal bleeding.

Irritable bowel syndrome (IBS)—Female > male; intermittent episodes of abdominal pain, cramps, diarrhea, and weight stable.

Ischemic bowel:
- Nonocclusive—*Treatment: No laparotomy*. Risk of anesthesia worsens ischemia.
- Occlusive—*Treatment: Laparotomy*.

Ischemic colitis—Not same as mesenteric ischemia. Elderly, diffuse or lower abdominal pain, (80%) associated with diarrhea, and (60%) often with blood. Not caused by large-vessel occlusive disease. Angiography not indicated. See mucosal/submucosal sloughing to full thickness. *Endoscopy.*

Large bowel obstruction on x-ray—Colonic distention and haustra not across the entire bowel width. (Figure 3-37)

Mesenteric ischemia—Scenario: Abdominal pain out of proportion to physical examination; history of atrial fibrillation or digoxin use. *Do angiogram.* X-ray findings: pneumointestinalis (air in bowel wall), "thumb printing" (edema of the bowel wall), submucosal hemorrhage, air in portal vein, and thickened bowel wall.

Nectar americanus (hookworm)—Hypochromic microcytic anemia with marked eosinophilia. Patient presents with abdominal pain, diarrhea, and guaiac-positive stool.

Ogilvie's syndrome—Dilated colon. Simulates a large bowel obstruction. Caused by tricyclics, antimotility drug, etc. *Do colonoscopy.*

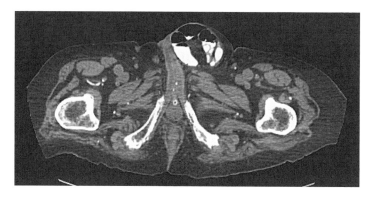

Figure 3-36 (bottom): CT scan: Left inguinal hernia in scrotal sac

Osteomyelitis of vertebral body—
Found in sickle cell disease and
salmonella.

**Pain out of proportion to physical
examination**—Mesenteric
ischemia. Acute mesenteric
arterial occlusion: embolism
(superior mesenteric
artery often). Nonocclusive
mesenteric infarction: low
cardiac output.

Parahaemolyticus—Associated with
oysters.

Perianal abscess—Throbbing pain
exacerbated by defecation.
- Incision and drainage in
ED—Perianal and perirectal
abscesses.

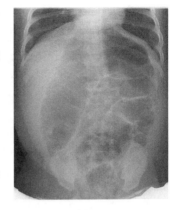

Figure 3-37: Large bowel ileus
from impacted stool in a 2 month
old infant

- Incision and drainage in OR—Ischiorectal, submucosal, and
supralevator abscess.

Procidentia—Rectal prolapse. Associated with cystic fibrosis or
malnutrition.

Pseudomembranous colitis—Diarrhea caused by *Clostridium difficile.*
See yellow plaques. *Treatment: Discontinue all antibiotics.*

Pseudotumor sign—Presence of a fluid-filled loop of bowel resembling
mass. Small bowel obstruction on x-ray.

Salmonella enteritis—Leukopenia and relative bradycardia.

Salmonella gastroenteritis—Associated with eggs, pet turtles, etc.
Treatment: Avoid antidiarrheals and antibiotics.

Scombroid poisoning—Facial flushing (histamine), cramps, diarrhea,
throbbing headache, and bitter or "peppery" taste. Fish include mahi
mahi, tuna, etc. Heat stable toxin. *Treatment: Antihistamine.*

Sentinel pile—Post-midline skin gathering in anal fissure. Resembles
external hemorrhoid.

Serum LDH level—Consistently elevated in early development of acute
intestinal ischemia.

Shigella—Explosive watery diarrhea and fever >101°F. Patient with altered
mental status (lethargy, coma, or convulsion), reactive arthritis,
Reiter's syndrome, or hemolytic-uremic syndrome (HUS). A child
may present with fever and seizures before there is any diarrhea or
other GI symptoms.

Shigellosis—Absolute band count >800/uL.

Small bowel obstruction

x-ray—Dilated bowel loops, air–fluid level, and see haustra across entire bowel width. (Figure 3-38)

Toxic megacolon—Complication of ulcerative colitis, pseudomembrane colitis, or Crohn's disease. >6 cm dilation of transverse colon is considered abnormal. Complications of ulcerative colitis.

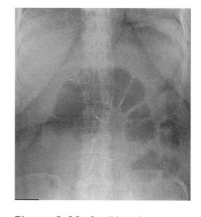

Figure 3-38: Small bowel obstruction

Tumors of colon—Left side mass causes obstruction. Right side mass causes bleeding and diarrhea.

Traveler's diarrhea (enterotoxigenic *E. coli*)—Scenario: patient returned from vacation in Mexico with frequent loose stools and no blood or fecal WBCs.

Typhoid fever—Intractable fever with bradycardia. Caused by *Salmonella* (subtype). See rose spots.

Ulcerative colitis—Rectum invasion, continuous, crypt abscesses, and bloody diarrhea. Antidiarrheals may cause toxic megacolon. Most common complication: hemorrhage. Associated with pyoderma gangrenosum, erythema nodosum, and aphthous stomatitis.

Vibrio cholera—"Rice-water" stool.

Vibrio parahaemolyticus—Oysters, clams, and crabs. Has 2 to 12 hour latency period. *Treatment: Tetracycline. Fulminant course often seen in alcoholics.*

Volvulus:

- Cecal—15%. Young adult with symptoms of bowel obstruction. Incomplete embryonic fixation of cecum, ascending colon, and terminal ileum. Abdominal x-ray: U-shaped sausage like loop toward RUQ. "Central stripe." *Treatment: Surgery for detorsion and bowel fixation.*

- Sigmoid—85%. Debilitated and bedridden elderly with abdominal pain and distention. Abdominal x-ray study: Kidney-shaped bowel loop toward left pelvis, "coffee-bean." *Treatment: Sigmoidoscopy, but if this does not produce detorsion (and it often does with explosive expulsion of colonic contents) or if necrotic mucosa seen, the patient will require surgical detorsion and colostomy.*

Vomiting—Bilious: obstruction distal to pylorus. Feculent: distal small or large bowel obstruction.

Yersinia—Pseudoappendicitis gastroenteritis associated with erythema nodosum. May cause mesenteric adenitis or terminal ileitis.

▶ GENITOURINARY

Acute kidney rejection—7 to 14 days posttransplantation. *Treatment: Corticosteroids. Patient will probably require admission to the transplant service.*

Acute renal failure (ARF)—Associated with erythema marginatum. Hyperkalemia is of concern.

Acute urinary retention—Causes: anticholinergic drug ingestion, benign prostatic hypertrophy (BPH), phimosis, postoperative pelvic floor repair, and urethral stricture. Epididymitis does not cause urinary retention.

Azotemia (pre-renal)—Elevated BUN–creatinine ratio and decreased urine sodium.

Balanitis—Inflammation of the foreskin. *Treatment: Clean with mild soap, antibiotics, and elective circumcision.*

Balanoposthitis—Candida in diabetic patients. Erosive lesions on prepuce and glans. *Nystatin cream.*

Behçet's syndrome—Vasculitis triad: chronic oral ulcer, genital ulcer, and relapse iridocyclitis.

Chancroid—Haemophilus ducreyi. Gram-negative rods in chains. Painful genital ulcer and painful inguinal nodes. *Treatment: Azithromycin, erythromycin, or cipro.*

Creatinine phosphokinase (CPK)—Most sensitive test to detect rhabdomyolysis (not myoglobin).

Dialysis:
- Dysequilibrium syndrome—Following dialysis, headache, nausea, vomiting, muscle cramps, and possible seizures. From osmolar imbalance between the brain and blood. *Treatment: Stop dialysis and give mannitol.*
- Intradialytic hypotension—*Treatment: NS IV 100–200 mL boluses.*
  — Early in dialysis session—From preexisting hypovolemia.
  — Late in dialysis session—From excessive ultrafiltration.

Epididymitis—<40 years of age, sexually transmitted disease (STD); >40 years of age, E. coli.

Fournier's gangrene—Edematous and infected scrotum with life-threatening necrotizing infection. The organism is usually anaerobic. *Treatment: Antibiotics, surgery, hyperbaric oxygen.*

Fractional excretion of Na (FENa)—Urine sodium/serum sodium/ urine creatinine/serum creatinine × 100. <1, prerenal; >1, renal or postrenal.

Interstitial nephritis—Proteinuria and pyuria.

Glomerulonephritis—Proteinuria, hematuria, and RBC casts.

Goodpasture's syndrome—Glomerulonephritis and hemoptysis.

Granuloma inguinale—Sexually transmitted lesions in inguinal areas. Under microscope see donovan bodies, which are purple safety-pin–shaped objects inside light-colored capsules.

Hematuria and papillary necrosis—Often seen in patients with sickle cell trait.

Hemoglobinuria (from severe hemolysis)—Reddish brown serum. Hemoglobin but no blood cells in urine.

Hemorrhagic cystitis—Adenovirus.

Hepatorenal syndrome—Oliguric renal failure. Complicating cirrhosis with ascites due to altered renal vasoregulation. Low urine sodium.

Hyperkalemia (severe)—Give calcium gluconate. Cardioprotective.

Hypothermic or sickle cell patients—Unable to concentrate urine.

Lymphogranuloma venereum—Chlamydia. Painless ulcer with tender unilateral inguinal nodes.

Myoglobinuria—Clear serum. Hemoglobin but no cells in urine. Black dark urine.

Nephrolithiasis—70% calcium oxalate or PO_4 and 15% struvite. (Figure 3-39)

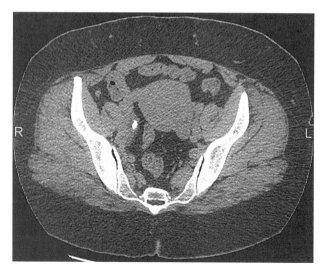

Figure 3-39: Non-Contrast CT scan—1 cm right ureteral stone

Paraphimosis—True emergency. Unable to reduce retracted foreskin over glans. Can progress to arterial compromise and gangrene. Manual reduction if possible, or a dorsal slit.

Perinephric abscess—Obscured psoas shadow on *CT. Treatment: Antibiotics and decompression.*

Peyronie's disease—Thickened plaque involving tunica albuginea resulting in curvature of penis.

Phimosis—Unable to retract foreskin from urethra toward shaft/base. *Treatment: Dorsal slit followed by circumcision after swelling and inflammation have subsided.*

Pregnant with complicated urinary tract infection (pyelonephritis)—*Treatment: Admit all third-trimester patients; first-trimester can be treated with IV antibiotics in the ED, and if able to take oral fluids, and are pain free, can be treated with oral antibiotics (14 days) as outpatients.*

Prehn's sign—In epididymitis, pain abates with elevation of scrotum (not reliable).

Priapism—*Treatment: Terbutaline subcutaneous, corpora aspiration, and phenylephrine irrigation.* Low flow: impaired venous outflow. High flow: increased arterial flow.

Prostatitis—Elderly man with fever, urinary frequency, and low back/perineal pain. Tender boggy prostate on examination. *May need suprapubic catheter. May not be able to insert a plain foley for drainage; best accomplished with liberal lubrication, and a Coude foley (curved distal tip of the catheter).*

Pyelonephritis (complicated urinary tract infection)—Fever, flank pain, and costovertebral area tenderness. *Indication for admission: third-trimester pregnancy, toxicity, immunocompromised, urologic emergencies, inability to intake orally, and lone kidney.*

Renal cortical abscess—Staphylococcus aureus. Hematogenous spread. May not have urinary symptoms.

Renal stones—90% radiopaque.
- Calcium oxalate stone—Sarcoidosis
- Cystine stone—Familial disease
- Struvite stone—Proteus urinary tract infection
- Uric acid stone—Glucose-6-phosphate dehydrogenase (G6PD) deficiency and Lesch-Nyhan syndrome; common in patients taking uric acid–excreting diuretics such as hydrochlorothiazide.

Renal transplantation—Common infection cytomegalovirus.

Scrotal nontender with painless mass—Urology consult to assess for malignancy.

Sterile pyuria—Urinalysis showing WBCs but no bacteria. Positive leukoesterase dip. Suspect Chlamydia urethritis.

Struvite stones—Contain Mg, NH_4, or PO_4. Chronic urinary tract infection.

Testicular cancer—Young male with painless distinct mass, or irregular enlarged testicle.

Testicular torsion—Puberty, unilateral pain, absent cremasteric reflex, and horizontal lie. Elevated testicle in the scrotum. May be seen in older patients; key is acute onset of pain. *Manual detorsion: open book. Need STAT ultrasound. Surgical emergency.*

Uremia—Rapid increase of BUN causes brain cell dehydration and buildup of cerebrotoxin metabolism.

Urethral prolapse—"Cherry red doughnut" or prolapsed cervix-like mass at introitus.

Urethral stricture—*12 or 14 French Coude catheter with copious anesthetic lubrication intraurethrally, or emergency suprapubic cystostomy via Seldinger technique.*

Urolithiasis and fever—*Treatment: Antibiotics and admit.* Other indications for urolithiasis admission: intractable pain, stone >5 mm, decreased renal function, urinary tract infection, no visualization of kidney on intravenous pyelogram, and extravasations of dye.

Varicocele—"Bag of worms." Painful vascular mass in scrotum caused by varicosity of the testicular vein in the spermatic cord.

▶ HEAD, EYES, EARS, NOSE, and THROAT (HEENT)

▶ *EYE EXAMINATION*

Corneal reflex—Cranial nerves (CN) V and VII.

Legally blind— Vision less than 20/200.

Pupillary constriction—Horner's syndrome, nontraumatic iritis, pontine hemorrhage, and pilocarpine.

Pupillary reflex—CN II and III.

▶ *HEAD AND FACE*

Cavernous sinus thrombosis—From dental extraction, sinusitis, etc. Toxic, high fever, eyelid edema, proptosis, chemosis, and pupillary dysfunction. CN III and VI palsy.

Ethmoid sinusitis—Complications: orbital cellulites, and cavernous sinus thrombosis. Proptosis.

Frontal sinus—Complications: forehead abscess (Pott's puffy tumor).

Sinuses:
- Frontal—Aerated by 8 years of age.
- Maxillary and ethmoid sinuses—Aerated soon after birth.
- Sphenoid—Aerated between third and fourth year.

▶ INFECTION

Acute iritis—Painful red eye, photophobia, miotic pupil, ciliary flush, and flare or cell in anterior chamber. *Treatment: Cycloplegics and steroid.*

Allergic conjunctivitis—Chemosis, cobblestone papillae under upper lid, stringy discharge, and pruritus. Staphylococcal infection.

Blepharitis—Lid margins. Staphylococcal or seborrheic dermatitis. *Treatment: Scrubbing with selenium shampoo.*

Chalazion—Chronic inflammation of meibomian gland on eyelid.

Chorioretinitis in AIDS—Caused by cytomegalovirus (CMV) in 5% to 10% of cases.

CMV retinitis—Cotton wool spots "tomato-cheese pizza" on eye examination.

Conjunctivitis—Most common: staphylococcus, most severe: gonococcus (GS).
- Bacterial—Mucopurulent discharge. Initially monocular.
- Chlamydia trachomatis—Infants 5 to 14 days post-delivery. Can cause blindness.
- GC—Infants 3 to 5 days post-delivery with copious eye discharge. Can perforate cornea.
- Herpes zoster—Ophthalmic branch of trigeminal nerve (ciliary branch).
- Staphlococcus aureus—White ulcers at limbus.
- Vernal—Males, family history of atopy, and cobblestone papillae under upper lid.
- Viral—Adenovirus.

Contact lens—Pseudomonas. Corneal ulceration. *Do not use eye patch.*

Corneal ulcer—Painful, localized white infiltrate on cornea. Hypopyon (pus anterior chamber).

Dacryocystitis—*Treatment: Warm compress and antibiotics.*

Epidemic keratoconjunctivitis (EKC)—Red painful eye with discharge. Contagious, photophobia, blurred vision, and erythematous sclera. Viral keratitis. Subepithelial corneal infiltrate. *Treatment: Steroids.*

Herpes simplex keratitis (HSK)—Ocular pain, photophobia, and dendritic corneal lesions. *Treatment: Topical antiviral and mydriatic. No steroids!*

Herpes simplex virus (HSV)—Recurrent, eye irritation, and dendrite epithelial defect.

Hordeolum (stye)—Acute. Hair follicle or meibomian gland. *Treatment: Antibiotics.*

Hutchinson's sign—Herpes keratitis. Lesion at tip of nose. Nasociliary branch of ophthalmic nerve.

Mucormycosis—Associated with diabetes and immunocompromised patients.

Needlestick exposure (for patient with three series of hepatitis B vaccine)—Draw blood for titer of the injured patient.
- If adequate titer (>10 mIU)—no vaccine or immunoglobulin required.
- Titer subtherapeutic—Administer hepatitis B vaccine (20 μg IM) and 2 doses of hepatitis immunoglobulin (0.6 mL/kg IM). First as soon as possible and second at 30 days.

Neonatal conjunctivitis—Rules of five:
- 0 to 5 days—Herpes or gonococcus
- 5 to 5 weeks—Chlamydia
- 5 weeks to 5 years—Streptococcus or Haemophilus flu

Nontraumatic iritis—Eye pain, injected, blurred vision, photophobia, miosis, ciliary flush, cells and flare, and pain in affected eye when light pointed to the other eye. *Treatment: Cycloplegics. If no post synechia (adhesions between iris and lens), then steroids.*

Optic neuritis—Young white woman, usually painful, and disc may be swollen. Commonly caused by multiple sclerosis.

Orbital cellulitis in children—Associated with ethmoid sinusitis. Painful ocular motility. Penetrates septum and pain with ocular movement. *Urgent CT. Treatment: IV antibiotics.*

Periorbital cellulites—Preseptal, erythema, warmth, and edema. Vision ocular movement normal. Fever and swelling more common with periorbital cellulitis. Staphylococcus aureus.
- *Treatment—Any orbital involvement, admit.*
    - *—<5 years of age—Admit and IV antibiotics.*
    - *—>5 years of age—Augmentin.*

"Pott's puffy tumor"—Complications of frontal sinusitis by osteomyelitis of frontal bone/abscess.

Pseudomonas—From contact lens or nail perforation through a tennis shoe.

Retrobulbar neuritis—Loss of central vision with preservation of peripheral vision. Multiple sclerosis.

Sinuses—Maxillary and ethmoid at birth. Sphenoid and frontal aerated by 6–8 years of age.

Staphylococcal allergic conjunctivitis—Multiple ulcers at limbus.

Subperiosteal abscess—Extension from orbital cellulitis. Surgical emergency.

Temporal arteritis—Elderly with decreased vision in ONE eye, temporal headache, and myalgia. Markedly increased erythrocyte sedimentation rate (ESR). *Treatment: Steroids.*

Ultraviolet (UV) keratitis—Diffuse punctate corneal lesion. *Treatment: Mydriatic agents, analgesics, eye patch, but no topical anesthetics.*

Vernal conjunctivitis—Seasonal. Cobblestone papillae.

Viral conjunctivitis—Conjunctival injection, chemosis, and preauricular lymphadenopathy.

White limbic ulcers (marginal)—Staphylococcal conjunctivitis.

▶ *TRAUMA*

Corneal abrasions—Suspect pseudomonas. Fluorescein shows white
spot on cornea. *Treatment: Mydriatics, but no patch or topical
anesthetics. Emergent ophthalmology consult.*

Corneal laceration—Teardrop-shaped pupil and black pigment
fragments at wound edges.

Eclipse burn—"Gun-barrel." Central visual field defect.

Ophthalmic burns—Alkali: irrigate, irrigate, and irrigate. Acid burns: less
destructive.

Foreign body:
- Bulbar or palpebral conjunctiva—*Sweeping with moist cotton-tipped
  applicator.*
- Corneal surface—*Topical anesthesia, use eye spud or 25-gauge needle
  under magnification. Topical steroids for allergic response to the foreign
  body. Emergent referral if unsuccessful or object deeply embedded.*

Globe perforation—Positive Seidel test. When fluorescein is applied to
damaged cornea, it becomes diluted with aqueous fluid from trauma
and turns bright green under blue light.

Hyphema—Blow to the eye with hemorrhage in the anterior chamber and
swollen eye. Complications: rebleeding and anterior or posterior
synechia formation.

Lens dislocation—History of trauma. Vision corrects with pinhole.

Mandibular dislocation or fracture:
- Dislocation—Jaw deviates toward the opposite side in unilateral
  dislocation.
- Fracture—Jaw deviates toward the fracture side. (Figures 3-40 and
  3-41)

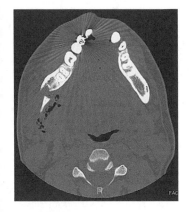 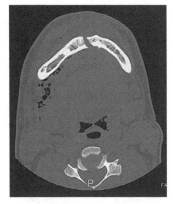

Figure 3-40 (left): Right
mandibular (angle) fracture

Figure 3-41 (right): Mandibular
(mentum) fracture

Marfan's syndrome—Predisposes to spontaneous lens dislocation.

Orbital blowout—Orbital blow, enophthalmos, restriction of upward gaze, and diplopia. Cloudy maxillary sinus on Water's view. *Treatment: Antibiotics and ophthalmology referral for repair.* (Figure 3-42)

Orbital emphysema—Orbital trauma. If vision loss, do a *lateral canthotomy.*

Orbital x-ray—For detecting metallic foreign bodies in patients with eye pain working with metal. It is also possible to use an orbital ultrasound study.

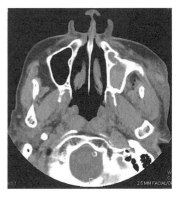

Figure 3-42: Left orbital floor fracture with fluid in maxillary sinus

Retinal detachment—Painless, flashing lights in peripheral, and curtain coming down. Most common in inferotemporal quadrant.

Retinal injury—No light perception.

Retrobulbar hematoma—Blow to the eye, painful, progressive irreversible vision loss, eye proptotic, pale fundus, and optic nerve ischemia. *Treatment: Do a lateral canthotomy.*

Ruptured globe—Most suggestive sign: teardrop pupil (points to rupture). Also bulging chemosis.

Schiotz tonometry—Used to detect glaucoma. Inversely related. The lower the number on the numerical scale, the higher is the intraocular pressure. The test is contraindicated in suspected globe perforation.

Seidel's test—Fluorescein streaming blue light in a river-like pattern seen with a ruptured globe.

Septal hematoma (nose)—*Treatment: Immediate drainage, otherwise may cause septal necrosis.*

Subconjunctival hemorrhage—Spontaneous or traumatic. Look for a ruptured globe if history of trauma, circumferential, dense, or elevated hemorrhage. *Treatment: None if benign, and the vast majority follow a sudden increase in intraorbital pressure, for example, after a sneeze, are spontaneous, need no workup, and do not recur.Emergent ophthalmologic consultation for a ruptured globe.*

Teardrop shaped pupil—Ruptured globe.

Teardrop sign—Orbital blow-out fracture as seen on facial x-ray.

Traumatic exophthalmus—*Treatment: Lateral canthotomy to relieve orbital hypertension with pressure necrosis of the optic nerve if the orbit is not emergently decompressed.*

Traumatic iritis—Orbital blow; severe orbital pain with motion but also with constriction of the pupil in a bright light; orbital pain, sluggish pupil, decreased visual acuity, cell and flare in anterior chamber, ciliary flush, miosis, and photophobic. Poorly dilated pupil. Glaucoma as complication. *Treatment: Cycloplegics and steroids.*

Vision corrects with pinhole—Lens dislocation or myopia.

Vitreous hemorrhage—Painless vision loss. Unable to see the red reflex due to blood "floaters": clumps of red cells in the visual field.

"Welder's flash"—Ultraviolet keratitis from tanning, eclipse viewing, or snow blindness. Slit-lamp: diffuse punctate keratopathy. *Treatment: Patch and topical NSAIDs. Steroid drops help. Topical anesthetic should be used only for initial eye examination.*

▶ NEURO-OPHTHALMOLOGY

Amaurosis fugax—Momentary blindness. Hollenhorst plaques (atheromatous emboli containing cholesterol crystals in the retinal arteries as seen on funduscopic examination). These warn of impending stroke.

Bell's palsy—Peripheral CN VII. Paralysis of ipsilateral forehead and lower face. *Treatment: Tapering steroids.*

Multiple sclerosis—Double vision. Optic neuritis (dull pain worsens with movement of eye) is many times the initial presenting symptom in multiple sclerosis.

Optic nerve pathology—Marcus Gunn pupil and red vision desaturation.

Red desaturation test—Associated with optic neuritis after staring at red, which becomes less red or pink.

Retrobulbar neuritis—Suspect multiple sclerosis. Loss of central vision with peripheral preserved.

Temporal arteritis—Same as giant cell arteritis. Involves external or internal carotid and vertebral branches. Painless vision loss, jaw claudication, fever, headache, temporal artery tenderness, and shoulder pain. *Treatment: Check ESR and start on steroids.*

Uveitis (iritis)—Painful eye with flare and cells in anterior chamber. May be followed by synechiae formation.

Vertigo:
  • Central—Insidious, nonfatigable, and nystagmus in any direction. Cause: Central nervous system (CNS) lesions.
  • Peripheral—Acute onset, fatigable, nystagmus horizontal or rotary, nausea, and vomiting.

▶ VISION LOSS

Central retinal arterial occlusion (CRAO)—Sudden painless vision loss in one eye. "Descending nightshade." "Box cars," pale fundus with bright red macula, or "cherry red spot" may be seen on funduscopic examination. *Emergency treatment: digital massage (probably won't help). Carbogen (95% O_2, 5% CO_2) to dilate artery; while worth trying, probably no benefit.*

Central retinal venous occlusion (CRVO)—Sudden painless loss of vision in one eye. Diffuse retinal hemorrhage, fundus "blood and thunder," or cotton wool spot may be seen on funduscopic examination. *Treatment: Ophthalmology referral. Aspirin daily.*

Functional blindness—No light perception (says can't see) with normal pupillary response. No afferent pupillary defect.

Glaucoma:
- Acute angle closure glaucoma—Painful. May be triggered in darkened movie theater; dilated pupil, fixed in mid-position, abdominal pain, nausea, vomiting, bradycardia, and cloudy cornea. *Treatment: Acetazolamide, timolol, glycerol, mannitol, and pilocarpine. Often it is confined to one eye.*
- Open angle glaucoma—Painless. Chronically increased intraocular pressure (IOP), optic nerve damage, arcuate scotomas, gradual loss of peripheral vision with central sparing.

Intraocular pressure (IOP)—Increased when >50 mm Hg.

Painful acute visual reduction—Acute angle closure glaucoma and optic neuritis.

Retinal detachment—Described as "curtain coming down."

Temporal arteritis—Scalp tenderness and blindness. *Treat with prednisone. Check erythrocyte sedimentation rate (ESR).*

Vitreous hemorrhage—Floaters with inability to visualize fundus. *Treatment: Elevate head of the bed and avoid valsalva. Ophthalmology consultation.*

▶ EAR

Bullous myringitis—Bullae on tympanic membrane. Mycoplasma. *Treat with erythromycin.*

Bullous myringitis and anemia—Hemolytic anemia secondary to cold antibody hemolysis. *Dress warmly.*

Cauliflower ear—Deformed auricle following a blunt cartilage injury with subsequent necrosis. If the auricular hematoma is seen before the necrosis develops, do incision and drainage of auricular hematoma and apply a compression dressing.

Cholesteatoma—Complication of chronic otitis media. Collection of keratin producing squamous epithelium in middle ear, and may result in bone erosion. *Treatment: Surgery.*

Conductive hearing loss:
  • Rinne's test—Test hearing with tuning fork on mastoid process and then next to the ear. If bone conduction > air, this is a positive test indicating a conductive hearing loss. If air > bone, the hearing is normal or there is a sensorineural loss.
  • Weber's test—Place the tuning fork in the middle of the patient's forehead; if hearing greater on one side, that is a positive test, and indicates conductive hearing loss. If heard better in the normal ear, then there is sensorineural loss.

Foreign body in ear—*Treatment: Do not flush vegetative matter with saline. Will expand. Live insects: drown with oil, lidocaine solution, and suction out. Solid foreign body may sometimes be removed with an ear curette; if not possible, refer to ENT for removal with operating microscope.*

Furunculosis of external ear canal—*Treatment: Cephalexin for staphylococcal infection with incision and drainage.*

Hearing loss:
  • Conductive—Lesions in external auditory canal, earwax, middle ear fluid, or Paget's disease.
  • Sensory-motor:
      — Brainstem lesion—Acoustic neuroma and vascular.
      — Inner ear—Ménière's, labyrinthitis, and syphilis.
      — Ototoxic drugs—Gentamicin, streptomycin, salicylate, and vancomycin.

Malignant otitis externa—Diabetic, immunocompromised, and debilitated patients with fever, pain, swelling, and granulation tissue. Pseudomonas, Staphylococcus aureus. *Treatment: Aminoglycosides and penicillin.*

Mastoiditis—Complication of untreated otitis media. *Treatment: Requires x-ray and IV antibiotics, and admission for possible mastoidectomy.*

Otitis externa—*Treatment: Acetic acid drops or hydrocortisone–polymyxin– neomycin drops.*

Otitis media—Streptococcus pneumoniae, Haemophilus flu, Mycoplasma pneumoniae, and moraxella catarrhalis. *Treatment: Amoxicillin.*

Pinna hematoma—*Treatment: Do incision and drainage of hematoma to prevent cauliflower ear.*

Post-traumatic perichondritis—Pseudomonas.

Ramsey-Hunt syndrome—Herpes zoster (varicella), CN VII involvement, ear pain, and vesicle on eardrum with CN VII palsy.

Swimmer's ear—Staphylococcus or pseudomonas. *Treatment: Corticosporin otic solution.*

▶ *NOSE*

Cribriform plate fracture—*Moraxella catarrhalis.* Litmus paper (or
    Kleenex) to nose collects fluid with a halo; this is a positive test
    and indicates a cerebrospinal fluid leak. *This requires a neurosurgery
    consultation. It does not require prophylactic antibiotics.*
Epistaxis—Need dry area for silver nitrate use (anterior bleed).
    • Anterior—90% of nosebleeds. Kiesselbach's area with local trauma.
      *Treatment: Use direct pressure, vasoconstrictors, cautery and nasal
      packing, outpatient antibiotics, and referral.*
    • Posterior—Sphenopalatine arterial bleed. *Treatment: Nasal packing,
      admission, and antibiotics.*
Septal hematoma—*Treatment: Will require incision and drainage.* Left
    untreated causes avascular necrosis of septum.
Sinusitis:
    • Acute—gram positive cocci and Haemophilus flu. If it involves
      only the antrum, the patient is not toxic, not immunosuppressed,
      nondiabetic, and with good social circumstances, the sinusitis can
      be treated with oral antibiotics and with outpatient follow-up. If
      the ethmoid or frontal sinuses are involved, the patient must be
      admitted for IV antibiotics, and possible surgical drainage. These
      sinuses are never involved singly.
    • Chronic—Gram negatives and anaerobes.

▶ *MOUTH*

Acute necrotizing ulcerative gingivitis (ANUG)—Also known as
    Vincent's angina or "trench-mouth". Fusobacterium and spirochete.
    Gray pseudomembrane, foul-breath, bacteria invading nonnecrotic
    tissue, fiery red edematous gingiva, metallic taste, and painful.
    Treatment: Saline rinse, penicillin, and follow-up.
Alveolar osteitis—Dry socket, foul odor, and pain free; 3 to 4 days after
    tooth extraction, sudden onset of excruciating pain and loss of clot
    occur. *Treatment: Nerve block, irrigate, packing, and antibiotics.* Follow-
    up with dentist within 24 hours.
Gingivitis—Painless, no bacterial invasion, and inflamed gingivae in
    response to the plaque.
Grayish membrane—On gingivae: Vincent's angina. On pharynx:
    diphtheria.
Group A beta-hemolytic streptococci (GABHS)—After strep
    infections, glomerulonephritis is not prevented with antibiotics.
    Rheumatic fever is *preventable with antibiotics.*
Hand-foot-mouth disease—Coxsackievirus. Vesicles on soft palate,
    tongue, and buccal membrane. Ulcers surrounded by red halos. Also
    on fingers and toes.

Herpangina—Ulcers on soft palate, uvula, and tonsillar pillars. Not on buccal mucosa.

Ludwig's angina—Often follows dental procedure and is associated with poor dentition and teeth caries. Dysphagia, dysphonia, cellulites in the floor of the mouth, and brawny neck. *Treatment: Intensive care unit, active airway management, and antibiotics.*

Masticator space infection—Infection from lower molar teeth invading space between pterygoid and masseter muscles. Toothache and trismus. *Treatment: Antibiotics and surgical drainage.*

Periapical abscess—Sharp severe pain on tooth percussion. Infection within the alveolar bone. Percussion tenderness. *Treatment: Penicillin and urgent dental referral.*

Periosteitis—Toothache within 24 hours of tooth extraction.

Peritonsillar abscess—Ill-appearing adolescents and young adults with hot potato voice, trismus, and drooling. Affected tonsil anteriorly and medially displaced. Uvula and soft palate displaced away from the affected tonsil. *Treatment: Needle drainage and antibiotics. For very young may need drainage in the operating room.*

Pharyngitis—Viral more common than bacterial.
- Adenovirus—Follicular lesion and unilateral conjunctivitis.
- Diphtheria—Pharyngeal erythema and gray pseudomembrane.
- Herpes—Vesicles.
- Influenza—High fever, myalgia, and headache.
- Mononucleosis—Tonsillar exudates, lymphadenopathy, and splenomegaly.
- Streptococcus—Temperature >38.3°C, exudates, cervical adenopathy, but no cough.
- Viral—Cough, rhinorrhea, myalgia, and headache.

Pre-dental space—Normal space: Children <5 mm; adults <3 mm.

Pyogenic granuloma—Gingival warty tumor. Seen in pregnancy. Can occur on digits or other extremities.

Ranula—Cyst in the floor of the mouth from salivary duct obstruction. *Treatment: Excision of cyst. Some association with hyperparathyroidism.*

Retropharyngeal abscess—In children <3 years of age. X-ray: C_2 retropharyngeal space 2 times diameter of vertebral body. Caused by Staphylococcus, Streptococcus, and oral flora. *Treatment: Antibiotics and ENT consult for incision and drainage.*

Stenson's duct—Parotid gland to opposite of maxillary molars.

Tooth avulsion:
- Primary—<5 years of age. *Do not replace.* Causes fusion to bone and deformity.
- Permanent—*Treatment: Replantation within 2 to 3 hours. Carry in mouth, or in milk.*

Wharton's duct—From submandibular or sublingual gland to floor of mouth.

▶ *THROAT*

Coin in x-ray—Trachea: Sagittal plane. Esophagus: Coronal plane.

Croup—6 months to 3 years of age. Parainfluenza. Barking cough, upper respiratory infection (URI) prodrome, and steeple sign. Nontoxic.

Epiglottitis—2 to 6 years of age. Haemophilus flu. Abrupt onset, fever, sniffing position, and toxic looking. Thumbprint sign on lateral neck x-ray. Now more common in adults since Haemophilus influenzae immunizations. Viral etiology also more common. *Treatment: Second- and third-generation cephalosporin, or ampicillin plus chloramphenicol. No racemic epinephrine.*

Prevertebral space:
- Adults—6 mm at C_2 22 mm at C_6.
- Children—14 mm at C_6.

"Steak stuck in throat"—*Treatment: IV glucagon, sublingual nifedipine, or oral gas-forming agents. No oral proteolytic enzymes due to risk of perforation.*

Steeple sign (x-ray)—Narrowing of the trachea in the anterior–posterior view. Associated with croup.

Thumbprint sign (x-ray)—Epiglottitis.

Tracheoinnominate artery fistula—Bleeding following tracheostomy. *Local digital pressure and tracheostomy tube cuff hyperinflation.*

Uvulitis—Febrile, difficulty breathing, and swollen uvula.

▶ HEMATOLOGY and ONCOLOGY

10,000 rule—1 unit platelets will increase platelet count by 10,000.

1-mL fresh frozen plasma (FFP)—Has 1 unit factor VIII and IX.

1-mL cryoprecipitate (CryoPPT)—Has 6 units factor VIII but no IX.

Acanthosis nigricans—Hyperpigmentation and velvety hyperkeratosis of axillae, neck, and groin. Associated with intra-abdominal malignancies, especially adenocarcinoma of stomach.

Autotransfusion—Only use intrathoracic blood. Contraindication: possible contamination with abdominal blood.

Blood transfusion and temperature spike—*Treatment: Stop the infusion.*

Brain abscess—Well-defined mass with low-density center and contrast-enhancing ring. With edema mass effect common. *Lumbar puncture not helpful, may be followed by herniation.*

Cancer patient with fever and confusion—*Needs lumbar puncture.* In neutropenic may not see WBC in CSF.

Cancer with encephalitis—Herpes zoster or Toxoplasma gondii. Lumbar puncture shows pleocytosis with increased protein but no organisms.

Cord compression—Patient with cancer and back pain.

Cryoprecipitate (CryoPPT)—To treat factor VIII and fibrinogen deficiencies. Risk of disease transmission. One unit or bag of CryoPPT has 80 to 120 units of factor VIII, and 200–300 mg of fibrinogen.

Dermatomyositis—Reddish purple skin changes of eyelids and periorbital area. Progressive muscle weakness. Associated with leukemias and Hodgkin's disease.

Disseminated intravascular coagulopathy (DIC)—Elevated prothrombin time (PT), elevated partial thromboplastin time (PTT), elevated thromboplastin time (TT), and elevated fibrin split products (FSP), decreased platelets, and decreased fibrinogen.

Epidural metastasis—Focal or radicular back pain is initial symptom in 95% cases.

Factor VIII concentrate—Treatment of choice for hemophilia A with hemorrhage. Shelf life is several months. Heated or detergent-treated concentrate eliminates HIV but has hepatitis risk. 1 unit/kg increases factor VIII by 2%. 1 unit of coagulation factor in 1 mL of plasma. $T_{\frac{1}{2}}$ 8 to 12 hours. *Treatment: Give half the initial dose every 8 to 12 hours.*
- Mild—12.5 µ/kg; skin laceration and hematuria.
- Moderate—25 µ/kg; dental extraction and joint or muscle hemarthrosis.
- Severe—50 µ/kg; intracranial hemorrhage (ICH), GI bleeding, and abdominal trauma.

Factor IX—Treatment of choice for hemophilia B.

Felty's syndrome—Triad of rheumatoid arthritis, neutropenia, and splenomegaly.

"Fish mouth"—H shape or "Lincoln log vertebrae." May be seen in sickle cell patients.

Hand-foot syndrome—Bilateral, symmetrical, and cylindrical swelling of soft tissue of hands and feet. First sign of sickle cell disease in infancy. (Not same as hand-foot and mouth disease.)

Hemolytic-uremic syndrome (HUS)—Diarrhea progresses to renal failure, hemolysis, fever, and low platelets. Precursor: E. coli O157:H7.

Hemophilia—*Treatment: CryoPPT or factor VIII-C concentrate.*

Hemophilia A (classic hemophilia)—Factor VIII-C deficiency. Abnormal PTT. Normal PT.

Hemophilia B (Christmas disease)—Factor IX deficiency. Abnormal PTT. Normal Factor VIII-C, PT, and TT.

Hemophilia with ICH—*Needs 50 U/kg factor VIII concentrate.*

Hemophilia with HIV—HIV risk incidence 3.6 per 10,000.

Heparin—Binds antithrombin III. *Reversal: protamine 1 mg per 100 U.*

Human immunodeficiency virus (HIV)—Opportunistic infections if CD4 <200 cells/mL. *Admit: Pneumocystis carinii pneumonia (PCP) with hypoxemia, cryptococcal meningitis, newly diagnosed tuberculosis, and CMV retinitis.*

Hypercalcemia:
- *Level <14 mg/dL—oral rehydration and ambulation.*
- *Level >14 mg/dL—saline, diuretics when urine output adequate. Treatment: Bisphosphonates for cancer induced hypercalcemia.*

Hypercalcemia in malignancy—Clinical triad of back pain, constipation, and CNS depression.

Hyperparathyroidism—Skull with ground glass appearance. See periosteal reaction and cysts in bones.

Hyperuricemia—Caused by thiazide and lasix diuretics.

Hyperviscosity syndrome (HVS)—Triad: bleeding, visual disturbance, and altered mental status. Anemia, "sausage-linked" retinal vessels, rouleau formation in peripheral smear, serum stasis, and clogs analyzer (laboratory unable to do tests). *Treatment: IVF, leukapheresis, and plasmapheresis.*

Hypothermia—Potential complication of multiple units of transfusion (also low calcium, low magnesium, and low platelets).

Idiopathic thrombocytopenic purpura (ITP):
- Acute form—Children, viral prodrome, and platelets <20,000/uL. *Treatment: 1 g/kg IV immunoglobulin.*
- Chronic form—Adults, female >male, no prodrome, and platelets 30,000/uL to 100,000/uL. *Treatment: Steroids.*

Inferior vena caval (IVC) syndrome—Secondary to pancreatic cancer, hepatic tumor, or deep vein thrombosis. May present with lower extremity edema and tachycardia.

Internal malignancy sign—Acanthosis nigricans, dermatomyositis, erythema multiforme, and erythema nodosum. *Treatment: Plasma exchange with FFP, steroids, splenectomy, and immune suppression.*

Kidney rejection:
- Hyperacute—Immediately due to ABO compatibility.
- Acute—First 3 months due to prior sensitization. Diagnosis: need a graft biopsy. Low urine output, generalized malaise, low grade fever, and tenderness over the graft.
- Late acute—In 6 months due to withdrawal of immunosuppressive therapy.
- Chronic—After 1 year due to immunologic factors. Progressive loss of renal function.

Lactic dehydrogenase (LDH)—Increased in hemolytic, thalassemic, sideroblastic, and megaloblastic anemia.

Leptomeningeal carcinomatosis—Headache. Lumbar puncture findings: increased pressure, high protein, low glucose, and positive cytology. *Treatment for impending herniation: Steroids and osmolar agents.*

Lupus anticoagulant—Increased risk of thrombosis as well as hemorrhagic diathesis.

Massive transfusion—Possible complication: bleeding from deficiencies of clotting factors.

Mediastinal mass—(Figure 3-43) Three compartments:
- Anterior compartment—Thymoma and lymphoma
- Middle compartment—Cysts and lymphoma
- Posterior compartment—Mostly neurogenic tumors

Meigs syndrome—Ascites and hydrothorax associated with pelvic tumor.

Methemoglobinemia—Cyanosis not relieved by O_2. *Treatment: Methylene blue.*

Microscopic hematuria—Prostatitis, sickle cell trait, tuberculosis, or coumadin use. Not myoglobinuria.

Multiple myeloma—See hypercalcemia, hyperviscosity, and pain in back and ribs.

Myoglobinuria—No RBCs in urine, just pigment.

O-Negative—Universal donor.

Pancoast's tumor—Lung apex epidermoid tumor with C_8, T_1, or T_2 neuropathy. First or second rib involvement.

Partial thromboplastin time (PTT)—Involves all factors but VII and XIII.

Parvovirus—Aplastic crisis in sickle cell crisis (SCC).

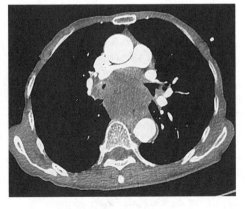

Figure 3-43: Mediastinal mass on CT scan

Pericarditis:
- Acute form—Inflammatory or effusive. Self limited. No complication.
- Chronic form—Lead to tamponade and death.

Pheochromocytoma—*Treatment: α-blocker (phenoxybenzamine) first, then β-blocker.*

Platelet transfusion—Indicated if <10,000 platelets or serious bleeding.

Polycythemia vera—Primary: involves all cell lines. Secondary: only RBC (normal WBC count and platelets). Full blown syndrome: hypervolemia, hyperviscosity, and platelet dysfunction.

Priapism—Sustained painful erection. *Treatment: Terbutaline 0.25 to 0.50 mg subcutaneously every 4 to 6 hours.*

Prothrombin time (PT)—To assess degree of hepatic dysfunction.

Reiter's syndrome—Triad: arthritis, conjunctivitis, and nongonococcal urethritis.

Rubin syndrome—Superior vena caval (SVC) syndrome with spinal cord compromise.

Salmonella osteomyelitis—More common in children with sickle cell disease.

Schizocyte—Typical cell in intravascular hemolysis.

Serum:
- Clear—In myoglobinemia.
- Pink—In intravascular hemolysis (from free hemoglobin).
- Yellow—In extravascular hemolysis (from increased bilirubin production).

Sickle cell crisis (SCC)—Types:
- Aplastic—Bone marrow suppression, low hematocrit (Hct), low reticulocyte count, and associated with Parvovirus.
- Hemolytic—Low Hct and high reticulocyte count.
- Sequestration—Sudden painful liver or spleen enlargement and hypotension.
- Vaso-occlusive—Pain in back, chest, and extremities.

SCC admission—Intractable pain, fever without source, unexplained leukocytosis, or priapism.

Spherocyte—Typical cell in extravascular hemolysis.

Spinal cord tumor compression—*Treatment: Steroids and radiation.*

Stokes' sign—Tightness of shirt collar in SVC.

Sulfhemoglobinemia—Not reversible with methylene blue. *Treatment: Supportive care.*

Superior vena cava (SVC) syndrome—Jugular venous distention (JVD), headache, facial plethora, feeling fullness in arms, tachypnea, shortness of breath, periorbital edema, and facial swelling. Worse in early morning and subsides later in the day. Squamous cell carcinoma (46%). *Treatment: Keep head of the bed elevated, chemotherapy, diuretics, and steroids.*

Temporal arteritis—Headache, fever, anemia, and elevated ESR. *Treatment: Steroids and biopsy.*

Thrombotic thrombocytopenic purpura (TTP)—Purpura, microangiopathic hemolytic anemia, neurologic signs, mild renal dysfunction, and fever (40% classic pentad). *Treatment: Plasma exchange with FFP. Steroids and splenectomy in refractory cases.*

Transfusion (massive)—Hypothermia. Use blood warmer.
- Type specific blood: 10 to 15 minutes availability.
- Fully cross-matched: 45 to 60 minutes availability.

Tumor lysis syndrome—Hyperkalemia, hyperuricemia, hyperphosphatemia, and hypocalcemia following treatment with chemotherapy. *Treatment: Hydration and dialysis.*

Vitamin K—Factors II, VII, IX, and X.

Von Willebrand disease—Autosomal dominant. Epistaxis, menorrhagia, or GI bleeding. *Treatment: CryoPPT 1 bag/10 kg weight. Type I: desmopressin. Type II, III: cryoPPT.*

Warfarin—Inhibits vitamin K factors II, VII, IX, and X. *Reversal: Vitamin K over 4 to 24 hours. FFP: Immediate reversal but short-lived.*

Whole blood storage—20 to 40 days stored at 4°C.

▶ INFECTIOUS DISEASE

Acyclovir—For herpes simplex encephalitis, herpes zoster in immunocompromised and ophthalmic branch, and primary genital herpes.

Aeromonas hydrophila—Seen with laceration in fresh water.

Amebiasis (Entamoeba histolytica)—Involves cecum, mimics ulcerative colitis, and causes liver abscess (chocolate cyst).

Ascariasis (ascaris lumbricoids)—Fever, cough, and hemoptysis.

Aseptic meningitis—Associated with mumps.

Babeosis—Prologia babesia. Malaria-like protozoan parasite syndrome. *Treatment: Clindamycin and quinine.*

Acillary angiomatosis—Osteolytic bone lesions in HIV patients.

Bacillus cereus:
- Emetic (like staphylococcal)—Fried rice.
- Diarrhea (like *Clostridium perfringens*)—Meats and vegetables.

Bell's palsy and complete heart block—Lyme's disease stage II.

Blackwater fever—Complication from falciparum malaria. Intravascular hemolysis causing renal pigment injury.

Botulism—Reflexes present and descending paralysis. (Opposite of Guillain-Barré: reflexes absent, ascending paralysis.)

Bubonic plague—Toxic, high fever, delirium, and generalized lymphadenopathy (buboes).

Cellulitis:
- Causes:
  - Plasmodium multocida—Dog or cat bite.
  - Aeromonas hydrophilia—Fresh water.
  - *Vibrio vulnificus*—From warm salt water. More common in alcoholics.
- Mechanism of spread:
  - *Staphylococcus aureus* and *Streptococcus pyogenes*—Locally.
  - Haemophilus flu—Hematogenously.

Cellulitis vs erysipelas—Rash margin sharply demarcated in erysipelas.

Cerebrospinal fluid (CSF):
- Bacterial meningitis—>150/uL WBC, polymorphonucleocytes (PMNs) predominate, low glucose, and elevated protein.
- Viral meningitis—<100/uL WBCs, monocytes predominate, and normal glucose.
- Brain abscess—As in bacterial meningitis.
- TB or fungal meningitis—High pressure, elevated protein, low glucose, and lymphocytes.

Chagas' disease—Caused by Trypanosoma cruzii. Fever, conjunctivitis, myocarditis, and megacolon. Meningoencephalitis in kids.

Chancroid—Painful necrotic ulcers of genitalia or perianal tissue. Haemophilus ducreyi.

Chicken pox—Incubation 14 to 21 days. Rash 1 to 2 days after prodromal (fever, malaise) symptoms. Communicability begins 5 days prior to appearance of rash and ends with crusting of all lesions.

Clostridium perfringens—Ingestion of improperly refrigerated cooked meat.

Colorado tick fever—Self-limited, severe viral syndrome, and retrobulbar headache. *Treatment: Supportive care.*

Condyloma acuminata—Pedunculated lesion. Herpes papilloma virus (HPV).

Condyloma lata—Secondary syphilis. Painless, moist, flat, and pale lesions in perianal region.

Congenital syphilis—Affects long bones. Osteochondritis and periosteal new bone formation.

Crepitus on extremity—Bad prognosis. Gas gangrene. *Treatment: IV antibiotics and surgery.*

Crohn's disease—Perirectal abscess with weight loss, diarrhea, abdominal pain, and fever.

Cysticercosis—Tissue invasion by larvae of Taenia solium after ingestion of eggs. Seizures. Endemic in Mexico. Not same as eating undercooked pork, which has intestinal tapeworm infestation from ingesting tapeworm.

Cytomegalovirus (CMV)—Associated with kidney transplantation.

CMV retinitis—Fluffy, white, and perivascular retinal lesions.

Diphyllobothrium latum—Fish tape worm. Causes pernicious anemia.

Disseminated gonorrhea—Hot, red, and painful posterolateral malleolar area with pustular lesion.

Disseminated toxoplasmosis—Associated with heart transplant.

Diphtherias, pertussis, tetanus (DPT) vaccine—Prevents pertussis epidemic, not lifelong immunity; 80% to 90% effective.

Enterobius vermicularis—Causes pruritic ani because the worms are excreted nocturnally.

Epididymitis—Gradual onset of pain and fever.
- < 35 years of age: gonorrhea and chlamydia.
- > 35 years of age: E. coli.

Epidural abscess—Presents with fever, back pain, and weakness in legs. *Treatment: Lumbar puncture contraindicated.*

Epiglottitis—Haemophilus influenzae is the most common bacteria in children and adults causing epiglottitis, but virus more common in adults. Epiglottitis is rare in children vaccinated against this bacteria.

Erysipelas—Streptococcal cellulites. Usually involves face. Demarcated area.

Functional asplenia—Treat for encapsulated organisms (Haemophilus inf, Streptococcus pneumoniae and Neisseria meningitidis).

Furuncular myiasis—Recent travel to tropics. Furuncle like nodules with central puncta, intermittent brownish drainage, or visible moving spiracles. Apply bacon fat to remove larvae with forceps while peeling off the bacon. Discard bacon.

Giardiasis (Giardia lamblia)—From fecally contaminated water. Affects duodenum and upper jejunum. F's—foul-smelling diarrhea, flatus, fatigue, fever, and fat (weight) loss.

Gonococcal proctitis—Diffuse hyperemia of anal mucosa with purulent drainage from rectum.

Granuloma inguinale—Small papule expands into extensive granulomatous and ulcerative lesions.

Gray Pseudomembrane on the posterior pharynx—Corynebacterium diphtheriae.

Hepatitis B—Associated with arthralgia or arthritis.

Herpetic whitlow—Periungual redness with vesicle formation. Risk to immunocompromised.

Hookworm (Nectar americanus)—Chronic anemia.

Impetigo:
- Bullous—Honey-colored crusted lesions with blisters. Caused by *Staphylococcus aureus.*
- Nonbullous—Smaller lesions with erythema and lymphadenopathy. Caused by Staphylococcus aureus or Group A streptococcus.

Hydradenitis suppurativa—Recurrent axillary abscess.

Intravenous drug abuse (IVDA)—Joints at greatest risk for infection: Sternoclavicular, sacroiliac, and intervertebral.

Intravenous immunoglobulin (IVIG)—Reduces mortality in Kawasaki's disease.

Jarisch-Herxheimer reaction—Marked fever spike reaction when organisms released after penicillin treatment (syphilis).

"Kissing lesions"—Chancroid.

Leptospira—Sudden headache, myalgia, and conjunctivitis. Avoid rat urine.

Lyme disease—*Borrelia burgdorferi*. Annular erythematous lesion with central clearing. Photophobia, headache, atrioventricular (AV) block, and facial nerve (Bell's palsy). *Treatment: Doxycycline or tetracycline.*

Lyme disease—Stages:
- Stage I—Rash (erythema migrans), malaise, fatigue, headache, and fever. 3 to 30 days.
- Stage II—Cardiac and neurologic symptoms. Weeks to months.
- Stage III—Migratory oligoarthritis of large joints. Months to years.

Malaria—Spiking fevers and chills after returning from foreign travel (i.e., Africa). Enlarged spleen. Normochromic normocytic anemia, Giemsa-stained parasite. *Treatment: Quinine and pyrimethamine-sulfadoxine or doxycycline, or both. Assume chloroquine resistance. Admission for >5% parasitemia, and for falciparum malaria.*

Maltase cross—Babeosis. Intraerythrocytic ring forms on Giemsa stain in peripheral smear.

Meningitis in >3 months of age—Haemophilus influenza>Streptococcus pneumoniae>Neisernia meningitidis. *Treatment: Ceftriaxone.*

Meningococcemia— >100 skin lesions (petechial or maculopapular); 55% have meningitis.
- Poor prognostic signs: Absence of meningitis, WBC <500, platelets <100,000/uL seizure on presentation, hypothermia, hyperpyrexia, low erythrocyte sedimentation rate (ESR), shock, purpura fulminans, petechiae within 12 hours of admission, and extremes of age.

Mononucleosis—Hepatitis, encephalitis, aseptic meningitis, Guillain-Barré, and splenic rupture.

Mumps—Viral, affects parotid gland, and <10% develop meningitis. Orchitis in 15–25% men with mumps.

Mycobacterium tuberculosis—Respiratory precautions.

Needlestick exposure—Risk of HIV through needlestick is 0.3%.

Osteomyelitis x-ray finding—Lytic lesions, periosteal elevation, and cortical irregular destruction. Seen 7 to 14 days after onset of symptoms.

Pancreatitis (acute)—Hypocalcemia and hypoglycemia. Caused by: gallstones, alcohol, hyperlipidemia, trauma, mumps, coxsackievirus, thiazide, and lasix.

Pilonidal cyst—*Treatment: Definitive treatment requires excision. Will recur.*

Pneumothorax in AIDS—Suspect Kaposi's sarcoma.

Post-streptococcal glomerulonephritis—Group A beta-hemolytic streptococcus. Tea-colored urine with RBC casts.

Postoperative fever:
- Day 1—Atelectasis
- Days 2 and 3—Pneumonia, superficial thrombophlebitis
- Days 4 to 5—Urinary tract infection (UTI)
- Day 6—Deep vein thrombosis (DVT), pulmonary embolus
- Day 7 to 10—Wound infection

Prostatitis—Fever, chills, perineal pain, irritative voiding, and boggy prostate. *Do not massage.*

Q fever (*Coxiella burnetii*)—Flu-like illness.

Quinsy—A synonym for a peritonsillar abscess. Complication of bacterial tonsillary infection.

Rabies—Viral. Affects all mammals. From peripheral to CNS. *Treatment: Active immunization with human diploid cell vaccine (HDCV) (Days 0, 3, 7, 14, and 28). Also passive immunization with human rabies immune globulin (HRIG) 20 IU/kg (one-half at site, one-half at gluteus).*

Rabies—Bats>skunks>raccoons>cows>dogs>foxes>cats (not squirrel, chimp, rats, or Easter Bunny).

Relapsing fever—Borrelia. Spirochete. Intermittent fever. *Treatment: Tetracycline or erythromycin.*

Reye's syndrome—Mitochondrial function disruption in brain and liver. Hypoglycemia, elevated serum ammonia, and abnormal liver function tests (LFTs). Fever, coma, hepatic failure; thought to be associated with aspirin therapy of fever.

Rocky Mountain spotted fever (RMSF)—Rickettsia rickettsii. *Treatment: Tetracycline or chloramphenicol IV or oral.*

Romaña's sign—Chagas' disease. Painless unilateral periorbital edema.

Scarlet fever—Exudative pharyngitis with diffuse papular (sandpaper) rash, but spares perioral region.

Schistosomiasis—Africa or South America. Painful or painless hematuria. Portal hypertension or obstructive hydroureter.

Scombroid poisoning—Histamine-like symptoms (improper preservation or refrigeration).

Septic hip—Referred knee pain with fever, cannot walk, hip tenderness, and elevated WBC count. *Treatment: Joint aspiration under fluoroscopy.* Overall: *Staphylococcus aureus.* Infants: *E. coli.* 6 months to 24 months: *Haemophilus influenza.*

Shingles in renal transplantation patients—*Treatment: IV acyclovir. Corticosteroid therapy controversial.*

Sleeping sickness—*Trypanosoma brucei rhodesiense* and T*rypanosoma. brucei gambiense.*

Staphylococcal scalded-skin syndrome (SSSS) versus Toxic epidermal necrolysis (TEN)—See Table 3-11.

***Staphylococcus aureus* food poisoning**—Dairy products and potato salad.

Steroid for *Pneumoncystis carinii* pneumonia (PCP)—If PaO_2 < 70 mmHg or A-a gradient > 35 mmHg.

Streptotoxic shock-like syndrome—Similar to toxic shock syndrome (TSS), but here source is skin infection or infected wound.

Strongyloides stercoralis threadworm—Cutaneous larval migraines.

Sulfur granules—Actinomyces. Affects external sinus.

Swimmer's itch—*Schistosome cercariae.* Acute pruritus.

Syphilis—Stages:
- I: Chancre—Painless papule on penis or labia.
- II: Pink rash 4 to 6 weeks later. Papulosquamous rash spreads from trunk to palms and soles.
- III: Tertiary—Neurosyphilis 6 months to 10 years later, meningitis, and stroke.
  - Tabes dorsalis: Progressive demyelinization with ataxia, incontinence, and leg pain.
  - Cardiovascular: 20–40 years later. Causes aortic valve insufficiency as well as aortitis and aneurysm formation.

Table 3-11: SSSS versus TEN

	SSSS	TEN
Age	Infants	Older children and adults
Etiology	*Staphylococcus aureus*	Drugs
Skin tenderness	Present	May be absent
Exfoliating skin	White	Necrotic
Skin split	Upper epidermis	Full-thickness epidermis
Nikolsky's sign	Positive	Negative
Mortality	Rarely seen	30%

SSSS, staphylococcal scalded skin syndrome; TEN, toxic epidermal necrolysis.

Tenosynovitis—Usually flexor tendons. *Treatment: Surgery if no improvement after 2 days of antibiotics.*

Tetanus immunization—Td = tetanus toxoid. TIG = tetanus immunoglobulin.
- *Td for dirty wound if last tetanus between 5 and 10 years.*
- *Td for clean or dirty wound if last tetanus >10 years.*
- *No Td or TIG if complete series (3) < 5 years.*
- *No TIG for clean wounds.*
- *TIG in contaminated wounds ONLY if uncertain history or 0 to 2 doses of Td.*

Tetanus—Trismus (lockjaw), risus sardonicus (sustained spasm of jaw muscles), and autonomic dysfunction: hypertension, tachycardia, and hyperthermia. *Treatment: Antibiotics choice metronidazole. TIG and toxoid, benzodiazepine, surgical débridement and airway management.*

Tick-borne—Lyme disease, Rocky Mountain spotted fever (RMSF), relapsing fever, Q-fever, tularemia, babeosis, and Colorado tick fever.

Tick paralysis—Restlessness and paresthesia of hands and feet progressing to ascending paralysis. Deep tendon reflex absent. *Treatment: Remove the tick.*

Toxic shock syndrome—Toxic, hypotensive, febrile, and tachycardiac with diffuse rash and erythroderma with peeling of skin around nails. May have sore throat, nausea, or vomiting. Pulmonary and peripheral edema, but no elevation of central venous pressure pressure. *Treatment: Anti-staphylococcal antibiotics and pressors.*

Trichinellosis—Ingestion of infected pork or beef. Presents with periorbital edema and has elevated creatine phosphokinase (CPK) level.

Tuberculosis meningitis—CSF finding: lymphocytic pleocytosis, low glucose, and high protein.

Tularemia—Ulceroglandular > typhoidal. Ticks. Gives life-long immunity. *Treatment: Streptomycin.*

Vibrio vulnificus—Seawater and contaminated seafood. Cellulitis with hemorrhagic bullae.

Water chestnuts—*Fasciolopsis buski.* Endemic in Far East. Intestinal fluke.

Waterhouse-Friderichsen syndrome—Shock, petechiae, and adrenal infarction secondary to adrenal hemorrhage.

Weil's syndrome—Severe hepatorenal disease due to leptospirosis.

▶ NEUROLOGY

Elderly—Basically everything decreases except for increased adipose tissue and increased peripheral vascular resistance. Unchanged hemoglobin and red cell indices.

Vertigo or dizziness:

- Central—*Treatment: Neurologic consult and admission except for multiple sclerosis and migraine. Outpatient follow-up.*

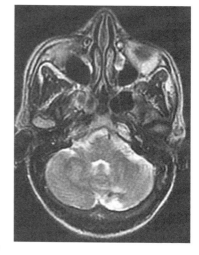

Figure 3-44: Cerebellar hemorrhage

  - Cerebellar hemorrhage—Acute vertigo. Ataxia, nausea, vomiting, and positive Romberg's (swaying on closing eyes while standing upright). (Figure 3-44)
  - Vertebrobasilar insufficiency (VBI)—New onset vertigo, old age, double vision, dysarthria, ataxia, weakness, and facial numbness.
  - Wallenberg's syndrome—Posterior-inferior cerebral artery (PICA) occlusion. Nausea, vomiting, ataxia, hoarseness, and paralysis of larynx, palate, and pharynx. Loss of pain and temperature same side of face, and opposite in body. Horner's syndrome: ipsilateral ptosis, miosis, and anhydrosis.
  - Others: Neoplasms (fourth ventricle), multiple sclerosis, and migraine.
- Peripheral—Abrupt onset. Worsened by rapid movements with nausea and severe vomiting. (Table 3-12)
  - Benign positional vertigo (BPV)—Positional episodes; no specific causes. Precipitate by sudden head movements. Hallpike maneuver: Bring the patient from sitting to lying position with head turned to 45° on one side and slightly extended backward. This causes nystagmus, and the test is then considered positive. *Treatment: Symptomatic (antiemetics).*
  - Cerebellopontine angel tumors—Acoustic neuromas and meningiomas. Deafness, ataxia, ipsilateral facial weakness, loss of the corneal reflex, and cerebellar signs.
  - CN VIII lesions—Gradual and preceded by hearing loss. Meningiomas, acoustic schwannomas, and Ramsey-Hunt syndrome are usual causes.

Table 3-12: Peripheral vertigo

	Hearing Loss	**Tinnitis**	**Vertigo**
Acoustic neuroma	Yes	Yes (gradual onset)	Yes
BPV	No	No	Yes
Labyrinthitis	Yes	No	Yes
Ménière's disease	Yes	Yes (sudden onset)	Yes
Perilymph fistula	No	No	Yes (sudden)
Vestibular neuronitis	No	No	Yes

BPV, benign positional vertigo.

— Labyrinthitis—Sudden vertigo and hearing loss, but no tinnitus or middle ear findings. Viral or bacterial infection of labyrinth. *Treatment: Symptomatic. Antibiotic if bacterial.*
— Ménière's—Rapid onset vertigo, unilateral hearing loss, recurring tinnitus, nystagmus, and nausea and vomiting lasting for hours to days. *Treatment: Symptomatic.*
— Perilymph fistula—Opening in the round or oval window. Sudden vertigo following severe straining, scuba diving, or heavy lifting. Positive Hennebert sign: nystagmus elicited by pneumatic otoscopy. *Treatment: Bed rest, ENT referral for surgical repair.*
— Vestibular neuronitis—Sudden, severe vertigo (3–5 days), nausea and vomiting, nonrecurring, and upper respiratory infection (URI) symptoms. No hearing loss or tinnitus. *Treatment: Symptomatic.*
— Others—Toxicity, posttraumatic vertigo, etc.

▶ *CENTRAL*

African sleeping sickness—Trypanosoma brucei rhodesiense.
Altered mental status (AMS)—Any degree of AMS with an acute onset should have a blood sugar determination.
Amaurosis fugax—Transient painless loss of vision.
Amyotrophic lateral sclerosis (ALS)—Upper motor neuron (UMN), spasticity; also lower motor neuron (LMN), atrophy. Death due to respiratory failure.
Anterior cerebral artery (ACA) strokes—Legs > weaker than arms (contrast with middle cerebral artery strokes: arms and faces weaker than legs).
Back pain admission—Cauda equina.

Barbiturate—Lowers intracranial pressure (ICP).

Basilar migraine—Migraine headache where aura is associated with symptoms as in VBI. Includes vertigo, decreased hearing, tinnitus, bilateral visual symptoms, dysarthria, diplopia, and decreased LOC.

Bitemporal hemianopsia—Optic chiasm lesion with loss of both lateral visual fields.

Botulism—Progressive, symmetric, and descending weakness or paralysis affecting cranial nerves first. Signs and symptoms include: ptosis, extraocular muscle (EOM) palsies, dilated fixed pupil, dysarthria, dysphagia, difficulty lifting head, and descending paralysis.

Brainstem lesion—Crossed findings (e.g., right facial weakness with left arm weakness).

"Burning hands"—C_6 to C_7 injury in a football player. Painful dysesthesia.

Cauda equina syndrome—L_5 dermatome loss, buttock pain, bowel or bladder incontinence, and saddle anesthesia. *Treatment: Neurosurgical emergency.*

Central nervous system (CNS) tumors—Headache worsens upon awakening, vomiting, and papilledema.
  • Frontal lobe—Uninhibited behavior.
  • Infratentorial—More common in children. Associated with occipital headache and cerebellar symptoms.
  • Supratentorial—More common in adults. Associated with frontal headache.
  • Temporal lobe—Behavioral symptoms.

Cerebellar degeneration—Limb ataxia and ataxic gait, but no incontinence.

Cerebellar hemorrhage—Sudden onset, headache, repeated vomiting, truncal ataxia, ipsilateral CN VI palsy, gaze paralysis to one side, and normal mental status with focal motor or sensory deficit.

Cerebellar strokes—Ataxia, nausea, vomiting, nystagmus, and inability to walk or stand.

Cerebral perfusion pressure (CPP):
  • Mean arterial pressure (MAP)–intracranial pressure (ICP). Keep ICP < 20 mm Hg.
  • Normal CPP is 40 mm Hg to 160 mm Hg.

Clumsy hand-dysarthria syndrome—Slurred speech, weakness, and ataxia of upper extremity. Anterior capsule lesion.

Cold calorics:
  • Cortex and brainstem intact—Slow toward the cold ear and fast toward center.
  • Only brainstem intact—Slow toward cold ear, but no fast component to midline.
  • Nothing intact—No movement.

Coma only from:
- Bilateral cerebral dysfunction—Hypoglycemia, hypoxia, toxin, or shock.
- Reticular activating system (RAS) lesion—Compression from lesion or tumor.

Concussion—Transient loss of consciousness with transient neurologic dysfunction.

Contusion—Organic brain intracerebral bleeding.

Conus medullaris injury—Injury at L_1 where spinal cord ends. Presents like cauda equina syndrome, central lesion, but no recovery potential.

Cord lesion—Upper extremities and lower extremities asymmetrical findings.

Corneal reflex—CN V (afferent) and CN VII (efferent). Touch the cornea with cotton wisp, and see eye blink.

Cortical lesion—Asymmetrical deep tendon reflexes (DTRs). Contralateral motor and sensory in limbs with contralateral cranial nerve findings (Right arm/leg and right facial neurological deficit with left cortical lesion).

Cranial nerve (CN) III paralysis—Ptosis.

Cranial nerve (CN) VI palsy—Impaired ability of that eye to move laterally past the midline.

Cranial nerve (CN) VIII and vestibular apparatus—Peripheral nervous system.

Cushing's triad—Hypertension, bradycardia, and irregular respiration seen with elevated intracranial pressure (ICP).

Cysticercosis—New onset seizure in patient from Mexico. CT head: calcific densities and cysts.

Deep tendon reflexes (DTRs):
- Absent—Guillain-Barré
- Decreased—Eaton-Lambert syndrome
- Present—Myasthenia Gravis

Diffuse axonal injury—Prolonged coma. CT head shows no mass lesion.

Diphtheria—Bulbar paralysis leading to generalized paralysis.

Diplopia—Brainstem ischemia.

Diplopia and vertigo—Central origin.

Doll's eye—When present means brainstem okay.

Drop attack—Cerebellar infarct. Sudden inability to walk or stand, vertigo, nausea, and vomiting. *Treatment: Surgery.*

Epidural abscess—Fever, back pain, and percussive tenderness. History of intravenous drug abuse (IVDA) or skin infection. *Diagnosis and treatment: MRI best imagining study, neurosurgery for incision and drainage, and antibiotics.*

Eye deviation—Toward stroke. Away from seizure focus.

Foot drop—Superficial peroneal nerve.

Funduscopic examination—Spontaneous pulsation implies normal function. No pulsation implies elevated ICP.

Grand mal seizure refractory to treatment—Suspect isoniazid poisoning. Treat with large quantity of vitamin B_6.

Guillain-Barré—Ascending paralysis and paresthesia.

Headache:

- Chronic subdural—Low-grade, diffuse, vague, and progressive cognitive dysfunction with focal neurologic signs.
- Classic migraine—Aura (visual scotomata), throbbing, and unilateral severe headache <3 weeks duration.
- Cluster—Unilateral, rhinorrhea, and lacrimation. Usually male patient.
- Glaucoma—Vomiting, abdominal pain, orbital pain, cloudy cornea, and dilated pupil.
- Meningitis—Fever, photophobia, and meningismus.
- Pseudotumor—Obese young female with papilledema.
- Subarachnoid hemorrhage—Sudden onset, syncope, nausea, vomiting, occipitonuchal.
- Temporal arteritis—Elderly with unilateral intermittent headaches and tenderness at temple.
- Tension—Across forehead and band-like that worsens through the day.
- Tumor—Headache upon awakening that worsens with Valsalva.

Herniation:

- Central—Slow decrease in level of consciousness (LOC). Downward and lateral shift of diencephalon and upper pons. Small reactive pupil, Cheyne-Stokes breathing (crescendic increase in rate and depth of breathing, followed by decrescendic decrease in both, followed by an apneic period), and no focal findings.
- Tonsillar—Rapid decrease in LOC. Cerebellum tonsils pushing through foramen magnum. Occipital headache, vomiting, hiccups, hypertension, and abrupt change in respiratory pattern.
- Uncal—Rapid decrease in LOC. Unilateral pupil dilation and ipsilateral hemiparesis. Lateral mass displaces temporal lobe, which compresses upper brainstem.

Herpes simplex virus (HSV)—Encephalitis that involves predominantly the temporal and frontal lobes. Frequent temporal lobe hallucinations (e.g., smelling something awful that no one else can smell).

Herpetic meningoencephalitis—Involves temporal lobes.

High protein and low glucose in spinal fluid—In bacterial, fungal, and tuberculosis meningitis. All other: see opposite.

Hollenhorst plaque—Cholesterol emboli seen on funduscopic examination.

Hydrocephalus:

- High pressure (CT slit like ventricles)—Increase intracranial pressure; if not relieved, can lead to blindness. Typically in obese

adolescent girls (pseudotumor cerebri). Do lumbar puncture.
Treatment: diamox.
- Normal pressure—Old person. Triad (confusion, urinary incontinence, and ataxia).

Hypertensive intracerebral bleed—
Putamen > thalamus > pons > cerebellum. (Figure 3-45)

Internuclear ophthalmoplegia—Associated with multiple sclerosis. Double vision with lateral gaze.

Intraventricular bleed—See Figure 3-46.

L₅—Great toe sensory, extension, dorsiflexion, and biceps femoris jerk reflex.

Lacunar infarct—Pure motor or sensory and associated with chronic hypertension. Location: pons or basal ganglia.

Lumbar puncture—Contraindicated in brain abscess.

Meningitis—Fever, stiff neck, headache, photophobia, altered mental state (AMS), and possible seizure.

Middle cerebral artery (MCA) strokes—Arms and face > weaker than legs. Contrast with anterior cerebral artery (ACA) strokes: legs weaker > arms and face. (Figure 3-47)

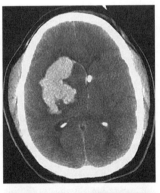

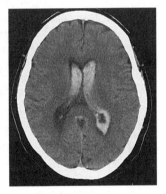

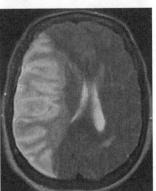

Figure 3-45 (top left): Right basal ganglia hypertensive hemorrhage with midline shift

Figure 3-46 (top right): Nontraumatic intraventricular bleed in a 76-year-old female

Figure 3-47 (bottom left): Acute right MCA infarct

Multiple sclerosis—Nystagmus persists, bilateral internuclear ophthalmologic ataxic eye movements, and vomiting with unrelated neurological deficit separated by time interval. Optic neuritis first symptom in 40%.

Myasthenia gravis with respiratory difficulty—Intubation first before diagnosis with Tensilon test (Physostigmine injection causes transient but quick resumption of normal motor function).

Nerve palsy:
- CN III—Eye does not go medially.
- CN VI—Eye does not go laterally.

Nerves (cranial):
- Corneal—CN V, CN VII
- EOM (external ocular movement)—CN III, CN IV, CN VI
- Pupillary reflex—CN II, CN III

Neurocysticercosis—Found in Mexico or Central America. Taenia solium (pork) eggs ingestion leading to intestinal tapeworm infestation, which enter bloodstream. CT calcific lesions and cystic lesions.

Normal pressure hydrocephalus—Mental confusion, ataxic gait, and urinary incontinence. CT shows ventricular dilation.

Osteochondritis desiccans—Knee locking, tender medial femoral condyle, and intraarticular loose body. *Treatment: Non-weight bearing with immobilization and follow-up.*

Paralysis:
- Botulism—Upper extremity and proximal weakness greater than lower extremity and distal weakness.
- Guillain-Barré—Ascending paralysis and paresthesia.
- Tick paralysis—Ascending paralysis, lack of eye involvement, and tick involved.

Parkinson's disease—Cogwheel rigidity, resting tremor, and akinesia or bradykinesia. Impairment in posture and equilibrium.

Pellagra—4 D's: dermatitis, dementia, diarrhea, and death.

Pontine lesion or hemorrhage—Pinpoint and minimally reactive pupils with sudden onset of profound quadriplegia and ataxic respirations.

Positive Nylen-Barany (Hallpike) maneuver—From sitting upright to supine position, turn head right to left quickly. This causes vertigo.

Posterior cerebral artery (PCA) strokes—Most common deficit contralateral hemianopia (e.g., with lesion in left PCA, cannot see right half of the visual field) or quadrantanopia.

Pseudomorphic or "hung up" DTRs—In hypothyroidism. Longer relaxation phase.

Pseudotumor cerebri (benign intracranial hypertension)—Obese young women, papilledema, elevated ICP, slit-like ventricles, and headache worse in the morning. *Treatment: Lumbar puncture and diamox.*

Pupil size:
- Small and constricted:
  - Argyll-Robertson—Reacts to accommodation but no light reflex. Tertiary syphilis.
  - Horner's syndrome—Miosis, ptosis, and anhydrosis. Sympathetic denervation. Often seen with Pancoast tumor (pulmonary apical lung cancer).
  - Iritis—Photophobia from inflammation of iris.
  - Metabolic encephalopathy—Light reflex okay.
  - Narcotic overdose—(with Demerol, can have a paradoxic dilated pupil.)
  - Pontine hemorrhage.
- Large and dilated:
  - Adie's pupil—Minimal reaction to light and impaired accommodation as well. Slow constriction and relaxation in change from near to distant vision. May have affected pupil greater than normal.
  - Anticholinergic syndrome—Large pupils that are minimally reactive.
  - Anoxia—Fixed pupil. Cardiac arrest.
  - CN III lesion—Fixed. Weakness of upward, medial, and lateral gaze.
  - Hypothermia—Fixed.
  - Uncal herniation—Fixed from compression of CN III.
- Variable: Alternating constriction and dilation of pupil when light pointed to the eye. From midbrain dysfunction.

Ring-enhancing lesion—Seen in toxoplasmosis. *Treatment: CT head with contrast.*

Romberg's test—Feet closely apposed with heels and toes together with arms at side. Defective proprioception (posterior column): If unable to stand with eyes closed. Cerebellar or labyrinthine defect: If unable to stand with eyes open.

Sacral nerve (S_1)—Fifth toe, lateral foot, plantar flexion, and ankle jerk reflex.

Subclavian steal—Central vertigo, syncopal with exercise, and diminished pulse on affected side.

Seizure versus syncope—In seizure have periods of lethargy and confusion (postictal). Not in syncope.

Spontaneous eye opening—Suggest reticular activating system (RAS) functioning, does not imply awareness.

Stroke blood pressure management:
- Hemorrhagic—Treat if systolic blood pressure (SBP) >160 to 180 mm Hg or diastolic blood pressure (DBP) >105 mm Hg.

- Ischemic—Treat if SBP>220 mm Hg, DBP>120 mm Hg, or mean arterial pressure (MAP)>130 mm Hg.

Stroke syndromes:
- Anterior cerebral artery—Contralateral paralysis. Legs weaker than arms.
- Basilar artery—"Locked in syndrome." Coma, quadriplegia, and bilateral upward gaze.
- Cerebellar hemorrhage—Rapid deterioration. Dizziness, nystagmus, and ataxia.
- Lacunar strokes:
  - "Clumsy hands"—Pontine.
  - Leg paresis and ataxia—Pons and internal capsule.
  - Pure motor—Pons and internal capsule.
  - Pure sensory—Thalamus.
- Middle cerebral artery—Contralateral paralysis. Arms, face weaker than legs. Broca's aphasia—unable to speak.
- Posterior cerebral artery—Homonymous hemianopsia (optic tract lesion), visual agnosia (unable to recognize objects), and cortical blindness.
- Vertebrobasilar artery—Vertigo, nystagmus, diplopia, dysarthria, dysphagia, and "drop attacks."

Syringomyelia—Delayed lesion of spinal cord. Incomplete cord lesion causing spasticity and incontinence.

Temporal lobe epilepsy—Memory impairment, hallucination, trance-like state, seizure, aphasia, or convulsion.

Thalamic infarct—Pure contralateral sensory loss.

Todd's paralysis—Focal postictal paralysis of varying location and degree of focality. Lasts minutes to days to weeks.

Toxoplasmosis—Most common cause of focal encephalitis in acquired immune deficiency syndrome (AIDS).

Transverse myelitis—Complete motor and sensory deficit below the level of the spinal cord lesion.

Tuberculous meningitis—Exudate at the base of the brain.

Uncal herniation—CN III compressed. Ipsilateral fixed and dilated pupils with contralateral hemiplegia. Most common cause for a unilateral dilated pupil (other than a recent eye examination with a dilating agent). Comatose, focal neurologic signs, and abnormal respiratory rate.

Unilateral dilated pupil—In alert patients: suspect glaucoma, mydriatic eye drops, or ocular trauma.

Ventriculoperitoneal (VP) shunt—Reservoir not compressible: distal occlusion. If fails to refill: proximal occlusion.

Vertebrobasilar migraine—Headache, vertigo, positive family history, begins in adolescence, and no residual neurologic deficit after ataxia.

Vertebrobasilar strokes—Crossed signs (ipsilateral cranial nerves and contralateral extremities).

Vertical nystagmus—Brainstem disease. Also seen in vertebrobasilar migraine and temporal lobe epilepsy.

Vestibular ataxia—Elderly with dysequilibrium, unsteadiness, vertigo, and broad-base gait.

Weakness:
- Eaton-Lambert syndrome—Muscle strength increases with exercise. Proximal muscles affected.
- Myasthenia gravis—Muscle strength decreases with exercise, eye signs prominent, and normal pupillary response.

Wernicke's—Confusion, ataxia, and nystagmus (CAN of beer). *Treatment: Give thiamine.*

Wernicke's and Korsakoff's psychosis—The preceding plus anterograde or retrograde amnesia. *Treatment: Admit, give thiamine. Wernicke's will improve; Korsakoff's is permanent.*

▸PERIPHERAL

Acute periodic paralysis—Sudden extreme weakness after exercise. *Treatment: Check potassium level.*

Botulism—Affects neuromuscular junction. Descending paralysis and positive deep tendon reflex (DTR).

Claw hand—Ulnar nerve neuropathy.

CN III palsy—Ptosis, mydriasis, and deviation of eye down and out.

CN VI palsy—Abduction deficit.

"Crutch palsy"—Compression of radial nerve in the axillae due to improper crutch use.

Hearing loss—Cerebropontine-angle tumor, excess cerumen, otitis media, and ototoxic drugs.

Horner's syndrome—Ptosis, miosis, and anhydrosis.

Lhermitte's sign—Seen in multiple sclerosis. Electric shock from back to arm and leg, and occasionally with neck flexion.

Lower extremity weakness:
- Ascending paralysis—Guillain-Barré
- Descending paralysis—Botulism

Lower motor neuron (LMN) lesion—Plantar reflex normal or absent, DTRs decreased or absent, and decreased to flaccid muscle tone. Guillain-Barré, diphtheria, porphyria, ciguatera, and puffer toxin.

Lyme disease—Peripheral CN VII palsy.

Mononeuropathy:
- Bridegroom's palsy—Radial nerve (bride sleeping on groom's arm). Also known as Saturday night palsy, from someone intoxicated falling asleep with arm over a chair back.

- Footdrop—Common peroneal nerve.
- Guyon's canal—Ulnar nerve passes through. Paper pinching tests function.
- LOAF weakness—Median nerve in carpel tunnel. Lumbricals, thumb **O**pposition, **A**bduction, and **F**lexion.

Myasthenia gravis—Extraocular and bulbar muscles involvement with proximal muscles weakness worsens with activity (contrast with Eaton-Lambert's) and improves with rest. *Treatment: Tensilon test.*

Nerve test:
- C_4—Spontaneous breathing.
- C_5—Shrugging the shoulders.
- C_6—Flexion at the elbow.
- C_7—Extension at the elbow.
- C_8 to T_1—Flexion of fingers.

Neuromuscular or muscle lesion—Plantar normal or absent, DTRs present, and decreased to flaccid muscle tone.

Neuromuscular junction—Myasthenia gravis, Eaton-Lambert's, botulism, periodic paralysis, tick paralysis, and electrolyte abnormalities.

Parkinson's—Pill rolling tremor.

Peripheral neuropathy due to ETOH—Lower extremity affected greater than upper extremity. Evolves over many months.

Polio—Asymmetric flaccid paralysis.

Sarcoidosis—Bilateral 7th nerve involvement.

Saturday night palsy—Radial nerve palsy from falling asleep with the arm over a chair or bench.

Transverse myelitis—Demarcated spinal cord level. Upper motor neuron (UMN) disorder.

Trigeminal neuralgia—Most common on right side of face.

Ulnar nerve dysfunction—Unable to pinch paper.

UMN lesion—Plantar upgoing, DTRs increased, and later spasticity. Found in transverse myelitis, polio, and multiple sclerosis

Wrist drop—Radial nerve.

▶ NUTRITION (DEFICIENCIES and OVERDOSE SYMPTOMS)

Vitamin A—Xerophthalmia and hyperkeratosis of skin. Used in treatment for measles. Overdose: hypervitaminosis A—blurred vision, appetite loss, abnormal skin pigmentation, dry skin, and long bone pain. Massive dose linked to pseudotumor cerebri. *Symptoms resolve when vitamin A discontinued.*

Vitamin B$_1$ (thiamine)—Beriberi, muscle weakness, tachycardia, and heart failure. Renal excretion, therefore no toxicity.

Vitamin B$_2$ (riboflavin)—Glossitis, angular cheilitis, and sore throat. No overdose adverse effects.

Vitamin B$_3$ (niacin)—Pellagra, glossitis, anorexia, weakness, and depression. Overdose: "niacin flush" from histamine release.

Vitamin B$_6$ (pyridoxine)—Sideroblastic anemia. Overdose: unstable gait, numbness of the feet, and loss of position and vibration sense. Best therapy for isoniazid induced seizures.

Vitamin B$_{12}$—Pernicious anemia, elevated lactate dehydrogenase (LDH), and macroanemia. Affects posterior column resulting in paresthesia. No overdose toxicity.

Vitamin C—Scurvy. Gum bleeding and tooth mobility. Overdose: Triggers gout and nephrolithiasis in patients with these diseases.

Vitamin D—Rickets. Overdose symptoms as in hypercalcemia.

Vitamin E—Cerebellar ataxia and areflexia. Overdose: bleeding tendencies (increased level inhibits platelet aggregation). Symptoms resolve when discontinued.

Vitamin K—Clotting abnormalities. Toxic effects: Hemolytic anemia, kernicterus, and hemoglobinuria in premature infants. Large doses can inhibit the effects of oral anticoagulants.

Folic acid—Developmental anomalies of fetal neural tube. No overdose toxicity.

▶ OBSTETRICS and GYNECOLOGY

Abortion:
- Complete—Product of conception passed, os closed, uterus firm, and bleeding stopped.
- Incomplete—Os open, vaginal bleeding, and products of conception at os or in vault.
- Inevitable abortion—Os open with vaginal bleeding.
- Missed abortion—Failure to pass product of conception beyond 2 months after fetal death.
- Threatened—Vaginal bleeding, closed cervical os, and intrauterine pregnancy (IUP); 25% of all pregnancies bleed, and 50% progress to miscarriage.

Abruptio placentae—Third-trimester painful bleeding. Accounts for 30% of third-trimester bleeding. Risk: hypertension, smoking, multipara, advanced maternal age, previous abruption, trauma, and drug use.

Adnexal torsion—Sudden onset of severe, sharp unilateral lower abdominal pain, nausea, vomiting, afebrile, and no previous history.

Amniotic fluid embolism—Thrombolytic no benefit. *Treatment: Supportive care, delivery.*

Antiphospholipid syndrome—Associated with recurrent spontaneous abortion.

APGAR:
- **A**—Appearance (color)
- **P**—Pulse
- **G**—Grimace (reflex)
- **A**—Activity (tone)
- **R**—Respiration

Asthma in pregnancy—*Treatment: Use albuterol, β blocker, and steroids.* Theophylline clearance is reduced.

Bacterial vaginosis—"Clue-cells" and positive sniff test. *Treatment: Flagyl or clindamycin.*

Bartholin's abscess—*Treatment: Incision and drainage. Antibiotics for concurrent vaginal, cervical, or urethral infection.*

Blighted ovum—In ultrasound study see a large intrauterine sac without yolk sac or fetal pole.

Calcium gluconate—Give for hypermagnesemia (loses reflex).

Cholestatic jaundice in pregnancy—Mild jaundice (bilirubin < 5 mg/dL) and pruritus in third trimester. *Treatment: Cholestyramine.*

Chronic hypertension in pregnancy—*Treatment: Bed rest, methyldopa, propranolol, and hydralazine.*

Cocaine—Third-trimester vaginal bleeding with snorting cocaine. Can cause placental abruption.

Congenital rubella syndrome—Cataracts, deafness, and patent ductus arteriosus (PDA).

Cord issues:
- Nuchal cord—*Treatment: If loose, slip over the baby's head. If tight, clamp and cut the cord and rapidly deliver the infant.*
- Prolapsed—*Treatment: Elevate the presenting part and wait for obstetrician for C-section delivery. If not available in timely fashion, do manual replacement of cord into the uterus.*

Dysfunctional uterine bleeding (DUB)—Continuous estrogen stimulation of the uterus. *If vital signs and blood parameters stable, follow-up outpatient.*

Dysuria-pyuria syndrome—*Treatment: In pregnancy, treat with nitrofurantoin.*

Eclampsia—Preeclampsia and seizure. *Treatment: Magnesium, hydralazine, or labetolol IV. Definitive treatment: Delivery for severe preeclampsia or eclampsia.*

Ectopic pregnancy—Clinical presentation at 5 to 8 weeks. Abdominal pain with or without vaginal bleeding, Beta-human chorionic gonadotropin (hCG)>1500 mIU/L (approximately), and transvaginal ultrasound showing an empty uterus. Work-up over if can identify ectopic pregnanc, which requires surgery, or can identify intrauterine pregnancy (IUP). (Figure 3-48)

ED cesarean section—Maternal demise with trauma after 10 minutes of profound shock and near term fetus.

Endometriosis—Constant pelvic pain associated with menses. Endometrial tissue outside uterus.

Endometritis after delivery—Fever, abdominal pain, and foul-smelling lochia. *Treatment: Admit for antibiotics.*

Fetal heart—Audible at 10 weeks by doppler and 20 weeks by fetoscope.

Fitz-Hugh-Curtis syndrome—Pelvic inflammatory disease (PID) with right upper quadrant (RUQ) pain and jaundice. *Treatment: Admission and antibiotics.*

Genital herpes—Tzanck's smear (herpes simplex virus, HSV inclusion bodies), culture, and enzyme-linked immunosorbent assay (ELISA). *Treatment: Daily oral acyclovir administered early during primary infection prevents recurrence.*

Gestational sac—Double decidua.

Groove sign—Lymphogranuloma venereum. Inguinal lymphadenopathy above and below the inguinal ligament.

HELLP—**H**emolysis, **E**levated **L**iver enzymes, and **L**ow **P**latelets. Seen in later pregnancy or postpartum.

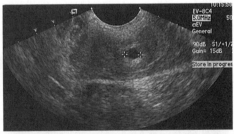

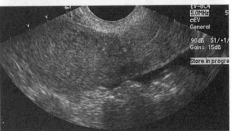

Figure 3-48: Empty uterus and free fluid in cul-de-sac. Beta Hcg 250.

Hemorrhage—>500-mL blood loss.

Immunoglobulin G (IgG)—Goes through placenta (G for go)

Labor:

- Failure to progress—No cervical change in 3 hours, cephalopelvic disproportion, and inadequate contractions. *Treatment: C-section.*
- Fetal distress—Tachycardia, decreased beat to beat variability, and late decelerations.
- Preterm labor—Labor starts <37 weeks of gestation. *Treatment: Admit, tocolytics.*
- Premature rupture of membranes (PROM)—Reports trickling of clear fluid from vagina. *Sterile speculum examination.* Nitrazine: If blue, test is positive for ruptured membrane. Test will also be positive if amniotic fluid is present.

Magnesium toxicity—Starts with decreased deep tendon reflexes (DTRs), leading to muscle weakness then apnea if left untreated. *Treatment: Give calcium gluconate.*

Mastitis—Staphylococcal. *Continue breastfeeding with the unaffected breast. Treatment: Cephalosporin or erythromycin.*

Methotrexate—Used for tubal mass <4 cm and no evidence of rupture. *Treatment: Follow up β-hCG 2 to 3 months until zero.*

Miscarriage:

- *Treatment: If Rh-negative and bleeding, give RhoGAM 300 μg within 72 hours.*
- *Treatment: If profuse bleeding, add oxytocin 20 units to IV fluids.*

Mittelschmerz—Mid-cycle pain due to ovulation bleeding from the ovary.

Molar pregnancy—Second trimester with bleeding, no fetal heart tones (FHTs), and snowstorm on ultrasound. Uterus appears much larger for age.

Mondor's disease—Superficial phlebitis of subcutaneous veins of the breast. *Treatment: Analgesics. Can also use coumadin.*

Motor vehicle crash (MVC) minor—*Treatment: Evaluate fetal heart rate (most sensitive).*

Nitrofurantoin and sulfonamide—Avoid in third trimester. Causes neonatal hyperbilirubinemia.

Nitroprusside—Contraindicated in pregnancy.

Nonclotted blood—Hemoperitoneum. Rupture of hemorrhagic ovarian cyst or ectopic pregnancy.

Obstetric bleeding:

- Abruptio placenta—Placenta separates from the site of uterine implantation before delivery of fetus.
- Ectopic pregnancy—Usually pain first then bleeding.
- Placenta previa—Placenta implants close to the cervical os.
- Spontaneous abortion—Usually bleeding first then pain.
- Uterine rupture—Uterus ruptures.

Ovarian cyst (Figure 3-49):
- Corpus luteum cyst—During the last two weeks of menstrual cycle.
- Follicular cyst—First 2 weeks of menstrual cycle (cycle starts the first day of menses).

Ovarian torsion—Severe unilateral lower abdominal pain and usually history of ovarian mass. *Treatment: Do ultrasound.*

Pelvic inflammatory disease (PID)—Need all three: Lower abdominal tenderness, CMT (cervical motion tenderness), and bilateral adnexal tenderness.

PID risk—Adolescent, multiple partners, intrauterine device (IUD), or recent instrumentation. Rare during pregnancy.

Physiologic anemia of pregnancy—Plasma volume increases by 45% with RBC mass unchanged.

Placenta percreta—Abnormal adherence of placenta to uterine wall with involvement of myometrium.

Placenta Previa—Third-trimester painless vaginal bleeding; 20% of third-trimester bleeding. Risk: prior C-section, multipara, previous placenta previa, and multiple gestations. *Treatment: No digital examination. Do ultrasound.*

Postmenopausal vaginal bleeding—If vitals and blood parameters stable, outpatient gynecologic referral for endometrial biopsy.

Postpartum hemorrhage—Blood loss >250 mL immediately or >500 mL within first 24 hours of delivery.

Preeclampsia—>20 weeks of gestation, hypertension >140/90 mm Hg, proteinuria (300 mg per 24 hours), and peripheral edema. Predisposition factors: primipara, older age, large placenta, diabetes, multiple pregnancies, family history, molar pregnancy, and renal hypertension. *Treatment: Systolic blood pressure (SBP) > 170 mmHg or diastolic blood pressure (DBP) > 100 mmHg. Treat with hydralazine.*

(Severe) preeclampsia—The preceding characteristics and any of the following: blood pressure >160/110 mm Hg, protein 5 g/day, or urine output (UOP) < 500 mL/day. Signs and symptoms include:

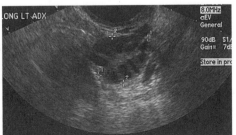

Figure 3-49: Multiple ovarian cyst

persistent headache, visual disturbance, epigastric pain, pulmonary edema, cyanosis, and liver dysfunction.

Pregnant with abdominal pain—Rule out ectopic pregnancy. May present with or without vaginal bleeding. Also consider appendicitis or cholecystitis.

Pregnant with complex urinary tract infection (pyelonephritis)—*Treatment: Admit for IV antibiotics during the third trimester.*

Pseudosac—See hypoechoic sac (instead of double decidua sign of normal IUP) inside uterus in patient with ectopic pregnancy.

Pulmonary embolism in pregnancy—Both CT scan and ventilation-perfusion (V/Q) scan can be performed safely during pregnancy. Use intravenous heparin, subcutaneous heparin, or low–molecular-weight heparin (LMWH) until therapeutic international normalized ratio (INR), then can be maintained on subcutaneous heparin or LMWH heparin. Coumadin is contraindicated.

Radiation risk—A dose of 1.0 rad is considered potentially dangerous to fetus.

Retained placenta—1 to 2 weeks postpartum. Sudden, brisk, and painless bleeding. Enlarged, boggy uterus. *Treatment: Oxytocin, and dilation and curettage.*

Rupture of follicular cyst—Adnexal pain occurs between days 12 and 16 in a cycle (12–16 days after menses start at the time of ovulation).

School of fish—Short gram-negative bacilli in linear or parallel formation in chancroid Gram staining.

Strawberry cervix—Punctate appearance of cervix in trichomoniasis.

Surgical emergency of pregnancy—Appendicitis more common than cholecystitis.

Trichomonas—Malodorous, frothy, and gray-white or greenish discharge. Strawberry cervix. *Treatment: In pregnancy: Clotrimazole suppository. Do not use flagyl in pregnancy.*

Tubal ring—In ectopic pregnancy see hypertrophy of the involved fallopian tube.

Ultrasound:
- At 5 weeks—See IUP per transvaginal ultrasound (US). See gestational sac. (Figure 3-50)
- At 8 weeks—See IUP per transabdominal US. See fetal pole.
- Ectopic—May see tubal ring.
- Transabdominal US—See IUP if beta-hCG >6500 mIU/L.
- Transvaginal US—See IUP if beta-hCG >1600 mIU/L.

Vaginal bleeding in third trimester—*Treatment: No pelvic examination (can do in OR with double set-up). Ultrasound.*

Vulvovaginitis—Dysuria in premenarche. Candida uncommon.

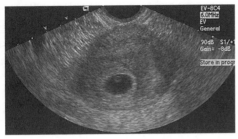

Figure 3-50: IUP at 6 weeks

▶ ORTHOPEDICS and MUSCULOSKELETAL

Table 3-13: Splints head to toe

Clavicular, scapular fracture	Sling
Shoulder	
Soft tissue, rotator cuff, AC joint	Sling
Dislocation, postreduction	Sling and swathe
Humerus	
Proximal fracture	Sling and swathe
Shaft fracture	Coaptation splint
Elbow	
Mild fracture	Sling or posterior mold
Moderate fracture	Posterior mold
Severe fracture	Double sugar tong
Forearm shaft fracture	Posterior mold or double sugar tong
Wrist	
Sprain, torus fracture	Volar splint
Colles' fracture	Sugar tong
Carpal or suspected fracture	Thumb spica
Hand	
1st metacarpal fracture	Thumb spica
2nd or 3rd metacarpal fracture	Radial gutter
4th or 5th metacarpal fracture	Ulnar gutter

Table 3-13: Splints head to toe *(continued)*

Finger

Proximal phalanx fracture	
1st digit (thumb)	Thumb spica
2nd (index) or 3rd (long)	Radial gutter or dorsal aluminum
4th (ring) or 5th (little)	Ulnar gutter or dorsal aluminum
Middle phalanx fracture	Dorsal aluminum or buddy tape
Distal phalanx fracture	U-Shaped aluminum
"Mallet" deformity	Short dorsal aluminum
Dislocation (postreduction)	Long dorsal aluminum

Pelvis fracture	Pneumatic antishock garment
Femur fracture (hip or shaft)	Traction

Knee

Soft-tissue injury	Knee immobilizer
Tendon rupture (quadriceps or patellar) or patellar fracture	Long leg posterior gutter or knee immobilizer
Patellar dislocation (post reduction)	Knee immobilizer
Femoral condyle fracture	Long leg posterior gutter
Tibial spine or tuberosity fracture	Knee immobilizer with compression dressing
Tibial plateau fracture	Knee immobilizer with compression dressing

Leg

Tibial or fibular shaft fracture	Long leg posterior gutter Long leg sugar tong
Gastrocnemius rupture	Short leg posterior

Ankle

Sprain	
1st degree	Air splint
2nd degree	Air splint or short leg posterior
3rd degree	Short leg posterior
Achilles tendon rupture	Short leg posterior (in equinus)

Table 3-13: Splints head to toe (continued)

Distal tibial or fibular fracture	Short leg posterior or sugar tong
Bimalleolar or trimalleolar fracture	Sugar tong with posterior splint
Dislocation (postreduction)	Short leg posterior or sugar tong with posterior splint
Foot	
Soft-tissue injuries	Postoperative shoe
Metatarsal fractures	
Minor or stable	Postoperative shoe
Major or severe	Short leg posterior or sugar tong with posterior splint
Calcaneal fracture	Short leg posterior
Talus fracture	
Avulsion	Air splint
Neck and body	Short leg posterior
Toe	
Soft tissue injury	Buddy taping
Fracture or dislocation (postreduction)	
Great toe	Postoperative shoe
2nd (index toe) to 5th (little/ pinkie toe)	Buddy taping with postoperative shoe

AC, acromioclavicular. (From Handbook of Orthopedic Emergencies)

▶ **SPINE**

Back pain in children—More serious and much less common than in adults. Get plain lumbar spine x-ray. Rule out vertebral tumors and discitis.

Bamboo spine—Ankylosing spondylitis, male > female, and associated with HLA b-27.

Bartolotti's syndrome—Unilateral fusion of either sacrum or L$_5$.

Paget's disease—X-ray: "Cotton-wool" skull, ivory picture frame of vertebral body, and "blade of grass" long bones.

► *UPPER EXTREMITY*

Acromioclavicular (AC) separation:

- Type I—Strain—partial tear of AC ligament. X-ray: normal
- Type II—Subluxation—complete AC tear. X-ray:<1-cm AC separation.
- Type III—Dislocation—complete AC and coracoclavicular (CC) tear. Step-off on examination. X-ray: >1-cm AC separation and >50% widening of CC space.
- Type IV—AC subluxation + posterior displacement of distal clavicle.
- Type V—Marked displacement of superior clavicle.
- Type VI—Distal clavicle inferiorly displaced.
- Treatment:
    - *Type I—1 to 2 weeks of immobilization.*
    - *Type II—2 to 4 weeks of immobilization.*
    - *Type III—Surgery if athlete or manual laborer for early mobilization.*
    - *Type IV to VI—Surgery.*

Anterior shoulder dislocation:

- Most common complications: Axillary nerve injury and recurrent dislocation.
- Mechanism: Abduction and external rotation. More common than posterior dislocation. *Treatment: Closed reduction then sling and swath.* (Figure 3-51)

Bankart's deformity—Glenoid rim fracture. Associated with anterior shoulder dislocation.

Bennett's fracture—Fracture of the ulnar base of the thumb. *Treatment: Surgery.*

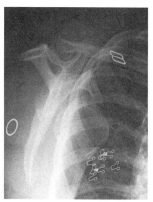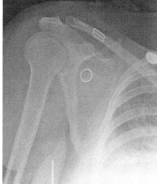

Figure 3-51: Anterior shoulder dislocation and post-reduction

Bicipital tendinitis—Point tenderness over bicipital groove.

Boutonniere deformity—Rupture of central slip of proximal interphalangeal (PIP) joint. *Treatment: Closed: Splinting in extension for 6 weeks. Open: Surgical repair.*

Boxer's fracture—Metacarpal neck of fifth digit. *Treatment: Reduction if angulation >15 degrees. Gutter splint.*

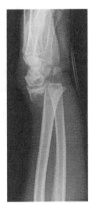

Figure 3-52: Colle's fracture with marked dorsal displacement

Carpal fracture—Scaphoid > triquetrum > lunate.

Claw hand—Distal ulnar nerve damage.

Clenched fist injury—Human bite injury as fist strikes opponent's tooth. Also known as a fight bite; often produces severe hand infection. *Treatment: Optimal management is open washout with IV antibiotics.*

Colles' fracture—Distal radial fracture with dorsal angulation and displacement. Fall on outstretched hand. (Figure 3-52)
- Stable—*Treatment: Splint or closed reduction and follow up for casting in 24 to 48 hours.*
- Unstable—*>20° angulation, ≥10 mm shortening, or intraarticular. Treatment: Open reduction with internal fixation (ORIF).*

"Drop arm test"—Passively raise the patient's arm to 90° of abduction and lower it slowly. If the patient is unable to maintain this position (the arm "drops"), this indicates rotator cuff pathology. Positive in rotator cuff injury.

Dupuytren's contracture—Inflammatory contracture of flexor mechanism of hand.

Fasciotomy for compartment pressure—If >35 mm Hg.

Flexor tendon sheath laceration—Check for tendon injury. *Treatment: If lacerated, consult hand surgeon.*

Galeazzi's fracture—Fracture of the distal radius with dislocation of the distal radial–ulnar joint. *Treatment: ORIF.*

Gamekeeper's thumb—Thumb ulnar collateral ligament torn due to forced hyperabduction. Also known as skier's thumb. *Treatment: Thumb spica splint. >20° laxity requires surgery.*

Hand tendon injury:
- Extensors—*Suture and splint wrist in extension.*
  - Closed boutonniere—*Splint in extension for 4 weeks.*
  - Mallet finger—*Splint distal interphalangeal joint in extension for 6 to 8 weeks.*

- Flexors—*Immediate orthopedic referral.*
- Partial tendon injury—*Immobilize in flexion (flexor tendon) and extension (extensor tendon).*

Hill-Sachs deformity—Posterior lateral defect of humeral head as it impacts on anterior rim of glenoid.

Humeral shaft fracture—Associated with radial nerve injury and brachial artery/nerve. *Treatment: Closed reduction with sling and swath, sugar tong, or hanging cast.* (Figure 3-53)

Hutchinson fracture—"Chauffeur fracture" trauma to radial side of wrist.

Kienböck's disease—Lunate collapse. Avascular necrosis. Lateral x-ray crescent lunate displaced.

Little finger sensation—C_8.

Little leaguer's elbow—Medial epicondyle avulsion from throwing too far or too hard.

Lunate dislocation—Posteroanterior (PA) view: piece of pie sign (triangular shape of lunate). Lateral view: spilled teacup sign, lunate tilting into the palm. *Treatment: Both lunate and perilunate fractures require emergent orthopedic consultation.*

Luxatio recta—Inferior shoulder dislocation. Patient's hand held behind the head with humerus fully abducted and elbow flexed. *Reduce: Traction in upward and outward direction in line with humerus and countertraction.*

Mallet finger—Disruption of extensor tendon at distal phalanx base → flexion of distal interphalangeal (DIP) joint. *Treatment: Dorsal splint in extension, allow motion at the PIP, but not DIP.*

Monteggia's fracture—Fracture of proximal and mid one-third of ulna with anterior dislocation of the radial head. *Treatment: ORIF.*

O.K. sign—Tests for median nerve function.

Perilunate dislocation—PA view: Subtle overlap of lunate and capitate. Lateral view: Lunate maintaining contact with the radius but capitate is dorsally displaced. *Treatment: Surgical reduction.*

Phalanx injury (Figure 3-54):
- Distal phalanx: *Protective splint.*
- Mid or proximal phalanx—Fourth and fifth: *ulnar gutter splint.* Index and long finger: *radial gutter splint.*

Posterior elbow dislocation—More common than anterior. Associated with ulnar nerve and brachial artery injury. *Treatment: Closed reduction and long arm splint in 90° flexion.* (Figure 3-55)

Posterior shoulder dislocation—Adduction and internally rotated (just like posterior hip dislocation).
- In x-ray see widening joint space, loss of overlap, and remains in same transverse plane. Requires more forceful mechanism of injury; often after a grand mal seizure.

Proximal humerus fracture—Elderly. Axillary nerve or artery most commonly injured. Neer's classification one-part versus two-part fracture. *Treatment: Closed reduction with sling and swath.* (Figure 3-56)

Radius and ulnar fracture (closed)—See Figure 3-57.

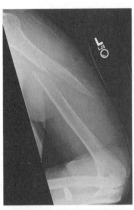
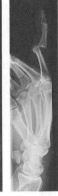

Figure 3-53 (left): Humeral shaft fracture

Figure 3-54 (right): Finger dislocation

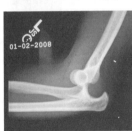
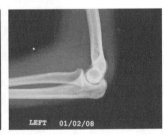

Figure 3-55 (top left and right): Posterior elbow dislocation and s/p reduction

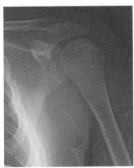
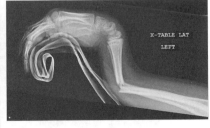

Figure 3-57: Distal radius and ulnar fracture s/p fall

Figure 3-56 (left): Proximal humerus fracture

Rolando fracture—Comminuted fracture of base of the thumb. *Treatment: Thumb spica. Later surgery.*

Rotator cuff tear—Weak abduction. Positive "drop arm test." *Initial treatment: Sling.*

Scaphoid fracture—Initial film misses 15%. *Treatment: Long- or short-arm spica cast.* Complication: avascular necrosis and nonunion. If the patient had a fall on an outstretched hand, and has tenderness in the anatomic snuff box, then thumb spica splint must be applied no matter what the x-ray shows. (Figure 3-58)

Scapholunate dislocation—"Terry Thomas sign"; also known as the David Letterman sign. A gap of >3 mm between scaphoid and lunate. Scaphoid appears shorter with a dense ring (cortical ring sign). *Radial gutter splint (posterior mold).*

Smith's fracture—Reverse Colles' fracture. Distal radial fracture volarly angulated. *Treatment: As Colles' fracture, except with reversed reduction forces.*

Snapping wrist—Diagnostic clue of scapholunate dislocation.

Supracondylar fracture—*Treatment: Reduction and may require hospitalization.* Complications: Volkmann's contracture. (Figure 3-59)

Tennis elbow—Lateral epicondylitis. Often caused by too small a grip; using a larger grip and a forearm brace will reduce the pain and relieve the recurrent inflammation.

Terry-Thomas sign—Widening of scapholunate joint.

Wrist drop—Radial nerve injury.

▶ *LOWER EXTREMITY*

Anterior collateral ligament (ACL) tear—Follows a varus blow to the lateral leg at the knee. There is often a hemarthrosis; the patient often hears a pop.

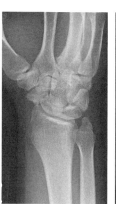 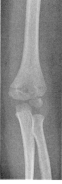

Figure 3-58 (left): Scaphoid fracture

Figure 3-59 (right): Supracondylar fracture

Achilles tendon rupture—From forced dorsiflexion. Positive Thompson's test. Palpable defect at the insertion of gastrocnemius and soleus tendons. *Treatment: Posterior splint in passive equinus.*

Ankle joint (mortise)—Tibia, fibula, and talus.

Ankle sprains—*Treatment: RICE: rest, ice, compressive dressing, and elevation.* Most lateral sprains(inversion injury) involve the anterior talofibular ligament. Medial sprains involve the deltoid ligament, which is very strong, and, therefore, often there is a medial malleolar fracture.

- 1st degree—Microscopic tear of a ligament. Able to bear weight and minimal swelling. *Treatment: Crutches, analgesics, and follow up in 1 to 2 weeks with primary care.*
- 2nd degree—Partial tear of ligament. Marked tenderness and edema with significant pain with and without weight bearing. *Treatment: Rigid splinting, and follow up with orthopedics in 1 week.*
- 3rd degree—Complete rupture of ligaments. There may be less edema than with a second-degree sprain, because the joint is open. Marked tenderness and unable to bear weight. *Treatment: As in 2nd degree, but an orthopedic consultation is often useful because young athletic patients will do better with a surgical repair.*

Anterior compartment—Deep peroneal nerve is at risk from swelling.

Anterior compartment syndrome of lower leg—Fracture of proximal tibia.

Baker's cyst ruptured—"Crescent sign": bluish discoloration around ankle.

Bertolotti's syndrome—Unilateral fusion of either sacrum or L_5.

"Bucket handle tear"—Tear of medial meniscus. See double posterior cruciate ligament (PCL) sign on x-ray.

Calcaneal fracture—Fall from a height. Boehlert's angle 20° to 40°. Most often fractured of the tarsal bones. Associated with lumber compression injuries (10%). May also be associated with cervical vertebral injury because of the S-shaped curvature of the spine.

Chopart's fracture—Talonavicular and calcaneocuboid joints.

Compartments—Four in lower leg: peroneal, anterior, deep, and superficial.

Compartment syndrome—Pain, pallor, paresthesia, pulselessness, and paralysis. Complaints of pain and area tender. Pulses, and neurologic examination may be normal. *Treatment: If the compartment pressure is > 30 mm Hg, the fascial compartment needs emergent decompressing fasciotomy.*

Dorsiflexion—Anterior muscles (tibialis anterior, extensor digitalis, and extensor hallices).

Eversion or plantar flexion—Lateral muscles of ankle (peroneus longus and brevis).

Femoral neck fracture—Elderly women. Shortened, externally rotated, and slight abduction. *Treatment: Displaced fractures require surgery.* Complications: avascular necrosis (AVN), nonunion, and pulmonary emboli. (Figure 3-60)

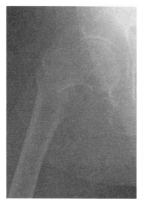 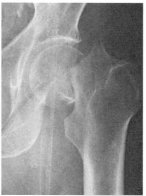

Figure 3-60: Impacted intertrochanteric fracture

Figure 3-61: Proximal femoral neck fracture

Greater trochanteric fractures—Avulsion at the gluteus medius insertion. Pain with abduction and extension Patient limps. *Conservative treatment with orthopedic consultation.*

Intertrochanteric fracture—Elderly and women. Extremity markedly externally rotated and shortened. (Figure 3-61)

Inversion—Medial muscles (tibialis posterior, flexor digitorum, and flexor hallucis).

Jones' fracture—Transverse fracture at base of 5th metatarsal. Not an avulsion fracture. Higher incidence of nonunion or delayed union. *Treatment: Internal fixation or cast.*

Lachman's test—Best clinical test for anterior cruciate ligament integrity. Lay patient supine in bed. With knee in 20° to 30° of flexion, place one hand on patient's thigh and other hand behind tibia. On pulling anteriorly on tibia, an intact anterior cruciate ligament (ACL) should prevent anterior translational movement of tibia on femur.

Lateral compartment—Superficial peroneal nerve injuries.

Lesser trochanteric fractures—Avulsion at the iliopsoas insertion. Pain with flexion and internal rotation. *Treatment: Orthopedic consultation.*

Lisfranc fracture—(Tarsal-metatarsal joint). Most common midfoot fracture. Fracture base of 2nd metatarsal with separation of 1st and 2nd metatarsal. *Treatment: Surgery.*

Locking of knee—Meniscal tear.

March fracture—Metatarsal shaft stress fracture.

Maisonneuve fracture—Proximal fibula fracture with an associated ankle fracture or deltoid ligament tear. *Treatment: Long leg cast if no malleolar fracture or mortise joint disruption.*

McMurry's test—For meniscal tear. Knee is flexed to 90°. Place one hand on the lateral side of knee and with other hand rotate the foot externally while extending the knee. If pain or "click" is felt, the test is considered positive.

Meniscal injury—Hear knee pop.

Metatarsal fracture—Most common: base of the little toe (5th metatarsal). *Treatment: Buddy taping, postoperative shoe, and crutches.*

O'Donoghue's terrible triad—ACL tear, medial cruciate ligament (MCL) tear, and medial meniscus tear.

Ortolani's test—Checks for hip dysplasia in infant. With infant in supine position, the examiner places his hands around the infant's knees. With knees abducted (moving away), the examiner would be able to discern a distinct "clicking" sound with the motion.

Osteochondritis dissecans—Knee locking and separation of bony segment from overlying cartilage.

Ottawa ankle rules—X-ray if tenderness on posterior edge, or tip of distal 6 cm of either malleolus, or unable to bear weight four steps after injury or in ED.

Patellar dislocation—High-riding patella that displaced laterally. Reduce by hyperextending the knee, flexing the hip, and applying a varus force to the patella (push the patella from the lateral to the medial leg while extending the knee); this will slide the patella back in place.

Patellar fracture—Transverse most common. X-ray: AP, lateral, and sunrise views. *Treatment: Cylindrical cast. For comminuted fracture: Surgery.*

Patellar tendon injury—<40 years of age.

Peroneal nerve injury—Paresthesia dorsal foot, foot drop, and decreased sensation between great and index toes.

Plantar flexion—Posterior muscles of ankle (soleus and gastrocnemius).

Posterior compartment—Posterior tibial artery and nerve.

Posterior drawer test—For posterior collateral ligament injury. With the patient in supine position, place the knee in 90° of flexion. Grasp the anterior aspect of the tibia over the tibial tuberosity and push forward. If the tibia moves posteriorly more than normal (compare with the uninjured leg), the test is positive.

Posterior hip dislocation (acute)—Posterior >> anterior. Extremity shortened, internally rotated, and adducted. Immediate closed reduction in ED. Complication: avascular necrosis (AVN) and sciatic nerve injury. The length of time the hip is dislocated is directly related to the incidence of AVN of the femoral head.

Quadriceps tendon injury—>40 years of age.

Ricketts—A calcium or vitamin D deficient disease in which the x-ray shows the metaphyses are capped, frayed, and splayed.

Spinal stenosis—Elderly, pseudoclaudication pain in lower extremities with walking, and improved with lying down. Feet may become numb on standing, and bending forward relieves the discomfort.

Stand, but cannot walk—Suspect patellar or quadriceps tendon rupture.

Talus—Only bone in lower leg with no muscular attachment.

Valgus—Deformity angled away from midline (bowlegged).

Varus—Deformity toward midline (knees almost touching).

▶ PEDIATRICS

▶ *CARDIAC*

1-day-old infant with respiratory distress that worsens with O₂—Suspect hypoplastic left ventricle.

1-week-old with shock, feeding difficulty, and decreased O₂ saturation, not corrected with O₂—*Treatment: O_2, prostaglandin E, septic work-up, antibiotics, and defer lumbar puncture. Prostaglandin E is used to keep or reopen the ductus arteriosus in infants with congenital ductal-dependent heart disease (tetralogy of Fallot [TOF], transposition of the great vessel, or coarctation of aorta).*

1-year-old with congestive heart failure (CHF) and recent upper respiratory infection (URI)—Suspect myocarditis.

Coarctation of aorta—Noncyanotic and decreased or absent pulses in legs. Associated with Turner's syndrome (ovarian agenesis) and bicuspid aortic valve. Chest x-ray: Rib notching. Upper extremity hypertension.

Complete heart block in infant—Resting pulse with crying, murmur, and canon A wave dissociation.

Congenital heart disease:
- Cyanotic:
  - Hypoplastic left heart syndrome—First few days. Low output cardiac failure. Grave prognosis.
  - Tetralogy of Fallot (TOF)—Presents in first few months. Episodic and unresponsive while feeding, cyanotic, tachypnea, single second heart sound, O_2 saturation not improved with O_2 and spells in which the child kneels to obtain more breath.
  - Transposition of great vessels—First few days. Cyanosis and tachypnea. *Treatment: Urgent balloon atrial septostomy until definitive surgical repair.*

- Noncyanotic:
  - Coarctation of aorta—Decreased or absent pulses in the legs. Presents in abrupt onset of CHF at the time of closure of the ductus arteriosus approximately second week of life. *Treatment: Give prostaglandin E to keep ductus open.*
  - Patent ductus arteriosus—Premature infant who presents in CHF.
  - Ventricular septal defect (VSD)—Presents in CHF.

CHF in a 6-month-old—Suspect large VSD.

CHF to occur—Need increased flow to pulmonary vessels or obstruction to left ventricular (LV) outflow.

Cyanosis—Causes:

- CNS—See apnea. Responds to O_2.
- Heart disease—See tachypnea. Responds to O_2.
- Methemoglobinemia—No symptoms. Does not respond to O_2.
- Pulmonary disease—See tachypnea, grunting, and retraction. Responds to O_2.

Cyanosis and CHF—Transposition of great vessels with VSD.

Digoxin—Treatment of choice for CHF in infants.

Eisenmenger's syndrome—VSD with pulmonary hypertension and reversal of right-to-left shunt in TOF.

Hypoplastic left ventricle—First few days, low output cardiac failure, globally diminished pulse, and grave prognosis.

Hypoplastic left heart, tricuspid atresia, and critical coarctation of the aorta—Rapid onset cardiogenic shock, acidosis, and hypotension.

Kawasaki—Need five of six criteria. Fever, mucous membrane change, rash, conjunctivitis, extremity edema, and lymphadenopathy. *Treatment: High-dose aspirin (ASA), gamma-globulin, and admit.*

Metaphyseal chip or "corner" fracture—Associated with child abuse.

Patent ductus arteriosus (PDA)—Common in the premature infant, large left-to-right intracardiac shunt. Presents as CHF. Not cyanotic. Continuous murmur at second left intercostal space.

Presentation with:

- CHF—Transposition of great vessels, hypoplastic left-heart syndrome, left-to-right shunts, and PDA. Presents with feeding difficulties and increased sweating. *Treatment: Digoxin.*
- Cyanosis—Right-to-left shunts, pulmonary atresia, and preductal coarctation.

Prostaglandin infusion—1- to 2-week-old infant presents with CHF after ductus arteriosus closes.

Sail sign—Enlarged thymus on chest x-ray.

Shunts:
- Right-to-left—Cyanosis. No improvement with O_2.
- Left-to-right—No cyanosis. Improvement with O_2.

Snowman—Total anomalous pulmonary venous return.

Tetralogy spells—From pulmonary spasm right-to-left shunt. Knee-chest position. *Treatment: Morphine relaxes pulmonary infundibulum and the infant. Also give O_2.*

TOF—Cyanotic, tetralogy spells, right ventricular (RV) outflow obstruction, VSD, overriding aorta, and RV hypertrophy. Single heart sound. On 100% O_2 PaO_2 ~95 mmHg. Right–to-left shunt continues.

Transposition of great vessels—Most common cause of death first year of life. Symptoms first few days, generalized cyanosis, no respiratory distress, and tachypnea becomes worse. Chest x-ray: Aortic valve anterior to pulmonic valve. *Treatment: Give prostaglandin E to keep ductus open. Balloon septostomy between atria.*

Verapamil—Contraindicated in <1 year of age for supraventricular tachycardia (SVT). Causes hypotension and cardiac depression.

X-ray findings:
- Boot-shaped heart—Tetralogy of Fallot.
- Box- or funnel-shaped heart—Ebstein's anomaly.
- "Egg on a string"—Transposition of the great arteries.

▶ CHILD ABUSE: NONACCIDENTAL TRAUMA (NAT)

Battered child syndrome—Metaphyseal "corner" and bucket-handle fractures.

NAT—Lack of history, abuse in sibling, injury inconsistent with mechanism, and conflicting histories. Injuries at various stages of healing, multiplanar injuries.

Failure to report suspected child abuse—Misdemeanor charge.

Prepubertal sexual abuse—No speculum. Call social service even if examination is normal.

Shaken baby syndrome—Retinal hemorrhages.

▶ DERMATOLOGY

Candidal rash—Sharply demarcated rash with satellite lesions.

Dermatomyositis—Erythematous scaly rash and facial heliotrope (reddish purple patch on eyelids).

Group A beta-hemolytic streptococci (GABHS)—Scarlatiniform rash and pharyngitis.

Hair tourniquet syndrome—Hair wrapped around the digit. Cries inconsolably.

Hand-foot-mouth disease—Approximately 2-year-old, well hydrated with shallow whitish ulcers on soft palate. Also grayish vesicles and erythematous papules on palms, back of hands, soles of feet, and diaper area.

Headlight sign—Nose is spared in infantile atopic dermatitis. Cheeks involved.

Rashes on palms and soles—Rocky Mountain spotted fever (RMSF), syphilis, psoriasis, and hand-foot-mouth disease.

▸ DEVELOPMENT

- 7 to 10 days—Regain birthweight.
- 4 months—Holds head steady, recognizes human face, and grasps voluntarily.
- 6 months—Sits up with propping. First tooth. Transfers object from one hand to the other.
- 8 months—Independent sitting.
- 1 year—Head circumference is 35 cm (average) at birth and increases an average of 1 cm/month during first year. Length: Grows 10" longer by first year. 5" second year, and 2–3"/year during school years.
- 3 years—Walks downstairs alternating foot; names 2 to 3 colors.
- 5 years—Counts 10 objects and catches ball.
- 6 years—Ties shoelaces and skips alternating feet (boys too).
- Birth weight—Doubles by 6 months and triples by 1 year.

Congenital adrenal hyperplasia (CAH)—Growth stops early due to virilization and speeding up of epiphyseal closure.

Constitutional growth delay—Lags behind in growth maturation. Bone age is also delayed. Small for age. Delayed puberty but ultimately catches up.

Cushing's syndrome—Excessive weight gain but retardation of linear growth.

Down's syndrome—Associated with duodenal atresia, congenital heart disease, and atlantoaxial instability.

Familial short stature—Bone age normal. 3rd to 5th percentile in growth curve. Ultimate height below average. Bone age parallels chronologic age rather than height.

First molar—First permanent teeth to erupt.

Ortolani maneuver—Check for hip click in congenital hip dislocation. With child in supine position, the examiner's fingers placed over the greater trochanter and thumb over the inner thigh. When both hips are flexed at 90°, a "click" is heard or felt when the hips are abducted slowly from the midline.

Physiologic gynecomastia—Normal in adolescent boys, but may occur in girls. Do not biopsy the mass in girls, because it is probably a breast bud, and this will destroy the breast. It is often unilateral in both genders.

Turner's syndrome—XO. Phenotypic female with short webbed-neck. Coarctation of aorta. Ovarian agenesis. Frequent gastrointestinal (GI) bleeds from intestinal angiomata.

▶ *ENDOCRINE*

Cherry spot in macula—Niemann-Pick (hepatosplenomegaly) or Tay-Sach's diseases.

Child with diabetic ketoacidosis (DKA)—Slow IVF. Cerebral edema may occur 6 to 8 hours after apparent clinical improvement.

Congenital hypothyroidism—Associated with prolonged neonatal hyperbilirubinemia, constipation, and umbilical hernia.

Kawasaki's—*Treatment: Admit and start intravenous immunoglobulin (IVIG) and aspirin.*

▶ *GASTROINTESTINAL*

10-10-20 fluid resuscitation:
- First 10 kg—100 cal/kg and 100 mL/kg
- Second 10 kg—50 cal/kg and 50 mL/kg
- >20 kg—20 cal/kg and 20 mL/kg

Anal fissure—Healthy infant with no abdominal pain and single episode of rectal bleeding or smear.

Annular pancreas—Vomiting. Congenital defect in which the pancreas encircles the duodenum.

Bilious vomiting in newborn—Suspect malrotation with midgut volvulus.

Botulism—Infant with worsening constipation, weak cry, poor tone, absent deep tendon reflexes (DTRs), and feeds poorly.

Bronze baby syndrome—Dark, grayish-brown discoloration of the skin in babies with elevated conjugated bilirubin when they are treated with phototherapy.

Button battery ingestion—*Treatment: Endoscopy if in esophagus. If past esophagus, surgical consultation.*

Cystic fibrosis—Suspect in patient with chronic cough, clubbing, and rectal prolapse.

Dance's sign—Elongated right upper quadrant (RUQ) abdominal mass with no bowel sounds in right lower quadrant (RLQ) in intussusception. On x-ray see loss of bowel gas in RLQ.

Diaphragmatic hernia—Newborn with severe respiratory distress.

Double bubble sign—Classic radiologic finding in duodenal atresia. In ultrasound of fetus, see two round circles in the abdomen.

Duodenal atresia—Newborn with bilious vomiting. Associated with Down's syndrome and polyhydramnios. See "double-bubble" sign on x-ray: air in stomach and duodenum without gas in distal bowel.

Esophageal atresia with tracheoesophageal fistula—Newborn with respiratory distress with feeding. Failure to pass nasogastric (NG) tube.

Failure to thrive—"Wary" and "wide-eyed." Weight gain in hospital is sine qua non of failure to thrive.

Gastroschisis—No sac. Defect in abdominal wall.

Giardia—Watery diarrhea and abdominal cramps.

Grunting—Sound produced by glottic closure during exhalation in an attempt to provide physiologic positive end-expiratory pressure (PEEP).

Hirschsprung's disease—Empty rectum, palpable colonic stool, and constipation since birth. Male>female. Congenital megacolon. Scenario: full-term infant with abdominal distension and failure to pass meconium.

Intussusception—3 months to 5 years of age. Paroxysms crying, vomiting, currant jelly stool, sausage-shaped mass in right midquadrant (RMQ), and no bowel sounds in RLQ. "Coiled spring" in barium enema. Ultrasound: donut, target or concentric ring on transverse view; "sandwich sign"; pseudo-kidney on longitudinal view. Most common location: ileocecal valve. *Treatment: Barium or air contrast enema.*

Iron deficiency in a 2-year-old child—Intake of large amount of unmodified cow's milk.

Juvenile polyps—Painless rectal bleeding.

Malrotation with midgut volvulus—First month of life, abrupt onset, bilious vomiting, ill appearing, pale, and in distress. *Treatment: Surgery consult.*

Meconium ileus—Full-term newborn with triad of bilious vomiting, abdominal distention, and failure to pass meconium. Associated with cystic fibrosis. X-ray: small bowel with "soap-bubble" appearance. Contrast enema: "Rabbit pellet" appearance.

"Meckel's rule of twos"—In 2% of population, 2% with symptoms, 2 feet proximal to terminal ileum, and 45% with symptoms <2 years old.

Midgut volvulus—First month (<1 year of age), bilious vomiting, abdominal palpable mass, and blood-streaked stool. Associated with malrotation of intestine. Ladd's bands. *Treatment: Surgery.*

Niemann-Pick disease—Hepatosplenomegaly and cherry-red spot in macula.

Omphalocele—Umbilical sac with defect in umbilical ring.

Pancreatic insufficiency in childhood—Cystic fibrosis.

Pneumatosis intestinalis—Diagnostic of necrotizing enterocolitis (NEC) in premature neonate. Child may have Hirschsprung's disease.

Pneumoperitoneum with NEC—*Treatment: Absolute indication for surgery.*

Portal vein thrombosis—Portal hypertension without cirrhosis. Seen in children.

Pyloric stenosis—"Olive" mass in RMQ abdomen, nonbilious vomiting, and hypochloremic hypokalemic metabolic alkalosis; 2 to 6 weeks of age, male>female, and elevated conjugated bilirubin. Metabolic abnormalities will not correct without potassium.

Reyes' syndrome—Hypoglycemia with increased liver function tests (LFTs); coma and liver failure.

Rotavirus—Upper respiratory infection (URI), fever, vomiting, and watery diarrhea.

Salmonella—Foul odor stool, which is rarely bloody, and may present with or without fever.

Shigella—Fever and bloody odorless diarrhea. May present with fever and seizures.

"String sign"—Narrow pylorus in pyloric stenosis.

Trichurid trichiura—Rectal prolapse in children.

Volvulus—First year, palpable mass, and bilious vomiting (contrast with: pyloric stenosis: mass and nonbilious vomiting).

Yersinia—RLQ pain and mimics appendicitis.

▶ HEAD, EARS, EYES, NOSE, and THROAT (HEENT)

Aniridia—Congenital absence or hypoplasia of iris. Associated with Wilms tumor.

Bacterial tracheitis—<3 years of age with URI symptoms, featuring both croup and epiglottitis, barky cough, and high fever. *Staphylococcus aureus*. Superinfection to croup. X-ray: fuzziness of tracheal air column border. Thick tracheal secretions. *Treatment: Antibiotics, intubate.*

Croup—Steeple sign. Narrowing of trachea on anteroposterior view of neck.

Cystic hygroma—Benign lymphangioma in head and neck.

Epiglottitis—Abrupt onset, 2 to 6 years of age, *Haemophilus* influenze, high fever, toxic, sits forward, drools, no cough, muffled voice, stridor, and dysphagia. Thumb-print sign on lateral neck x-ray. Thickened aryepiglottic folds.

Foreign body aspiration—Most commonly, right mainstem bronchus. Segmental atelectasis after complete bronchus obstruction. Decubitus view: Foreign body on the side with increased relative lung volume. Any child with history of choking, needs evaluation and probably bronchoscopy no matter how well the child looks, and no matter how normal the chest x-ray looks.

Hand-foot syndrome (dactylitis)—Sickle cell disease. Swelling of all or one extremities seen <2 years of age.

Grunting—Sound produced by glottic closure during exhalation in an attempt to provide physiologic positive end-expiratory pressure (PEEP).

Mastoiditis—Severe pain behind the ear and decreased hearing. On CT scan see fluid in mastoid cells. *Treatment: IV antibiotics. Mastoidectomy if any evidence of bony destruction.*

Laryngeal fracture—Elevation of hyoid bone above C_3.

Neonatal conjunctivitis—See within first 24 hours. *Treatment: Silver nitrate.*

Retropharyngeal abscess—<6 years of age. "Tracheal rock sign" and duck quack (cri du canard).

Sinuses:
- Frontal and sphenoid—Become aerated by 6 to 7 years of age.
- Ethmoid and maxillary—Present at birth.

Steroids and epinephrine—Use for croup and bronchiolitis. Not needed for epiglottitis or bacterial tracheitis.

Stridor:
- Inspiratory stridor—Above carina.
- Expiratory stridor—Below carina.

Uveitis (anterior)—Associated with juvenile rheumatoid arthritis.

White pupillary reflex—Retinoblastoma.

X-ray findings:
- Croup—Steeple sign with mild degree of subglottic narrowing.
- Epiglottitis—Thumb-like projection and aryepiglottic folds thickened. Subglottic and prevertebral space normal.
- Retropharyngeal abscess—Epiglottis normal (triangular) and subglottic space normal.

▶ INFECTION

Antibiotics—For salmonella with sickle cell trait. Not for just plain salmonella.

Beaus' lines—Transverse grooves of nails (Kawasaki's lines).

Foreign body—Foul-smelling discharge either from one nostril or vagina in a preschool child.

Hypovolemic shock from vomiting and diarrhea—Most common cause of preload disorders in children.

Irritable child with URI and petechiae—*Treat for meningitis and isolate.*

Meningococcemia—Absence of meningitis is a poor prognostic indicator.

Minors—Can consent for STDs and drug-abuse treatments.

Non-toxic 18 month old, T 40.5°C with no focus for fever—*Treatment: Blood, urine culture, and ceftriaxone. Lumbar puncture (LP) based on judgment of the child as well as immunization history (if the child had Haemophilus influenza and pneumococcal vaccines, probably doesn't need an LP).*

Omphalitis—Infection of umbilical cord. *Treatment: Admit for erythema, purulent drainage, or circumferential erythema.*

Otitis media—Least diagnostic value is positive light reflex.

Retropharyngeal abscess—Toxic looking child, fever, neck stiffness and swelling, drooling, muffled voice, epiglottis normal, and cries with mouth wide open.

Reyes' syndrome:
- Stage I—Lethargy, normal posture, and brisk pupils.
- Stage II—Combative or stuporous, with sluggish pupillary response.
- Stage III—Coma, flexor posturing, and sluggish pupils.
- Stage IV—Extensor posturing.
- Stage V—Flaccid coma with unreactive pupils.

Staphylococcus impetigo—*Treatment: Give oral cephalexin and local wound care. Topical not effective.*

Urine for culture—*Treatment: Clean catch in an uncircumcised, toilet trained 5-year-old boy—no need to catheterize.*

▶ *NEONATAL*

2 week old, T 38°C, decreased feeding, and no other problems—*Treatment: Blood, urine culture, lumbar puncture, and admit for IV ampicillin and gentamicin.*

< 1 month—Do not use ceftriaxone (displaces bilirubin).

Apnea—No respiration for 20 seconds, associated with heart rate ≤80, or accompanied by cyanosis or pallor. Abnormal if present on first day of life. Always abnormal in term infants. Benign apnea of prematurity if occurs in premature infants >3 days old. *Treatment: Admit all infants with apnea. Give theophylline.*

Apt test—To determine presence of maternal blood. Mix small amount of baby's blood with tap water to cause hemolysis. The sample is then centrifuged and the pink supernatant is mixed with NaOH. Fetal hemoglobin is resistant to alkali denaturation so remains pink. Adult hemoglobin is denatured, turning yellow brownish color.

Bilateral choanal atresia—Respiratory distress in neonatal period.

Birthweight—28 weeks, ~1000 g.

Congenital hip dislocation—Unequal leg length and thigh skin crease. Hear "hip-click" on examination.

Disseminated varicella—If mom has varicella <5 days prior to delivery, antibodies have not had chance to go to fetus; 30% mortality rate.

Epiphyseal dysgenesis—Associated with hypothyroidism.

Erythema toxicum—First 2 days. Term baby with blotchy erythematous macula 2 to 3 cm in diameter. Eosinophils in Wright's stain.

Impetigo neonatorum—Staphylococcal. Pustules with erythematous margins in diaper area.

Ischemic injury:
- Preterm infants—Periventricular white matter.
- Term infants—Gray matter "water-shed" cortex.

Jaundice—If starts:
- First 24 hours—ABO or Rh incompatibility, sepsis, congenital infections (rubella, toxoplasmosis, cytomegalovirus [CMV], or excessive bruising from birth trauma. *Exchange transfusion for unconjugated bilirubin > 20 mg/dL first 24 hours.*
- Day 2 to 3—Physiologic. From breakdown of fetal RBCs. Resolves within the week. *Phototherapy if unconjugated bilirubin > 12 mg/dL first few days.*
- Remainder of 1st week—Septicemia or infections (syphilis, toxoplasmosis, and CMV).
- After first week—Sepsis, congenital atresia of bile ducts, hepatitis, congenital hemolytic anemia, hemolytic anemias due to drugs, rubella, hypothyroidism, and breast-milk jaundice.

Kernicterus—Direct toxic effect of unconjugated bilirubin on brain. Hypotonia and lethargy. Fever, seizure, and opisthotonos are late findings.

Mom with untreated Grave's disease—Thyrotoxicosis in infant the first day. Long-acting thyroid stimulator (LATS) crossing stimulating thyroid gland to produce hormone.

Mother with hyperparathyroidism—Infant likely to develop hypocalcemia. Suppression of fetal parathyroid gland by mom's parahormone.

Necrotizing enterocolitis (NEC)—Vomiting, abdominal distention, and bloody stools.

Neonatal acne— ~7 to 8-day-old with pustules on forehead and nose.

Neonatal jaundice:
- Biliary atresia—5-week-old infant with 2-week history of jaundice. Direct bilirubin >> Indirect bilirubin. Normal liver enzymes. Ultrasound: gallbladder not visualized.
- Crigler-Najjar syndrome—4-week-old with jaundice since 3-day-old; elevated indirect bilirubin.
- Physiologic—Healthy few days old. Indirect bilirubin >> direct bilirubin.

Neonatal mastitis—Low-grade fever, redness, streaking from breast, and pus from nipple. *Staphylococcus* or *Streptococcus*.

Newborn baby with whitish eye discharge following normal spontaneous vaginal delivery (NSVD) with mild URI— *Fluorescein stain.*
- *If negative: Gram stain and culture for gonorrhea (GC). If negative for GC, do nasopharyngeal aspirate for chlamydia; give parenteral antibiotics.*

Respiratory distress syndrome (RDS)—Tachypnea, retraction, cyanosis, and grunting in a premature infant.

Subcutaneous fat necrosis—Violaceous and circumscribed subcutaneous nodules immediately beneath fading forceps mark on one cheek.

Tracheoesophageal fistula—Respiratory distress first 24 hours after delivery.

Vaginal bleeding—In neonate from withdrawal of maternal estrogen at birth. Will stop spontaneously.

Vomiting, coma, and acidosis first week of life—Suspect genetic disorder of organic acid metabolism. Always check blood sugar.

Vomiting first day—Look for duodenal atresia, meconium ileus, volvulus, and annular pancreas.

▶ NEUROLOGIC

Absence seizure—3-second spike and wave pattern on electroencephalogram (EEG).

Breath-holding spell—Child <2 years of age, with rage, crying, cyanosis, loss of consciousness, and loss of motor tone. No postictal period. Benign.

Craniopharyngioma—Elevated intracranial pressure and suprasellar calcification.

Febrile seizure—6 months to 5 years of age. Generalized, lasts <20 minutes, no neurologic deficits, and recurs in 30% cases.

Focal neurologic findings—Separates viral meningitis from bacterial meningitis (bacterial meningitis has focal findings).

Hypertension and seizure—Look for hypertensive encephalopathy.

Infantile spasm (West's syndrome)—Bilateral symmetric clustered spasm. Most are central nervous system (CNS) disorders.

Neuroblastoma—Orbital mass and abdominal mass that crosses midline.

Pseudotumor cerebri—Benign intracranial hypertension. Seen with hypoparathyroidism.

Roseola—2 to 3 days of high fever; after defervescence, an erythematous rash develops on the trunk.

Seizure (due to hyponatremia)—Bottle-fed baby with gastroenteritis given diluted formula.

Shigella—Associated with seizure.

▶ ORTHOPEDICS

Ewing's sarcoma—Osteolytic lesion. Multiple layers of subperiosteal "onion peel" or "sunburst" on x-ray.

Legg-Calve-Perthes—Boys 4 to 9 years of age with hip and knee pain. Examination normal. Idiopathic, avascular osteochondrosis of

Table 3-14: Salter-Harris types	
I: Epiphyseal plate disruption	May not see in x-ray
II: Epiphyseal plate + metaphysis	No growth disturbance
III: Epiphyseal plate + epiphysis	Growth disturbance may occur
IV: Epiphyseal plate + metaphysis + epiphysis	Growth disturbance in high proportion
V: Crush injury to epiphysis	Growth arrest often

femoral head with stress fracture, and affected hip limited range of motion. Hip x-ray; smaller femoral head with resorption.

Osgood-Schlatter's disease—Pain and swelling of tibial tuberosity with negative x-ray. Apophysitis of tibial tuberosity. No actual avulsion. Short-term immobilization.

Osteogenic imperfecta—Blue sclera with generalized osteopenia and frequent fractures.

Painless limp in a 5-year-old—Seen in Legg-Calve-Perthes, but also in tenosynovitis.

Salter-Harris types—See Table 3-14.

Septic arthritis—<4 years of age. Staphylococcus aureus. Fever, toxic, and lying in supine position with leg flexed, abducted, and externally rotated. Refuses to walk. *Definitive diagnosis: needle aspiration. Will often require fluoroscopic assistance from radiology.*

Slipped capital femoral epiphysis (SCFE)—10- to 14-year-old obese boy with acute inability to walk. Pain in groin, thigh, and knee. Externally rotated thigh, male>female, and bilateral in 40%. Get lateral x-ray. Positive log roll. *Treatment: Emergent orthopedic consultation.*

Transient synovitis—Unilateral. Boys peak 5 to 6 years of age. Inability to walk, nontoxic, resists hip movement, and normal WBCs. Diagnosis by exclusion. Signs and symptoms as in septic hip but less toxic.

▶ **PULMONARY**

Aspirated foreign body—Decubitus chest x-ray: Lack of dependent atelectasis on foreign body side. No matter how good the imaging studies look, after a choking episode, the child should have a bronchoscopy.

Bacterial pneumonia—High fever and abrupt chills.

Breath-holding spell—Screams, falls to the ground, tonic-clonic movements, and nontoxic.

Bronchiolitis—Respiratory syncytial virus (RSV). *Treatment: No steroids or antibiotics. Use bronchodilator and racemic epinephrine.*

Chlamydia pneumonia—4 to 16 years of age. Conjunctivitis and staccato cough.

Croup—Parainfluenza virus.

Cystic fibrosis—Hypochloremic metabolic alkalosis.

Grunting—Lower respiratory tract.

Haemophilus influenza—Still leading cause of epiglottitis but very rare since immunization.

Methemoglobinemia—Normal PO_2. Blood does not turn red or pink. Does not improve with O_2.

Mycoplasma—Hacking cough nonproductive.

Pertussis—Staccato cough "whoop." Three stages- catarrhal (mild URI/cough), staccato, and whooping cough.

Pharyngeal infections:
- Croup and bacterial tracheitis—<3 years old. Peak 21 to 24 months of age.
- Epiglottitis—Bimodal: 2 to 6 years of age and 20 to 60 years of age.
- Peritonsillar abscess—Adolescents and young adults (rare in young children).
- Retropharyngeal abscess—<4 years old.

Respiratory syncytial virus (RSV)—Wheezing.

Spasmodic cough—Like viral, but suddenly without prodrome.

Stridor—Supraglottic: Inspiratory stridor. Subglottic: Expiratory stridor.

Sudden infant death syndrome (SIDS)—1 month to 1 year of age. Risk factors: maternal smoking and age<20 at first pregnancy, Native Americans. Baby sleeping prone.

Use of accessory muscles—Correlates best with obstruction in pediatric asthma.

Viral croup—6 months to 3 years of age, boys> girls, fall or winter, barky cough, and URI. Parainfluenza.

▶ RESUSCITATION

Children—Defibrillate: 2 J/kg initial, double the rest. Cardioversion: 0.5 J/kg initial, and double the rest. Compressions—infants ½" to 1", child 1" to 1½", >8 years of age 1½" to 2".

Cricothyrotomy—Contraindicated in <10 years of age.

Dehydration and shock—Isotonic bolus 20 mL/kg. May be repeated.

Intravenous fluids—<3 months: D_{10} at 2 to 4 mL/kg. >3 months: D_{25} at 2 mL/kg.

Maintenance fluid—100/50/20 or 4/2/1.

Pediatric arrest—Epinephrine 0.01 mg/kg of a 10,000 solution.

Rule of 6:
- Inotrope: 6 × kg of body wt = mg added to make 100 mL. 1 mL/hour delivers 1 mg/kg/min.

- Epinephrine, norepinephrine, and isuprel: 0.6 × kg wt = mg added to make 100 mL. 1 mL/hour delivers 0.1 mg/kg/min.

▶ *TRAUMA*

Cervical spine (C-spine) injury—Upper C-spine injury >> common than lower C-spine in children (big head acts as fulcrum).

Destot's sign—Superficial hematoma along inguinal ligament or scrotum. Pelvic fracture.

Earle's sign—Palpable bony prominence or large hematoma on rectal examination.

Minors with life or limb threatening injuries—*Treat per standard protocol. No need to wait for permission to treat.*

Spinal cord injury without x-ray abnormalities (SCIWORA)— Children <8 years of age.

Supracondylar fracture of the humerus—*Treatment: Splint arm in extension, orthopedic consultation. Often requires reduction.*

▶ PHARMACOLOGY

Adenosine—May cause bronchoconstriction in asthma.

Amiodarone—Associated with hypothyroidism.

Anticholinergics—Affects bronchi.

Antidysrhythmics:
- Class IA—Procainamide and quinidine.
- Class IB—Lidocaine and phenytoin.
- Class IC—Flecainide.
- Class II—β-Blockers.
- Class III—Bretylium and amiodarone.
- Class IV—Calcium channel blockers.

Anti-malarial agents—Side effects: corneal deposits and irreversible retinopathy.

β-Agonists—Affects smaller peripheral airways.

Chlorpropamide—*Treatment: Hypoglycemia after this drug requires admission for 24 hours. ($T_{1/2}$ 36 hours.) Glyburide shorter $T_{1/2}$, but both longer than effect of glucose, so recurrent hypoglycemia is common. It may require a glucose 10% continuous drip; Octreotide is also useful.*

Clonidine—Bradycardia, hypotension, and central nervous system (CNS) depression.

Clozapine—Causes agranulocytosis.

Conscious sedation monitoring—Increased respiratory depression in the absence of pain stimuli.

Cyclosporine treated patients—Avoid P_{450} inhibitors (toxicity), and inducers (rejection).

Demerol—CNS toxicity may occur due to the metabolite normeperidine. Anxiety, seizure, and psychosis. Avoidable by not giving repeated doses and avoiding more than 800 mg total dose.

Depression—Caused by aldomet, inderal, reserpine, guanethidine, birth control pills, and benzodiazepines.

Diazepam—Worsens hyperbilirubinemia.

Digoxin toxicity—Bradycardia, hypotension, lethargy, and hyperkalemia.

Drug elimination:
- First order—Decline in drug levels at a constant percentage of the remaining drug.
- Zero order—Constant quantity of drug is eliminated per unit of time.
- Michaelis-Menton—Mixture of first and zero order.

Drugs causing hypoglycemia—Pentamidine, antimalarials, propranolol, salicylate sulfonylureas, insulin, and alcohol.

Ethambutol—Retrobulbar neuritis and visual loss.

Etomidate—Drug of choice for intubation in multiple trauma.

Fentanyl—No histamine release. Board like chest rigidity with high dose. Also muscular and glottic rigidity. Not detected in urine.

First-phase metabolism—Orally ingested drug metabolized by liver before systemic circulation.

Flumazenil—Benzodiazepine reversal. Binds competitively and reversibly with (gamma-aminobutyric acid, GABA) GABA-benzo receptors. $T_{½}$ 40 to 80 minutes. Precipitates withdrawal and seizures.

Furosemide—In oliguric renal failure: 2 to 6 mg/kg to maximum of 400 mg.

Glyburide induced hypoglycemia—*Treatment: Use glucagon, D_{50}, diazoxide (insulin antagonist), or octreotide.*

Glycoprotein platelet IIb/IIIa inhibitor—Inhibits platelet activation by binding to receptors. (ASA inhibits platelet aggregation.)

Hemorrhagic cystitis—Associated with cyclophosphamide.

Hydralazine—Reflex tachycardia and lupus-like syndrome.

Indinavir—Causes symptomatic urolithiasis.

Isoniazid—Causes peripheral neuritis, hepatitis, and status epilepticus in overdose.

Ketamine—Dissociative anesthesia. Nightmares 50% in adults and 10% in children. Decreases reuptake of catecholamine. Choice sedative for patients without head injury.

Lidocaine—Increasing the concentration will increase the duration of anesthesia. Plain 3 to 5 mg/kg, with epinephrine 7 mg/kg. Adverse effects: drowsiness to coma, perioral paresthesia, twitching, sinoatrial and atrioventricular (SA/AV) dysfunction, seizures and hypotension.

Lidocaine with epinephrine—Not for end-arterial field (digits, pinna, nose, nipple, and penis). To reverse use local or IV, 1.5 to 5 mg phentolamine.

Lithium—Mimics iodine inhibits thyroid release. *Treatment: Lithium toxicity with coma needs dialysis.*

Local anesthesia—Amide class (has two ii)—Lidocaine, mepivacaine, bupivacaine, and etidocaine. Ester class (has one i)—Procaine and tetracaine. Allergy due to preservative.

Mellaril with nonsedating antihistamine—Predisposes to torsade de pointes.

Meprobamate—See bezoars with massive ingestion. Forced diuresis.

Morphine sulfate—Hypotension secondary to histamine release. Give IVF. Naloxone does not reverse vasodilation.

Naloxone—For opioid reversal, 0.1 to 0.2 mg initially to avoid with withdrawal. Total 2 mg.

Nitroprusside—Coronary steal syndrome (less diseased vessels dilate, thereby stealing blood from diseased vessels).

Nitroprusside toxicity—Hypoxia, tinnitus, and psychosis (chronic use may cause hypothyroidism).

Nitrous oxide—Flow controlled with inhalation. Contraindicated in altered mental status. Use 30% O_2 and scavenger device.

Neuroleptic malignant syndrome (NMS)—Fever, altered mental status, and muscle rigidity. *Treatment: Dantrolene.*

Phenytoin—Contraindicated in hyperosmolar hyperglycemic nonketotic coma (HHNC) seizure. It impairs endogenous insulin release.

Physostigmine—Only centrally acting anticholinesterases, that can cross the blood-brain barrier. In contrast neostigmine does not cross the barrier.

Primidone (mysoline)—Phenobarbital is active metabolite.

Prophylactic antibiotics—Not indicated in laceration repairs in healthy patients.

Psychotomimetic reaction—Producing symptoms resembling those of psychoses (visual hallucinations, distortion of perception, and schizophrenia-like behavior). Most significant side effect of pentazocine (Talwin). Agonist and antagonist.

Rifampin—Orange tears and saliva. Will permanently stain contact lenses. May cause renal failure.

Salicylates—Uncouples oxidative phosphorylation.

Succinylcholine—Increases intracranial pressure (use lidocaine), contraindicated in burn or trauma > days or weeks, but not in immediate burn or trauma.

Vasopressin—Noncatecholamine pressor. Alternative to epinephrine in shock-refractory ventricular fibrillation. Dose 40 units IV push once. Longer $T_{1/2}$ than epinephrine.

Vecuronium—Use 0.01 mg/kg as pretreatment to minimize elevation in intracranial pressure (ICP) for intubation.

▶ PULMONARY

200 mL—Amount of fluid on chest x-ray needed to diagnose pleural effusion.

A-a gradient—[150 – pCO_2/0.8] or [150 – PaO_2 – 1.2($PaCO_2$)] or [140 – PaO_2 – $PaCO_2$].

Acidic pleural fluid (< 7.0)—Esophagus rupture or empyema.

Acute respiratory distress syndrome (ARDS)—Activation of complement system causes damage to pulmonary vascular endothelium. In chest x-ray: See diffuse infiltrate with normal size heart. Most common cause sepsis.

Amniotic fluid embolism—Cardiopulmonary collapse followed by pulmonary edema.

Anti-cholinergics—Decreases cyclic GMP in asthma treatment.

Aspiration—Signs and symptoms occur within first hour in ~90% patients.

Asthma—To intubate use lidocaine (suppress cough), then ketamine, and then succinylcholine.

Asthma exacerbation—Bronchial smooth muscle contraction, calcium influx, mast cell, and edema.

Bornholm's disease—Prodromal symptoms, coxsackievirus, and paresthesia over ribs and sternum.

Chemoreceptors:
- Carotid body—Responds to hypoxia.
- Medulla—Responds to $PaCO_2$.

Chest tube:
- Simple pneumothorax: Use 24F to 28F chest tubes or Heimlich valve.
- Hemothorax: Use 32F to 40F chest tubes.

Chronic obstructive pulmonary disease (COPD)—Cor pulmonale. Correct O_2 to 90%. *Most appropriate initial treatment: Nebulizer.*

Coccidioides immitis—Soil, (bike riding), granulomas, and hilar adenopathy.

Cryptococcus—India ink stain of spinal fluid.

CXR in pneumonia (Figures 3-62–3-64):
- Cavitary lesions—Tuberculosis.
- Hilar adenopathy—Atypical pneumonia.
- Lobar segmental infiltrate—Pneumococcus.
- Lung abscesses—*Staphylococcus, Klebsiella.*
- Pleural effusion—Bacterial pneumonia

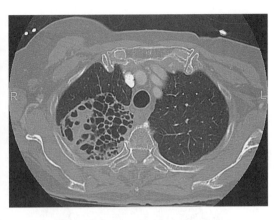

Figure 3-62:
Caviatary
lesions in right
apex

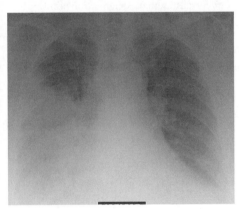

Figure 3-63:
Right middle and right
lower infiltrate

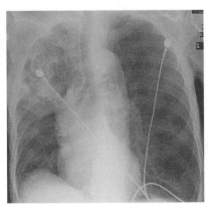

Figure 3-64:
Right upper lobe (RUL)
infiltrate

Cyanosis—Absolute amount reduced hemoglobin (Hgb) determine presence of cyanosis. Difficult to detect in anemia, easier to detect in polycythemia vera.
- Central:
    - Low O_2 saturation—Does not improve with oxygen.
    - Normal PO_2—Abnormal Hgb cannot bind normal amount O_2.
    - Low PO_2—Cardiopulmonary cause.
- Peripheral:
    - Decreased delivery to tissues. Responds to O_2. Caused by: cold, shock, or CHF.

Cytomegalovirus (CMV)—Most common pneumonia in transplantation patient.

Fat embolism—Dyspnea after a long bone fracture. Petechial rash on chest, axillae, and neck. *Treatment: No heparin.*

Hamman's crunch—Pneumomediastinum. Respiratory rub heard in posterior chest.

Hampton's hump—Wedge-shaped infiltrate (rounded border facing the hilus) seen in pulmonary embolism on chest x-ray.

Hanta virus—Pneumonia, ARDS, and shock in Southwestern United States.

Hemoptysis (Figure 3-65):
- >49 years of age—Most common causes: neoplasm and lung abscess
- <49 years of age—Most common causes: CHF, TB, bronchitis, or foreign body.

Histoplasmosis—"Coin" lesion. Associated with bird or bat excretion.

HIV and pneumonia—Mortality rate and symptoms same in HIV-positive community acquired pneumonia (CAP) and HIV-negative CAP.

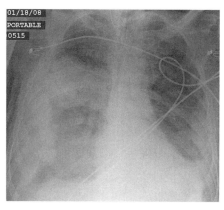

Figure 3-65: Metastatic lesions in lung with infiltrate

- CD4>800—Pneumococcus most common
- CD4 250 to 500—Mycobacterium TB
- CD4<200—Pneumocystis carinii (PCP)

Hydrocarbon ingestion—In chest x-ray see medial lower lobe opacities.

Inhaled albuterol—Used for exacerbation of cor pulmonale.

Inhaled β-agonist in asthma—It increases cyclic AMP.

Massive hemoptysis—Approximately 300 mL in 24 hours.

Mechanical ventilation—"Rules of ten":

- 10 breaths/minute
- Tidal volume 10 mL/kg
- FiO_2 of 1.0
- Others: Pulmonary end-expiratory pressure (PEEP) 2.5 to 5 cm H_2O, inspiratory to expiratory (I:E) ratio 1:2
- Pressure-cycled preferred in children to avoid barotrauma

Mediastinal emphysema—Esophageal perforation (spontaneous or traumatic). *Treat promptly as it could be fatal.* Asthma, cocaine or marijuana smoking, or spontaneous. Discomfort can be treated with 100% oxygen inhalation. This replaces the nitrogen bubbles with oxygen that is absorbed from the tissues.

Mycoplasma pneumonia—Bullous myringitis is often associated.

Noncardiogenic pulmonary edema—Seen in heroin abuse. Normal to decreased wedge pressure, leaky capillaries, and increased alveolar protein.

Phosgene—Forms white cloud with newly mown hay. In alveoli forms CO_2 and HCl leading to capillary leak.

Pleural effusion—Need >250 mL fluid to be seen on chest x-ray. (Figure 3-66)

Pneumoconiosis—Grain handler with progressive pulmonary fibrosis.

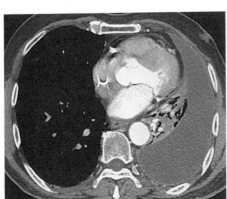

Figure 3-66: CT left-sided pleural effusion

Pneumocystis carinii pneumonia (PCP)—Classic triad of chronic dyspnea, fever, and nonproductive cough. Positive silver stain. Chest x-ray may be normal in 10% to 15% of cases. No hilar adenopathy.

Pneumomediastinum—Associated with pulmonary infection, asthma, and valsalva (marijuana or cocaine).

Pneumonia:

- Aspiration pneumonia—Cough, fever, tachypnea, and localized rales. *Treatment: Clindamycin.*
- Chlamydia trachomatis—<3 months of age. Afebrile, tachypneic, and mild conjunctivitis first. *Treatment: Erythromycin (EES).*
- Group A streptococci—Patchy multilobar (usually lower) and large pleural effusion. *Treatment: Ampicillin.* (Figure 3-67)
- E. coli—Patchy bilateral lower lobe infiltrate.
- Hanta virus—Ribavirus. Nausea, vomiting, and diarrhea leading to acute respiratory distress syndrome (ARDS) and shock. Elevated lactic dehydrogenase (LDH). The virus is often present in deer, mouse, and rodent feces.
- Haemophilus influenzae—Chest pain with worsening cough and sputum. Gram-negative pleomorphic rods. Patchy alveolar infiltrate, consolidation in >75%, bilateral in 25%, and pleural effusion. *Treatment: Ampicillin.*
- Legionella—Dry cough, watery diarrhea, bradycardia, altered mental status (AMS), and hyponatremia. *Treatment: Erythromycin.*
- Mycobacterium tuberculosis—Weakly gram-positive rod.
- Mycoplasma—Young, bullous myringitis, myalgia, dry cough, headache, and chest x-ray looks worse than the patient. Patchy infiltrate and bilateral perihilar (like viral) infiltrate.
- Pseudomonas—Patchy lower and middle lobe with abscess. Green sputum.

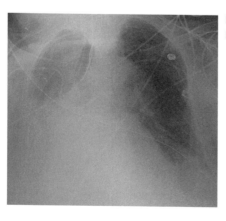

Figure 3-67: Right-sided pleural effusion/infiltrate

- Q fever—Hepatosplenomegaly. Coxiella brunetti.
- Staphylococcus aureus—Flu-like viral symptoms in nursing home or IV drug abusing patient. Abscess, lobar, patchy, pleural effusion, multicentric infiltrate, empyema, pneumothorax, or consolidation in chest x-ray.
- Streptococcus pneumonia—Most common community acquired pneumonia (CAP). Rusty sputum, single chill, and single lobe with small pleural effusion. Diplococcus. WBCs, 12,000 to 25,000 uL. Admit for immunosuppression, multiple lobe involvement, poor social situation, atoxicity (marked pain and inability to eat or drink). Local environments have varying recommendations for appropriate antibiotics ranging from penicillins to the floxacins.
- Tularemia—Glandular and typhoidal.
- Varicella—Cough, dyspnea, pleuritic chest pain, and hemoptysis few days after rash, fever, and malaise. Chest x-ray: diffuse miliary or nodular infiltrates.

Psittacosis—Bird vector. Nonproductive cough with infiltrate at base.

Pulmonary angiogram—Former gold standard for pulmonary embolism. Most institutions now utilizing CT angiography.

Pulmonary embolism:
- 40 rule—(in pulmonary embolism)
    - 40% mortality in massive pulmonary embolism (Figure 3-68)
    - 40% pulmonary vascular occlusion needed for hypoxia
    - 40% see EKG changes

Pulmonary embolism:
- Decreased probability + decreased clinical suspicion → 96% NPV.
- Increased probability + increased clinical suspicion → 96% PPV.
- EKG—Nonspecific ST-T changes most common abnormality, but

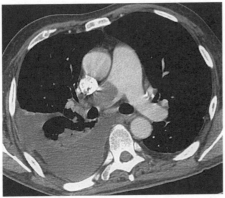

Figure 3-68: Large PE in right pulmonary artery

Table 3-15: Pulmonary embolism

Pulmonary Embolism	Sensitivity	Specificity
V/Q	98%	10%
Duplex US	95%	95%
Spiral CT	90%	96%

CT, computerized tomography; US, ultrasound; V/Q, ventilation-perfusion.

    sometimes see $S_1Q_3T_3$ suggestive of right ventricular strain; may
    see left V lead ST depression.
- Sinus tachycardia—Most common rhythm disturbance.
- Chest x-ray—Normal in 33%, atelectasis or infiltrate in 50%, and
  elevated hemidiaphragm in 40%.

Pulse oximetry—Measures hemoglobin saturated with O_2. Not same as
arterial blood gas (ABG) PaO_2.

Reexpansion pulmonary edema—Patient presents with hypoxemia,
hypotension, and hypovolemia following removal of chest tube. Seen
after very large pneumothorax, that has been present for 3 or more
days. *Treatment: IVF and O_2.*

Right upper lobe (RUL) lung collapse—Reverse "S" sign of Golden.

Septic pulmonary emboli—Multiple, rounded, and patchy lung
infiltrates with cavitation. Caused by tricuspid valve endocarditis or
septic thrombophlebitis. Organism: Staphylococcus aureus.

Silo gas—Nitrogen oxide. After inhalation this becomes nitric acid in
alveoli. Flu-like symptoms initially improves then worsens with
pulmonary edema.

$S_1Q_3T_3$—Classic EKG pattern with pulmonary embolism, but seen only
25% of the time.

Solitary pulmonary nodule—Most are benign. Patient requires close
follow-up. (Figure 3-69)

Steroids in pediatric asthma—Indicated if recent use, >4 attacks per
year, severe attack, not responsive to β-agonist, and history of
frequent hospitalizations.

Superior vena cava (SVC) syndrome—Throbbing headache and
hoarseness with face, neck, and hand swelling. *Treatment: Steroids,
diuretics, and radiation.*

(Elevated) Sweat chloride level—Cystic fibrosis. Serum electrolytes
normal. Normal sweat chloride is <40.

Tension pneumothorax—When suspected, do needle insertion followed
by chest tube. DO NOT OBTAIN chest x-ray first.

Thrombolytics—For massive pulmonary embolism with refractory
hypoxemia and circulatory collapse.

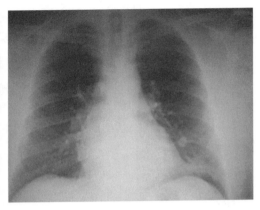

Figure 3-69:
Solitary lung nodule

Tube thoracostomy—Indicated for >20% pneumothorax.
Tuberculosis (TB)—Four drug treatment: RIPE—*Rifampin, INH, pyrazinamide, and ethambutol.* 90% with chest x-ray findings.
  • Primary TB—Parenchymal infiltrate with unilateral hilar adenopathy.
  • Reactivation TB—Lesions in upper lobe or superior segment of lower lobe.
Varicella pneumonia—Patient presents with pruritic rash and shortness of breath. Chest x-ray: bilateral interstitial pattern.
Ventilator adjustment:
  • To improve oxygenation: increase FiO_2 or add PEEP.
  • To improve ventilation: increase tidal volume, or increase rate.
Virchow's triad—Venous stasis, vascular endothelium trauma, and hypercoagulable state.
V/Q scan—If normal, rules out pulmonary embolism (PE). Any other reading is still compatible with a PE, and decisions for anticoagulation should be based clinically, or other imaging and diagnostic studies obtained.

▶ RESUSCITATION

ABC—In the absence of complete airway obstruction, do ventilation before intubation.
Awake oral intubation—For any patient who cannot afford to have respirations stopped; for example, distorted airway anatomy, epiglottitis, or morbid obesity. If oral intubation is not possible, go to cricothyrotomy.

Blind nasotracheal intubation—Apnea makes this procedure very difficult to impossible. Need a breathing patient.

Cricothyrotomy—Contraindicated in <10 years of age or with penetrating injury in upper zone 2 or 3 of the neck.

Endotracheal tube (ETT) drugs—NAVEL (Narcan, atropine, valium, epinephrine, and lidocaine).

Endotracheal tube (ETT) placement—Visualization of ETT passing through the cords is most reliable sign for successful intubation. (Figure 3-70)

Esophageal obturator airway—Complication: rupture of lower esophagus.

Hypotension and bradycardia—Seen in spinal cord lesions below T_4. *Treatment: Give atropine and α-agonist (e.g., phenylephrine).*

Hypotension nonhypovolemic:
- Dopamine: for BP <90 mm Hg.
- Dobutamine: for BP >100 mm Hg.

Intraaortic balloon pumps—Contraindicated in aortic insufficiency.

Intraosseous access—When venous access cannot be accessed. No age cut-off.

Mallampati classification—Determines difficulty of intubation.
- Grade I—All of faucial pillars, soft palate, and uvula are visualized.
- Grade II—Faucial pillars and soft palate are visualized.
- Grade III—Only the base of the uvula is visualized.
- Grade IV—Only see the tongue.

Military antishock trousers (MAST)—Contraindicated in pulmonary edema.

Nasotracheal intubation—Tube malposition is commonly palpated as a bulge in the piriform fossa.

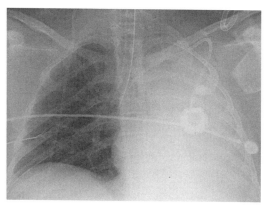

Figure 3-70:
ETT in right main bronchus

Table 3-16: Types of shock

Types of Shock	CO	SVR	PAWP
Anaphylactic	Decreased	Decreased	Decreased
Cardiogenic	Decreased	Increased	Increased
Early septic shock	Increased later decreased	Decreased	decreased
Hypovolemic	Decreased	Increased	Decreased
Neurogenic	Increased	Decreased	Decreased

CO (cardiac output); SVR (systemic venous resistance); PAWP (pulmonary artery wedge pressure)

Normal saline—Initial treatment of choice in hemorrhagic shock.

Packed cells—Resuscitative fluid of choice for persistent hemorrhagic shock.

Shock refractory ventricular fibrillation or pulseless ventricular tachycardia:
- Vasopressin 40 U IV × 1 as an alternative to epinephrine.
- Amiodarone—After epinephrine.

Succinylcholine—Contraindicated in >1 week of denervation (paraplegia, Guillain Barré, etc.), and >8 hours of crush or burn injury.

Tachycardia—Early signal of cardiogenic shock in an anterior MI.

Types of shock—See Table 3-16.

▶ RHEUMATOLOGY

Acute rheumatic fever—Group A streptococci. *Treatment: Penicillin, aspirin, and steroid.*

Angiotensin-converting enzyme (ACE) elevated—Seen in sarcoidosis along with bilateral hilar adenopathy.

Ankylosing spondylitis—Male <40 years of age, HLA B27, and symmetrical squaring of margins of the vertebrae. Only form of rheumatoid arthritis more common in men. Associated with aortic stenosis, aortic insufficiency, and aortic dissection.

Arthritis:
- Migratory—Gonorrhea, acute rheumatic fever, Lyme disease, viral arthritis, and systemic lupus erythematosus (SLE).
- Monoarthritis—Trauma, sepsis, acute osteomyelitis, gout, pseudogout, Lyme disease, and avascular necrosis.

- Oligoarthritis (two to three joints)—Lyme disease, Reiter's syndrome, ankylosing spondylitis, gonorrhea, and rheumatic fever.
- Polyarthritis—Rheumatic fever, systemic lupus erythematosus (SLE), viral, and chronic osteoarthritis.

Back pain (caused by):
- Infection—0.01%.
- Malignancy—1%.
- Serious pathologic condition—lumber pain: 10%; thoracic pain: 30%.

Behçet's syndrome—Young adults with oral and genital ulcers, arthritis, and uveitis.

Charcot's joint—"Bag of worms" ankle joint, boggy, and painless. In diabetes mellitus, chronic trauma due to denervation causing multiple small fractures.

Crohn's disease—Associated with peripheral arthritis, ankylosing spondylitis, and erythema nodosum.

DeQuervain's tenosynovitis—Involves extensor pollicis brevis and abductor pollicis longus.

Dermatomyositis—Swelling, pain, and shiny skin of fingers. Associated with dysphagia and telangiectasia.

Disseminated gonorrhea—Young patient, women>men, with single joint arthralgia, pustular rash, and fever.

Drugs causing lupus—Procainamide, hydralazine, methyldopa, and chlorpromazine.

Felty's syndrome—Triad of rheumatoid arthritis, neutropenia, and splenomegaly.

Finkelstein's test—DeQuervain's disease. Making fist over folded thumb causes pain means positive test.

Gout—Negative birefringent. "Punched out" erosions of bone. *Treatment: Colchicine acutely and allopurinol to prevent attacks.*

Hemolytic-uremic syndrome (HUS)—Abdominal pain, arthritis, hematuria, and palpable purpura.

Herniated disc—Positive straight leg test. Minimal tenderness on back. *Treatment: Activity as tolerated.*

Iliotibial band syndrome—High mileage runners. Thickened strip of fascia lata.

Junior rheumatoid arthritis (JRA)—30% are monoarticular. Knee most common joint involved.

Multiple myeloma—Slowly progressive back pain in the elderly, hypercalcemia, anemia, and acute renal insufficiency. Lytic lesions on plain films of skull and pelvis.

Osteoarthritis—Knee with effusion. Joint fluid: decreased WBCs, normal glucose, and normal mucin clot. Earliest imaging findings in bone scan.

Plural fluid:
- Rheumatoid arthritis—Glucose is decreased.
- SLE—Pleural fluid glucose is equal to serum fluid glucose.

Precordial catch syndrome—Short sharp anterior chest pain resolves with shallow respiration and rest.

Pseudogout—Positive birefringent. *Treatment: Do not use colchicine; use NSAIDS.*

Reflex sympathetic dystrophy—Pain syndrome following orthopedic surgeries or soft-tissue injuries. Distal end of affected extremity has burning pain, edema, and temperature, color, and hair growth change.

Reiter's syndrome triad—Nongonococcal (chlamydial) urethritis, conjunctivitis, and poly-asymmetrical arthritis. Associated with HLA-B27.

Rheumatic fever—Jones' criteria—Two major or one major and two minor.
- Major—Arthritis, carditis, chorea, erythema marginatum, or subcutaneous nodules.
- Minor—Fever, arthralgias, history of rheumatic heart disease, elevated erthryocyte sedimentation rate (ESR), elevated C-reactive protein (CRP), elevated antistreptolysin *O* (ASO), or increased PR interval.

Rheumatoid arthritis—Knee effusion. Joint fluid: Elevated WBCs, decreased glucose, and abnormal mucin clot test. Swan neck and boutonniere deformity.

Sarcoidosis—Lupus pernio skin findings. Hypercalcemia.

Scleroderma—Raynaud's pnenomenon with skin lesions and visceral involvement.

Septic arthritis:
- Infant—E. coli
- Children—Haemophilus influenza
- Adults—*Staphylococcus aureus*
- Sickle cell disease—*Salmonella*

Shigella—Organism isolated from stool in Reiter's syndrome.

Shoulder pain evaluation:
- Adhesive capsulitis—Decreased range of shoulder motion.
- Bicipital tendinitis—Tenderness when supinating or pronating the hand against resistance.
- Rotator cuff tear—Unable to hold arm up at 90° of abduction.
- Supraspinatus tendinitis (Impingement syndrome)—Audible click on passive abduction to 60° as the swollen tendon is caught under the acromion.

Sudeck's atrophy—Posttraumatic osteoporosis. Same as reflex sympathetic dystrophy.

Systemic lupus erythematosus (SLE)—Triad: fever, joint pain, and malar rash in child-bearing age woman. Hitchhiker's thumb.

Temporal arteritis—Headache, fatigue, fever, anemia, and elevated ESR. Treat with steroids.

Thoracic outlet syndrome—Positive elevated arm stress test (EAST). Patient brings hands up above head. With elbows slightly back, the patient then opens and closes the hands for 3 minutes. Any numbness, weakness, or heaviness indicate positive signs.

Tietze's syndrome—Pain and swelling usually of a single costochondral junction.

▶ TOXICOLOGY (Table 3-17)

Table 3-17: Antidotes

Drugs	Antidotes
Acetaminophen	NAC
Anticholinergic	Physostigmine
Arsenic/mercury/gold	Chelation with dimercaprol
Benzodiazepine	Flumazenil
β-Blocker	Glucagon
Calcium-channel blocker	Calcium, glucagon
CO	High-flow O_2, hyperbaric
Cholinergic	Atropine, pralidoxime
Cyanide	Amyl nitrite pearl → sodium nitrite → sodium thiosulfate
Digoxin	Fab fragments
Ethylene glycol	Ethanol, fomepizole, calcium, dialysis
INH	Pyridoxine (vitamin B_6)
Iron	Deferoxamine
Lead	Calcium disodium edentate
Methanol	Ethanol, fomepizole, folate, dialysis
Nitrites	Methylene blue
Opiates	Naloxone
Organophosphates	2-Pam, atropine

INH, isoniazide; NAC, N-acetylcysteine.

Acetaminophen toxicity—Children less vulnerable. Uses sulfate pathway (adults: glucuronide). Rumack-Mathew nomogram for acute and single ingestions. Plot at 4 hours post ingestion. *Treatment: N-Acetylcysteine (NAC) 140 mg/kg loading dose, then 70 mg/kg for a total of 17 doses.*

Activated charcoal—Dose 1 g/kg. sorbitol with the first dose.

Amanita muscaria—Not muscarinic. *Treatment: Supportive care. Atropine worsens.*

Amanita mushroom (cyclopeptide)—Heat stable; 90% death from mushroom poisoning.

Amphetamine toxicity—Agitation, restlessness, psychosis, seizure, coma, tachycardia, hypertension, and myocardial infarction (MI).

Arsenic—Causes acute hemolytic anemia. *Treatment: Dimercaprol, British Anti-lewisite (BAL).*

Arsine—Binds to sulfhydryl group of hemoglobin resulting in hemolysis.

Asphyxiant:
- Chemical—Binds chemically. Agents: carbon monoxide (CO), hydrogen sulfide (HS), arsine, and carbon disulfide.
- Simple—Displaces O_2. Agents: carbon dioxide (CO_2), methane, helium, nitrogen, and nitrogen oxide (NO).

Benzodiazepine overdose—CNS depression.

β-Blocker overdose—*Treatment: Atropine, β-agonist, and glucagon.*

Botulism—Same signs and symptoms as diphtheria (both ptosis, weakness, and cholinergic), but diphtheria has cardiac symptoms and a febrile course.

Breath odor:
- Bitter almond or silver polish—Cyanide
- Fruity—DKA and isopropanol
- Garlic—Organophosphate
- Rubbing alcohol—Isopropyl

Cadmium toxicity—Severe respiratory distress. Chest x-ray: noncardiogenic pulmonary edema.

Camphor poisoning—CNS excitation (seizure) with emesis, restlessness, confusion, and delirium.

Carbamate toxicity (Sevin)—*Treatment: Atropine. Not pralidoxime (2-PAM), it will worsen.*

Carbon Monoxide (CO) poisoning—Chemical asphyxiant. Hgb binds to CO greater than O_2. Headache symptoms relating to ischemia. Flame-shaped retinal hemorrhages and erythematous patches and bullae on skin. Head CT shows bilateral lesions of globus pallidus. Presentation: Early winter headache, dizziness, weakness, nausea, and normal examination. Multiple family members with same symptoms or personality changes.

Caustic ingestion—Lye. Liquefaction necrosis. Depends on nature, volume, concentration, time, and gastrointestinal content.

Cholinergic:
- Muscarinic—MUDPILES: **M**ethanol, **U**remia, **D**KA, **P**araldehyde, **I**ron/INH, **L**actic acid, **E**thanol, **S**alicylates. or DUMBELLS: **D**iaphoresis, **U**rination, **M**iosis, **B**radycardia, **E**mesis, **L**acrimation, **L**ethargy, and **S**alivation.
- Nicotinic—Hypertension, tachycardia, muscle fasciculation, and weakness.

CHAMP—Need GI decontamination. Camphor, Halogenated, Aromatic, Metals, and Pesticide.

Chinese restaurant syndrome (MSG)—Numbness and tightness of neck with headache.

CHIPS—Radiopaque: Chloral hydrate, Heavy metal, Iodide, Iron, Psychotropics, Phenothiazine, and Sustained-release potassium.

Cocaethylene—Combination of cocaine and alcohol. More toxic combined.

Cocaine toxicity—Give benzodiazepine. β-Blocker contraindicated (unopposed α effects).

Cyanide—Deep coma, bradycardia, and acidosis. NO cyanosis or hypoxia on ABGs. Binds to mitochondrial cytochrome oxidase and interferes with cell O_2 use and ATP production.
- Adults—300 mg 3% Na nitrate IV. Then 12.5 gm Na thiosulfate IV.
- Children—0.23 mL/kg 10% Na nitrate IV. Then 1.65 mL/kg Na thiosulfate IV.

Cyanosis:
- When methemoglobin >15%.
- When sulfhemoglobin >5%.

Cyproheptadine—Antiserotonin agent.

Darvon (propoxyphene hydrochloride)—Needs higher dose of Narcan. Death can be within 15 minutes.

Deferoxamine—Combined with iron and forms ferrioxamine. Water soluble. Urine turns pink. Indications: serum iron > total iron-binding capacity (TIBC), iron >350 μg/dL, or if significant ingestion suspected.

Digibind—Each vial binds 0.5 mg digoxin. *Treatment: Give 10 vials in life threatening toxicity.*

Digoxin toxicity:
- Classic—Sustained atrial tachycardia with artrioventricular (AV) block.
- Most common is PVC. Pathognomonic atrial tachycardia and AV block. Rare bi-directional block.
- Acute—Associated with hyperkalemia.
- Chronic—Normo- to hypokalemia.

Digoxin toxicity and hyperkalemia—*Treatment: Do not give calcium (give Fab, lidocaine, or dilantin). Avoid cardioversion, bretylium, procainamide, or inderal.*

Diphenoxylate (lomotil and atropine) ingestion—*Treatment: Naloxone. admit for 24 hours.* As little as 7.5 mg can be a fatal ingestion.

Disulfiram-ethanol reaction—Within 15 minutes of ethanol ingestion. Nausea, vomiting, and flushing. *Treatment: IVF and antiemetic.*

Doriden (glutethimide)—Combination of glutethimide and codeine. Heroin substitute.

Drug intoxication (alcohol, phencyclidine [PCP], and cocaine)— Agitation, confusion, hypertension, and tachycardia.

DUMBELLS—**D**iaphoresis, **U**rination, **M**iosis, **B**radycardia, **E**mesis, **L**acrimation, **L**ethargy, and **S**alivation. Seen in organophosphate, carbamate, and pesticide poisoning.

Ethanol—Zero order kinetics = 20 mg/dL/hour. 2 proof = 1% ethanol.

Ethanol and tylenol:
- Acute alcohol intake—Prognosis good. Alcohol decreases tylenol toxicity by competitive inhibition.
- Chronic alcohol intake—Prognosis bad. Through induction of P_{450}.

Ethylene glycol—Antifreeze. Urine may fluoresce under Wood's lamp. Calcium oxalate crystals in urine. *Treatment: Give 10% ethanol 0.8 mg/kg IV. Maintain blood ethanol 100 to 150 mg/L.*

Gamma-hydroxybutyric acid (GHB)—No response to naloxone. In deep coma but wakes up suddenly violent. Often intubated before awakening suddenly and extubating self. When clinical presentation suggests this toxin, intubate the patient but restrain as well.

Gasoline ingestion—If less than one mouthful, spits out, and asymptomatic, then discharge home.

Globus pallidus (bilateral lesions) edema and necrosis—Carbon monoxide (CO) poisoning.

Glutethimide (doriden)—Dilated pupils and coma. Sedative drug with atropine-like effects.

Hemodialysis—Treatment for SALT: **S**alicylates, **A**lcohols, **L**ithium, and **T**heophylline toxicity.

Heroin or clonidine overdose—Fixed miosis and hypoventilation.

Hydrofluoric (HF) acid—Tissue damage similar to strong alkali. *Treatment: Irrigate with calcium gluconate given topically, subcutaneous, and intraartery guided by pain relief.*

Hydrogen sulfide (HS)—Disrupts cytochrome P_{450}, preventing ATP formation.

Hyperbaric chamber treatment for CO—For pregnant, young, or if carboxyhemoglobin >25%.

Hypocalcemia—Caused by strychnine poisoning and tetanus toxin.
Ingestion of plants—Least lethal but most common poisoning.
Ingestion of strong acids (sulfuric acid)—Do gastric aspiration.
Lavage with milk may benefit.
Iron poisoning—Blood level > 350 µg/dL; four stages:
- Stage I—0 to 6 hours. Nausea, hematemesis, abdominal pain, lethargy, and bloody diarrhea leading to shock.
- Stage II—6 to 48 hours. Quiet stage.
- Stage III—12 to 48 hours. Shock.
- Stage IV—2 to 6 weeks. Gastric outlet obstruction.
- Iron poisoning—Treatment:
  - Symptomatic > 20 mg/kg, serious > 40 mg/kg.
  - Asymptomatic 6 hours after ingestion—*No treatment.*
  - 20 mg/kg—*Gastric decontamination, no ipecac.*
  - See pills in abdomen—*GoLYTELY until clean stools.*
  - Minimum GI symptoms—*Observe 3 to 6 hours. if iron level <350 µg/dL, discharge.*
  - Anion gap—Best indication of clinical severity.
- Deferoxamine—Urine changes to "vin-rose" color. Indications:
  - Moderate/severe symptoms regardless of iron level.
  - Patients with iron level > TIBC.
  - Patients with iron level > 350 µg/dL.
  - *Continue treatment until iron levels are normal, and the patient is symptom free.* Side effect may be hypotension
    - Dosing:
      Shock: 15 mg/kg/hr IV deferoxamine (daily maximum 6 g).
      No shock: 90 mg/kg IM (maximum 1 g).

Isoniazid (INH)—Status seizures refractory to anticonvulsant therapy.
Treatment: Pyridoxine (vitamin B_6) in equal dose. Often the overdose magnitude is unknown, and must give B_6 until seizures stop; may require entire supply of hospital pharmacy.
Isopropyl alcohol—Fruity odor. Ketosis (acetone) but no ketoacidosis.
Normal anion gap, mild acidosis and osmolar gap. Not in
MUDPILES. Causes hemorrhagic gastritis. Not every hospital
laboratory checks for isopropanol with routine alcohol level request.
Check with your laboratory if needed to order separately.
"Lead lines"—Blue-gray gingival line.
Lead poisoning—Basophilic stippling metaphyseal density.
- Acute—Focal weakness of finger and wrist extensors but rarely legs.
  - Conscious—Dimercaptosuccinic acid (DMSA) *10 mg/kg t.i.d.*

> —Unconscious—British Anti-lewisite (*BAL*) *4mg/kg every*
> *4 hours plus ethylenediamine tetraacetic acid (EDTA) 4 hours*
> *followed by 75 mg/kg IV over 24 hours.*

- Chronic—Lethargy, headache, abdominal pain, constiptation, and anemia.

Leucovorin (folic-acid derivative)—Enhance formic acid in methanol toxicity.

Lidocaine toxicity—Affects liver. Agitation, confusion, restlessness, muscle twitch, seizures, and respiratory depression.

Lindane (Kwell)—Can cause central nervous system (CNS) toxicity. Seizures in children. Not used in young or pregnant patient.

Low viscosity hydrocarbon—High mortality rate. Viscosities <60 Saybolt Seconds Universal (SSU) at greater risk.

Mercury—*Treat like lead poisoning.*

Metal fume fever—Flu-like symptoms. Hypersensitivity reactions to zinc oxide from welding.

Methanol—*Treat like ethylene glycol.*

Methemoglobinemia—"Blue skin," mild headache, cyanosis, and chocolate-brown blood. No change in cyanosis with 100% O_2. With a methemoglobin concentration >45% see seizure, coma, or death. Normal PO_2, normal calculated O_2 saturation, low measured O_2 saturation. *Treatment: Methylene blue: >30% methemoglobin level, angina, or hypotension.*

Methylene dioxymethamphetamine (MDMA)—Love pill or "ecstasy." Increases sexual enhancement.

Monamine oxidase inhibitor (MAOI) overdose—Delayed symptoms, seizure, coma, cardiovascular instability, hyperthermia, and respiratory distress.

N-Acetylcysteine (NAC)—*Treatment: 140 mg/kg followed by 70 mg/kg every 4 hours × 17 doses for acetaminophen toxicity.*

Nitrite—*Treatment: Methylene blue 1 to 2 mg IV of 1% solution over 5 minutes.*

Nomograms:
- Acetyl salicylic acid (ASA)—6 hour level.
- Acetaminophen (tylenol)—4 hour level.

Oil of wintergreen—Extremely toxic form of salicylate. 1 mL = 1.4 g ASA.

Opioid withdrawal—Yawning, lacrimation, nausea, vomiting, diarrhea, piloerection, tachycardia, and hypertension. No seizure.

Organophosphate—SLUDGE (**S**alivation, **L**acrimation, **U**rinary incontinence, **D**iarrhea, **GI** distress, and **E**mesis). Farmer or kid in garage with confusion, diaphoresis, drooling, pinpoint pupils, coma, muscle fasciculations, garlic breath, and bradycardia. Same as DUMBELLS. **D**iaphoresis, **U**rination, **M**iosis, **B**radycardia, **E**mesis, **L**acrimation, **L**ethargy, and **S**alivation. *Treatment: High-dose atropine* *until symptoms of dry mouth and flushing occur.* Muscarinic: miosis, bradycardia, and hypersecretion. Nicotinic: muscle weakness and tachycardia.

Paraquat poisoning—Only condition that worsens with O_2. *Treatment: Need lung transplantation.*

Phencyclidine (PCP)—See rotary nystagmus. Management not dependent on quantitative laboratory analysis.

Phenothiazine—In children can mimic meningitis, but no fever and child is alert. *Treatment: Benadryl and cogentin.*

Physostigmine—Contraindicated in tricyclics poisoning (may cause asystole).

Positive Phenistix test—Salicylate present.

Puffer fish (tetrodotoxin)—State of "suspended animation" simulating death. Heat stable. Muscular paralysis and flaccidity like botulism.

Pyridoxine (vitamin B₆)—*Use for isoniazid (INH) toxicity seizures.*

Red phosphorus—Not absorbed.

Salicylate—Hypokalemia, hypoglycemia or hyperglycemia, mixed respiratory alkalosis and metabolic acidosis, elevated triiodothyronine (T_3) or thyroxine (T_4), hyperthermia, tachycardia, altered mental status (AMS), and Kussmaul's breathing. Chest x-ray showing noncardiogenic pulmonary edema. *Treatment: Na HCO_3. Dialysis if level >100 mg/dL in acute ingestion, acidosis not improved, or patient worsens. Hypokalemia common and severe.*

Salicylate (chronic)—Unexplained CNS dysfunction and positive urine ferric chloride test (urine purple).

Salicylate in children—Hyperventilation, diaphoresis, and behavior change.

Seizure—Suspect lithium, wellbutrin, cyanide, and isoniazid (INH).

Serotonin syndrome—SSRI (selective serotonin reuptake inhibitor) drugs.

Simple asphyxiant gases—Displaces O_2. CO_2, methane, helium, nitrogen, and NO_2.

Strychnine poisoning—Symptoms similar to tetanus (tetanus affects presynaptic glycine receptors). Strychnine inhibits post-synaptic glycine receptors. May cause seizure.

Theophylline poisoning—Hyperglycemia, hypokalemia, and respiratory alkalosis.

Tricyclic antidepressant (TCA) overdose—3 C's: convulsion, coma, and cardiovascular collapse. Patient is unresponsive, with generalized seizures, hypotensive, and wide-complex tachycardia. *Treatment: No procainamide (widens QRS more). Use lidocaine, phenytoin, and NaHCO₃.*

Toxidromes:

- Anticholinergics—"Hot as hare, dry as bone, red as a beet, and mad as a hatter." Atropine effect. Jimsonweed.

- Cholinergics—SLUDGE or DUMBELLS. **S**alivation, **L**acrimation, **U**rinary incontinence, **D**iarrhea, **G**I distress, and **E**mesis; or **D**iaphoresis, **U**rination, **M**iosis, **B**radycardia, **E**mesis, **L**acrimation, **L**ethargy, and **S**alivation. Insecticides.
- Hypoglycemia—AMS, diaphoresis, tachycardia, and bizarre behavior.
- Opioids—Everything depressed and small. Depressed CNS, constricted pupils, bradycardia, and decreased respiratory rate. Heroin.
- Salicylates—Altered mental state (AMS), hyperventilation, hyperthermia, tachycardia, diaphoresis, tinnitus, anion gap, and metabolic acidosis. ASA, oil of wintergreen.
- Serotonin—AMS, increased muscle tone, hyperreflexia, hyperthermia, and "wet dog shakes". SSRIs + TCAs.
- Sympathomimetics—Excited. Tachycardia, hyperthermia, and hypertension. Cocaine or amphetamines.

Urine alkalinization—Promotes excretion of weak acid by ion trapping in renal tubules. *Treatment: IV NaHCO₃. Keep serum pH <7.55, urine pH >7.5 to 8.*

Vin rose wine—Iron toxicity.

Water hemlock—Seizure from neurotoxin cicutoxin.

▶ TRAUMA

▶ ABC

Belted MVC with abdominal pain, 99% on nonrebreather, hypotensive after 3 liters fluid bolus—*Treatment: Type specific packed red blood cells (PRBCs),foley, NG tube, then diagnostic peritoneal lavage (DPL), if CT not immediately available. May also utilize Focused Assessment with Sonography for Trauma (FAST) examination.*

Diagnostic peritoneal lavage (DPL)—For liver, spleen, stomach, and gallbladder injuries (not pancreas—retroperitoneal).

Emergent thoracotomy:
- Penetrating trauma patient who arrests during transport or in ED—Best chance.
- Not indicated—Blunt trauma with no signs of life before arrival at the hospital.
- Dismal prognosis—Blunt trauma who arrest in ED, and penetrating trauma with no signs of life.

Eyebrow wound—Do not shave before repair; need landmarks to approximate eyebrow accurately.

FAST examination shows free fluid and patient hemodynamically unstable— *Treatment: Patient goes to OR for laparotomy.* FAST examination has mostly replaced DPL. May initially be negative so perform serial studies along with serial reevaluation of abdomen. Useful to detect pericardial tamponade. Does not give any information about what are the injuries, or where. Not useful for retroperitoneal injuries.

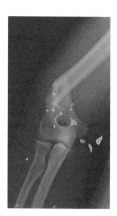

Gunshot wound (GSW) to extremity— Extremity pale, cool, no pulse palpable, and expanding hematoma. *Treatment: Emergent vascular surgery consult.* (Figure 3-71)

Figure 3-71: GSW to distal humerus

Hemorrhage classification:
- Class I—Up to 15% blood volume loss.
- Class II—15% to 30% blood volume loss. Tachycardia and increased diastolic BP.
- Class III—30% to 40% blood volume loss. Hypotension and decreased capillary refill.
- Class IV—>40% blood volume loss.

Jumping out of four-story building and landing on feet—*Treatment: Need cervical spine x-ray, chest x-ray, and x-ray of thoracolumbar spine and pelvis as well as calcaneal views once patient is stable.*

Left phrenic nerve—Most likely to be damaged during ED thoracotomy.

Tetanus—Can be given days to weeks after injury. Give toxoid and immunoglobulin, at different sites.

Trauma captain—Delegates duties.

Trauma patient hypotensive, low O₂ saturation, lungs clear, and jaw swollen and deformed—*Treatment: Do rapid-sequence intubation (RSI).*

▶ *HEAD*

Basilar skull fracture—Battle's sign (retroauricular ecchymoses), cerebro-spinal fluid (CSF) rhinorrhea, hemotympanum, and Raccoon eyes (periorbital ecchymoses).

Central cord syndrome—Upper extremity weaker>lower extremity. Patchy sensory deficit and decreased sphincter tone.

Contusion—In CT scan see small hemorrhagic foci (white areas).

CT head—Indicated for lacerations that might cover a depressed skull fracture.

Cushing's reflex—Hypertension, bradycardia, and respiratory irregularity (seen only one-third of time).

Epidural hematoma—Lucid interval seen only 30% of the time. Frequently associated with skull fracture. Lenticular shape affecting middle meningeal artery. Does not cross sutures.

Glasgow coma scale (GCS) scoring—A dead person will score 3.

- I—*Eye opening*:
    - — Spontaneous: 4
    - — To verbal: 3
    - — To pain: 2
    - — No response: 1
- II—*Verbal*:
    - — Oriented: 5
    - — Disoriented: 4
    - — Inappropriate words: 3
    - — Incomprehensible sounds: 2
    - — No response: 1
- III—*Motor*:
    - — Obeys commands: 6
    - — Localizes pain: 5
    - — Flexion/withdrawal: 4
    - — Decorticate: 3
    - — Decerebrate: 2
    - — None: 1

Halo or double-ring sign—CSF rhinorrhea.

Neurogenic shock—Hypotension and bradycardia.

Seizure prophylaxis—For intubated and paralyzed head injured patients.

Subarachnoid hematoma—Preceded by sentinel bleed. "Zipper sign": see blood in sulci and gyri. Sudden onset of severe headache with nausea and vomiting from meningeal irritation. Blood within CSF due to tears of subarachnoid vessels. Suspect ruptured saccular aneurysm. *CT then LP if the CT is negative.* (Figure 3-72)

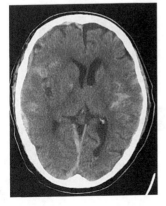

Figure 3-72: Subarachnoid bleed and small right subdural bleed

Subdural hematoma—See blood in falx cerebri. Crescent shape.
- Acute (24 hours), subacute (1 day to 2 weeks), and chronic (>2 weeks) to become symptomatic.
- Elderly or alcoholics due to longer bridging veins.
- Patient presents with right-sided pupillary dilation and left hemiplegia: Right subdural hematoma. (Figures 3-73–3-74)

Traumatic brain injury—See Table 3-18.

▶ *FACE*

Admission—For zygomatic, tripod, or posterior sinus wall fracture.
Angle—Most common fracture area of mandible. Ramus is least.
Ellis classification—Tooth fractures:
- Type I—Enamel.
- Type II—Enamel with exposed dentin.
- Type III—Pulp exposed.

Facial wounds—*May delay repair up to 24 hours after injury.*
Facial x-rays:
- Jug-handle or submental vertex view—For zygomatic arch.
- PA or Caldwell view—For upper facial bone.
- Townes view—For mandibular rami and basilar skull fracture.
- Water's view (occipital-mental view)—For mid-face.

Le Fort—Levels of Le Fort fractures are often mixed between sides of the face.
- Type I—Fracture alveolar ridge below nose; mobility of upper teeth and hard palate.

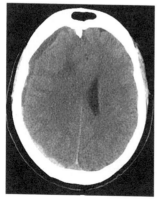

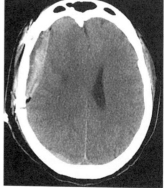

Figure 3-73: Right chronic subdural bleed

Figure 3-74: Acute and chronic right subdural bleed following craniotomy

Table 3-18: Traumatic Brain Injury

Symptoms	GCS	Mortality rate	Incidence
Mild	>13	—	70% to 80%
Moderate	9–13	20%	10%
Severe:	<9	40%	10%

GCS, Glasgow coma scale.

- Type II—Pyramidal area; maxilla, nasal bones, and medial orbits. Mid-face mobility and dish face.
- Type III—Fracture through zygomaticofacial sutures; complete craniofacial dislocation.

Lid laceration—*Do not repair if lid tissue loss, margin violated, or lacrimal gland damage. Refer to ophthalmology.*

Mandibular dislocation—Unilateral mandibular dislocation displaces jaw to contralateral side.

Mandibular fracture—Check for malocclusion.
- Alveolar fracture—Angulated but not avulsed teeth.
- Condylar fracture—Lateral crossbite.
- Injury to mental nerve—Anesthesia of the lower lip.
- Symphysis and body fracture—Malocclusion.

Orbital blowout fracture—Enophthalmos, inability to gaze up, and double vision. *Treatment: Repair in 10 to 14 days.*

Orbital emphysema—If decreased vision, do lateral canthotomy or intraorbital needle aspiration (air).

Saddle deformity of the nose—Complication of nasal fracture with septal necrosis following an undrained septal hematoma. Also seen in congenital syphilis.

Septal hematoma—Grape-like swelling at septum. *Treatment: Incision and drainage, and anterior packing.* Complication: avascular necrosis of septum.

Stenson's (parotid) duct injury—Bloody discharge while milking the gland implies injury. *Treatment: Refer for repair.*

Sublingual or buccal ecchymosis—Pathognomonic for mandibular fracture.

Zygomatic fractures:
- Tripod fracture—Depression of the malar eminence. Frontozygomatic suture, zygomaticotemporal suture, and through the infraorbital foramen. *Get Water's view*
- Zygomatic arch fracture—*Need submental vertex (jug-handle view).*

▶ NECK

Blind clamping of vessels—*Do not.*

Carotid artery thrombosis—Unilateral limb paresis or Horner's syndrome following trauma to the side of the head or face from stretching of the carotid artery against the vertebral bodies.

Endotracheal tube (ETT) balloon appears round on chest x-ray— Suspect tracheobronchial injury.

Esophageal injuries—Combination of contrast swallow and endoscopy: 100% sensitivity.

Flexion and extension view—Most effective in detecting ligamentous instability of C-spine.

Laryngeal fracture—Triad: hoarseness, subcutaneous emphysema, and palpable crepitus. *Treatment: Tacheostomy (enter lower than usual 4th or 5th tracheal ring) if unable to do orotracheal. Cricothyrotomy contraindicated.* Lateral c-spine x-ray shows prevertebral air.

Machinery-like murmur—Air embolism. Tachypnea, tachycardia, and hypotension. *Treatment: Direct pressure, Trendelenburg, and aspirate right ventricle.*

Neck injury—*Treatment: No IV ipsilateral side. If active arterial bleeding or bubbling in wound, patient goes to OR.*

Neck stab with airway intact, brisk bleeding—*Treatment: Apply external pressure first, not intubation.*

Neck stab with bleeding into oropharynx—*Treatment: Intubate and pack oropharynx prior to transfer.*

Neck stab wound with hematoma, distorted airway, and no stridor—Rapid-sequence intubation (RSI).

Neck zones of injury:

- Zone 1—Sternal notch to cricoid cartilage. Most lethal. *Treatment: Angiography, esophagogram, or esophagoscopy. Laryngoscopy or bronchoscopy if symptomatic.*
- Zone II—Cricoid to angle of mandible. *Treatment: Angiography, esophagogram, or esophagoscopy. Laryngoscopy or bronchoscopy if symptomatic, mandatory exploration in OR.*
- Zone III—Base of mandible to base of occiput. *Treatment: Angiography.*

Pulseless trauma pulseless electrical activity (PEA)—Suspect air embolism. *Treatment: Cross clamp aorta and aspirate from right ventricle.*

Stellate ganglion injury—Ipsilateral ptosis upper eyelid, elevation lower lid, facial anhydrosis, and miosis as in Horner's syndrome. Seen following penetrating injury to neck.

Zones I and III—*Treatment: Angiogram to rule out aerodigestive injuries. Nonsurgical management.*

Zone II—Easy to obtain proximal and distal control. *Treatment: Surgical exploration for platysma violation.*

▶ *SPINE*

Bilateral facet dislocation (BFD)—Unstable with neurologic deficit. Hyperflexion without rotation. Upper vertebrae pass over causing displacement more than one-half of diameter. Involves anterior longitudinal ligament.

Bulbocavernosus reflux—When present indicates absence of spinal shock. Pulling on the Foley causes rectal sphincter contraction.

Burning hands—Football player with painful dysesthesia (burning and tingling). Injury to C_6–C_7.

Burst fracture—From flexion. Distraction injury through lumbar spine body and pedicle. Stable.

Chance fracture—Lap belt injury in MVC. Unstable fracture. Vertebral burst injury almost always produces spinal cord permanent injury.

Clay shoveler's fracture—Spinous process injury cervical spine. Stable.

Complete cord lesion with sacral sparing—Same as central cord lesion.

Cord syndromes:
- Anterior cord syndrome—Motor paralysis and loss of pain and sensation distal to lesion.
- Brown-Sequard—Ipsilateral paralysis and loss of vibration and proprioception with contralateral loss of pain and temperature sensation. Hemisection.
- Central cord syndrome—Upper extremity weakness >> Lower extremity weakness. Hands weaker than proximal muscles. Quadriplegic with sacral sparing. Associated with arthritis and hyperextension. Ligamentum flavum encroaches into cord causing contusion of central cord.

C-Spine x-ray—See Table 3-19.

Diaphragmatic or abdominal breathing and absence of thoracic breathing—Lower cervical injury below C_5.

Fracture mechanisms of C-spine (Figure 3-75):
- Axial loading—Jefferson's and burst fracture.
- Extension—Hangman's of C_2, extension teardrop, and posterior arch of C_1 fracture.

Table 3-19: Cervical-Spine x-ray

X-ray	Sensitivity
Lateral	80%
Lateral and odontoid	90%
Lateral, odontoid, and anterior posterior	95%
All three views plus oblique	97%

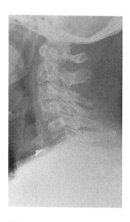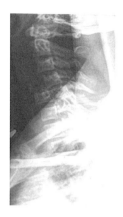

Figure 3-75: Fracture dislocation at C_5–C_6 seen in Swimmer's View on right

- Flexion—Anterior subluxation, bilateral facet dislocation (BFD), simple wedge, clay-shoveler's, and flexion tear drop.
- Flexion-rotation—Unilateral facet dislocation (UFD).

Hangman's fracture—Unstable, bilateral C_2 pedicle fracture, and hyperextension. Spinal cord injury often does not occur because spinal canal widest at this level.

Jefferson's fracture—Unstable but usually no spinal cord injury. Vertical compression. C_1 ring, and lateral mass involved. Widening predental space. Normal predental space: 3 mm in adults and 5 mm in children.

Lumbar spine compression fracture—Associated with fall and ankle or heel fracture. (Figure 3-76)

Neurogenic shock—Acute spinal cord injury disrupts sympathetic outflow. Unopposed vagal nerve causes hypotension and bradycardia.

Odontoid fracture—*All need surgical consultation.* (Figures 3-77–3-78)
- I—Tip. Stable about transverse ligament.
- II—Base. Unstable.
- III—Body of C_2. Unstable.

Orotracheal intubation—Preferred method of intubation in traumatic arrest with spinal cord injury.

Prevertebral soft tissue swelling:
- 6 mm at C_2
- 22 mm at C_6 (14 mm in children)

Sacral sparing—Good prognostic sign in spinal cord injury. Persistent perianal sensation.

Spinal cord injuries—Response will vary by degree of intactness. See Table 3-20.

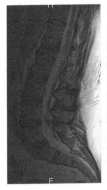
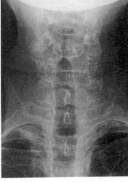
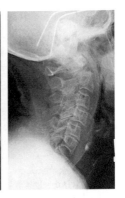

Figure 3-76: MRI—Compression fracture L1

Figure 3-77: Odontoid fracture

Figure 3-78: Type 2 odontoid fracture

Spinal shock—Complete loss of reflexes and paralysis. Neurologic deficits lasts < 24 hours. Warm, pink, and dry skin. Relative bradycardia. Adequate urinary output.

Spondylolisthesis—Slippage of one vertebral body forward on another.

Spondylosis—Defect in pars interarticularis.

Stable c-spine fractures—Burst fracture, clay shoveler's, wedge fracture, and isolated vertebral fracture.

Unilateral facet dislocation (UFD)—Flexion and rotation. < 50% stable and no neurologic deficit.

Unstable c-spine fracture—Jefferson's, Hangman's, bilateral facet dislocation (BFD), flexion teardrop, extension teardrop, and any fractures of C_1 or C_2.

Unstable spinal injury—Two or more column failure.
- Anterior column—Anterior longitudinal ligament + anterior half of vertebral body.
- Middle column—Posterior longitudinal ligament + posterior half of vertebral body.
- Posterior column—Pedicle, lamina, spinous process + posterior ligament complex.

Table 3-20: Spinal cord injuries

MOTOR	SENSORY
C_4 – Spontaneous breathing	Suprasternal notch sensation
C_5 – Shrugging of shoulders	Sensation below clavicle
C_6 – Flexion at the elbow	Thumb sensation
C_7 – Extension at the elbow	Index finger sensation
C_8 – Flexion of the fingers	Little finger sensation

▸ *CHEST*

Aortic aneurysm—Usually hypotension present.
Aortic rupture—Following a fall off ladder, interscapular back pain, and hoarse voice (laryngeal nerve). Transesophageal echocardiogram highly sensitive and specific. *CT highly sensitive.* Esophagus shifted to right.
Aortic transection—Hypertension present 25%.
Aortic transection distal to left subclavian take-off—*Treatment: β-blocker and nitroprusside.*
Aortography—Gold standard. Indicated in patient with mediastinal widening following decelerating trauma with possible aortic injury.
Beck's triad—Distant heart sounds, distended neck veins, and hypotension. Difficult to assess in ED.
Boerhaave's syndrome—Left longitudinal tear at posterolateral site of esophagus.
Bubbling from neck wound—Suspect airway injuries.
Cardiac contusion or concussion—Tachycardia out of proportion.
Cardiac rupture—Trauma with shock out of proportion with injury with poor response to volume and hemorrhage control.
Chest tube thoracostomy—Bilateral pneumothorax, hemothorax associated with small pneumothorax, increasing pneumothorax, and tachypnea and desaturation with pneumothorax.
Child falling on lollipop—Look for blunt internal carotid artery injury.
Chylothorax in right chest tube—Thoracic duct injury.
Diaphragmatic hernia—Epigastric pain worsens lying down following a stab wound of the left lower chest. *Chest x-ray diagnostic test.*
Diaphragmatic tear—Common after auto crash; left side more frequent than right because of the liver. Blunt injury 5 to 15 cm, penetrating injury <2 cm long. DPL need only 5000 RBC to be positive (not the standard 100,000 RBC). Chest tube for tension viscerothorax.
ED thoracotomy—*Treatment: Incise the pericardial sac median to phrenic nerve. Left-sided incision even for right-sided chest trauma. The incision can be extended across the midline and the sternum.*
Electrical alternans—Highly specific sign of chronic pericardial tamponade (rare in acute).
Elevated CVP, tachycardia, and hypotension—Most reliable sign of pericardial tamponade.
Fat embolism—Develops acute dyspnea and petechiae over neck after long bone fracture.
First or 2nd rib fracture—See 1st rib fracture in AP c-spine x-ray No mandatory angiography, unless direct evidence of neurovascular trauma.

Flail chest—Paradoxical chest movements. Seen when two or more ribs are broken in two or more places.

Hanging:
- Judicial hanging—Complete hanging with body freely suspended. High cervical fracture and cord transection. Must have drop at least the length of the body to produce the fracture.
- Nonjudicial hanging—Rare in suicide to have sufficient drop to fracture neck. In incomplete hanging some part of the body may still be in contact with the floor. Ligature causes venous congestion and stasis of blood flow resulting in arterial obstruction that leads to coma or death. No need to assess status of cervical spine unless there has been a drop at least the length of the body.

Hole repair (heart):
- Large atrial tear from blunt trauma—Put in Foley with purse string suture.
- Small penetrating wound of ventricles—horizontal mattress suture with pledgets.

Innominate rupture—Esophagus shifted to left.

Intubated patient with potential tension pneumothorax—Increased resistance to ventilate. *Treatment: Immediate needle thoracostomy followed by a chest tube; do not delay for a chest x-ray study.*

Intubation in flail chest—Shock, 3+ associated injuries, history of pulmonary disease, fracture 8+ ribs, >65 years of age , and O_2 saturation <92 %. *Otherwise, nonrebreather mask. If respiratory rate or pCO2 rise, then intubate.*

Laryngotracheal injuries—Tracheostomy at 4th or 5th tracheal ring (not cricothyrotomy or intubation).

Left lateral thoracotomy—Perform in patient with pericardial tamponade who suddenly becomes bradycardic. This is a sign of impending arrest.

Myocardial contusion—Difficult diagnosis to prove in ED. If a sternal fracture is present, or if the patient develops dysrhythmias post blunt chest trauma, a myocardial contusion is undoubtedly present. Most are benign and require only monitored observation.

Neurogenic pulmonary edema—Centrally mediated, massive sympathetic discharge.

Pericardial tamponade—Tachycardia, JVD, and hypotension (most reliable sign: hypotension). *Treatment: In cardiac arrest, do left lateral thoracotomy. Pericardiocentesis in pre-arrest.*

Phenytoin—For treatment of near hanging patients. Ameliorate development of neurogenic pulmonary edema. Used to facilitate catecholamine reuptake by CNS.

Pneumomediastinum—Subcutaneous emphysema over supraclavicular or anterior neck. *Treatment: 100% oxygen to relieve discomfort.*

Pneumothorax—More visible on end-expiration film. (Figure 3-79)

Postobstructive pulmonary edema—Forceful inspiration against extrathoracic obstruction removed causing pulmonary edema. Good prognosis.

Pulmonary contusion—Seen on the initial chest x-ray. *Treatment: Serial ABGs. If PO$_2$ <60% on room air, intubate.*

Pulmonary contusion versus ARDS:
- Pulmonary contusion—localized area on chest x-ray seen within 6 hours but may degenerate into adult respiratory distress syndrome (ARDS).
- ARDS—Diffuse and delayed within 24 to 72 hours.

Pulmonary edema—Absolute contraindication to military antishock trousers (MAST).

Sternal fracture—Seen on lateral chest x-ray. *Treatment: Needs admission. Can discharge if no cardiac, chest x-ray, or EKG abnormality.*

Sucking chest wound—From trauma. *Treatment: Apply occlusive dressing on three sides; leaving one side untaped allows air to escape from forming tension pneumothorax.*

Supraclavicular pain—Think of diaphragmatic irritation.

Tardieu's spots—Asphyxial death. Petechial hemorrhage in conjunctiva, mucous membrane, and skin cephalad to ligature.

Tension pneumomediastinum—*Treatment: Immediate pericardiocentesis with aspiration of air.*

Tension pneumothorax—Tachycardia, jugular venous distention (JVD), and absent breath sounds on affected side. *Treatment: Needle thoracotomy followed by chest tube. May not require intubation after decompression.*

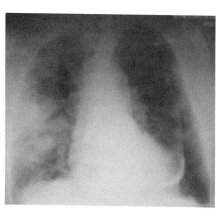

Figure 3-79: Left-sided pneumothorax

Thoracotomy—Indicated for:
- Initial chest tube drainage >20 mL/Kg of blood (or 1,000 ml of blood for adults).
- > 300 to 400 mL per hour for 4 hours, or >1500 mL in 12 to 24 hours (chest tube drainage).
- Patient hypotensive despite transfusion.
- Patient decompensates after initial response to resuscitation.

Tracheobronchial disruption—Continue bubbling after chest tube in place. Hemoptysis, dyspnea, and cyanosis.

Tracheobronchial fistula—*Treatment: Place chest tube. If still bubbling means persistent pneumothorax.*

Traumatic asphyxia—Severe thoracic compression. Deep violet color face and facial edema. Pulmonary injury.

Widened mediastinum—*Treatment: If stable, do angiogram. If unstable, patient goes to OR.*

▶ ESOPHAGUS

Boerhaave's syndrome—Left posterolateral aspect of esophagus. Longitudinal tear with mediastinal soiling causes mediastinitis.

Esophageal injuries—*Treatment: If suspected, do esophagogram using water-soluble contrast. If negative (has high false-negative rate) do barium study. Prophylactic antibiotics. <24 hours—primary closure. >24 hours—continuous drainage of stomach and adjacent mediastinum.*

Esophageal perforation—Cricopharyngeal muscle > aortic arch > gastroesophageal (GE) junction.

Gastrografin—Use for x-ray evaluation of esophageal perforation. Barium complicates mediastinitis.

▶ DIAPHRAGM

Diaphragmatic hernia—Nasogastric tube (NG) useful for diagnosis and therapy. Contrast studies helpful.

Diaphragmatic tear—Blunt trauma defect > penetrating. But penetrating (knives most common) more common > blunt.

DPL in diaphragmatic tear—Positive with 5000 RBCs (not 100,000). *Exploration indicated.*

Tension viscerothorax (from diaphragmatic tear)—*Treatment: Chest tube as in for tension pneumothorax but NO TROCAR.*

▶ ABDOMEN

Abdomen gunshot wound (GSW)—*Treatment: Laparotomy in > 90% required with penetration into peritoneal cavity.*

Anterior abdominal wall stab wound:
- One-third—Do not penetrate peritoneum.
- One-third—Penetrate peritoneum but do not require laparotomy.
- One-third—Require laparotomy.

Base deficit >−6 mEq/L—Look for intraabdominal injury.

Chest x-ray with shifting of gastric bubble to right—Expanding splenic hematoma.

DPL—Highly accurate for intra-abdominal trauma, poor for retroperitoneal trauma.
- DPL is positive—Lower chest stab wound; RBCs >5000.
- GSW to abdomen: RBCs >5000.
- Penetrating flank/abdominal trauma: RBCs >10,000–20,000.
- Blunt abdominal trauma: RBCs >100,000.

ED thoracotomy—Survival for penetrating>blunt. Thoracic>abdominal trauma.

Evisceration of bowel—Contraindications to DPL. *Treatment: Patient goes to OR.*

False positive DPL—Abdominal wall hematoma, inadequate hemostasis, and pelvic fracture.

Fluid in Morrison's pouch—*Treatment: Patient goes to OR.*

Free air—Rupture of hollow viscous. *Treatment: Patient goes to OR.*

Handlebar injury—Associated with traumatic pancreatitis. *Treatment: Get CT.*

Indications for celiotomy—If unstable, acute abdomen, evisceration, diaphragmatic injury, GI bleeding, and knife sticking out of abdomen. Gunshot wound of abdomen should be explored: 96% will have intraabdominal organ injuries.

Kehr's sign—Shoulder pain with splenic trauma.

Lap belt injury—Ecchymosis, duodenal hematoma, and bowel perforation. Chance fracture may affect spinous process, pedicles, vertebrae, and bladder.

Loss of renal or psoas shadow—Retroperitoneal injury.

Pancreatic injury—Physical examination improves initially then worsens over next 6 hours.

Penetrating trauma to abdomen—*Treatment: Local wound exploration. If anterior rectus fascia is intact, discharge. If entry into the fascia, further work-up required.*

Penetrating and blunt trauma:
- Adults—No correlation between degree of hematuria and injury severity.
- Children—Yes, there is correlation. *Treatment: Get CT of abdomen and pelvis if >50 RBCs in urine.*

Rectal injury—Usually no peritoneal signs.

Retroperitoneal injury—Pain in the testicle implies injury to duodenal or urogenital area.

Serial abdominal examinations—More accurate than serial H/H (hemoglobin/ hematocrit) in an abdominal trauma patient.

Shoulder pain:
- Left—Splenic injury.
- Right—Hepatic injury.

Stab wound exploration—*Treatment: With no violation of fascia, can discharge home.*

Surgical exploration if:
- >5000/uL RBCs in DPL following stab wound to lower chest.
- >5000/uL RBCs in penetrating abdominal wound.
- >100,000/uL RBCs in blunt abdominal trauma.
- GSW to back or flank.

Suspect rectal injury—*Treatment: Do sigmoidoscopy.*

Traumatic hemoperitoneum—Most sensitive: DPL needs 5 mL blood.

Traumatic pancreatitis—Look for in patient previously treated for "handle bar" injury. Patient returns with epigastric pain radiating to back and vomiting.

▸ GENITOURINARY

Adults GSW flank with or without hematuria—Cannot predict upper urinary tract injuries based on hematuria. Location determines injuries.

Children with trauma and hematuria—*Treatment: Complete urologic evaluation.*

Woman with blood at meatus—Urethrography not helpful. *Treatment: If unable to pass Foley, place suprapubic catheter.*

Bladder trauma:
- Bladder contusion—*Treatment: Manage expectantly.*
- Bladder neck, or proximal urethral injury—*Treatment: Primary surgical repair.*
- Bladder rupture:
    - Intraperitoneal or penetrating rupture. *Treatment: Patient goes to OR;* contrast material outlines intraperitoneal structures (bowel loops, liver, spleen).
    - Extraperitoneal rupture—*Foley catheter drainage;* contrast material seen in pubic symphysis and pelvic outlet.
- Retrograde cystogram—Follows exclusion of urethral trauma and presence of Foley.
- Sign of bladder injury—Gross hematuria alone or in conjunction with pelvic fracture.

Penile trauma:
- Penile fracture—Tunical albuginea torn, snapping sound, and slowly progressive penile hematoma. *Treatment: Surgery.*

- Peyronie's disease—Recurring microtrauma. Plaque-like fibrosis of dorsal tunica albuginea. *Treatment: Vitamin E.*
- Severed penis—*Treatment: Reanastomosis up to 6 hours. After that local reshaping.*
- Traumatic lymphangitis—After vigorous or prolonged sex. Palpable cord-like cartilage in subcutaneous tissue. *Treatment: NSAIDs and rest.*

Renal trauma:

- Blunt renal trauma discharge criteria—Adult: microhematuria (3 to 5 RBCs) and no shock. Pediatric: <50 RBCs in urine and no other injuries.
- Blunt renal trauma in adults—At risk if gross hematuria, microhematuria with shock, and history of sudden deceleration. *Treatment: Helical CT with contrast. If patient needs to go to OR, get OR film with intraoperative bolus.*
- Blunt renal trauma in children—Can occur with microhematuria without shock.
- Hematuria and IVP with nonvisualized kidney—*Treatment: Next step renal angiogram.*
- Microscopic hematuria, vitals stable—*Treatment: Does not need a workup, other than for concomitant injuries; safe to follow as outpatient if isolated finding.*
- Penetrating renal trauma—Location determines injury (not hematuria). *Treatment: If positive findings on CT, patient goes to surgery.*
- Renal injury:
    - Class I—Renal contusion. Normal IVP.
    - Class II—Cortical laceration. Extravasation of dye through cortical defect.
    - Class III—Caliceal laceration. Capsule okay. Intrarenal extravasation dye and pelvicaliceal disruption.
    - Class IV—Complete renal tear or fracture. IVP: intra- and extrarenal extravasation of dye.
    - Class V—Injury to the vascular pedicle. Kidney not visualized on IVP. *Treatment: Do angiogram.*
- Renal trauma—Most common of all urologic injuries. Blunt trauma five time more common than penetrating.
- Unilateral testicular pain—Suspect renal colic.

Testes trauma:

- Bilateral testicular pain—Retroperitoneal injuries can cause this, especially duodenum. Refer pain to testicles.
- Right testicular pain after trauma—Look for duodenal injury.
- Testicular trauma—*Treatment: Color Doppler ultrasound.*

Heterogeneous appearance is diagnostic of trauma.
— Contusion—*Treatment: Bed rest, ice pack, and NSAIDs.*
— Dislocation—Swollen, ecchymotic, and absent testis.
Treatment: OR repair for testes laceration or dislocation.

Ureteral trauma—Hematuria, flank pain similar to with renal colic, and flank mass. *Treatment: Contrast helical CT with delayed films or IVP bolus with delayed films. Surgery.*

Urethral trauma—Pelvic fracture, blood at meatus, high-riding or absent prostate with perineal, scrotal, and penile hemorrhage:
- Anterior urethral injuries—Due to straddle injuries, falls, GSW, and self-instrument.
- Complete urethral tear—No contrast seen in bladder.
- Partial urethral tear—See extravasation of contrast outside urethra and bladder filling.
- Posterior urethral injuries—Due to pelvic trauma.
- Retrograde urethrography—Gross blood at meatus: diagnosis of urethral injury. *Treatment: If negative, then Foley.*
- Suspect urethral injury—*Treatment: NO Foley.*
- Urethral injury:
    - Normal retrograde urethrogram—*Treatment: May pass foley, as urethra is intact.*
    - Partial anterior or posterior urethral tear—*Treatment: One attempt with foley for stenting or Coude catheter. If unable to pass foley, place suprapubic catheter.*
    - Complete urethral tear—*Treatment: Urologic consult and suprapubic catheter.*
- Urogenital diaphragm—Separates posterior urethra (membranous and prostate) from anterior urethra.

▶ ORTHOPEDICS (UPPER EXTREMITY)

Bennet's fracture—Thumb carpometacarpal joint.
Children < 15 years of age—Fracture more common than sprains.
Colles'and Smith's fractures—*Treatment: Closed reduction.*
Dislocations:
- Lunate perilunate junction—*Treatment: Emergent consult.*
- Scapholunate junction—*Treatment: Splint and refer.*

Elbow aspiration—Preferred position lateral.
Elbow dislocation—Posterior > anterior. Complication: injury to brachial artery and median nerve.
Extremity wound closure—*Treatment: > 12 hours, use delayed primary closure in 4 days.*
Fingertip avulsion injuries—*Treatment: If wound < 1 cm with no bone exposed, wound can heal itself without need for skin graft.*

Flexor digitorum profundus tendon injury (complete)—"Jersey finger"; *Treatment: Need surgical consult. Repair ~10 days.*

Galeazzi's fracture—Radial shaft fracture with dislocation of radioulnar joint.

Humerus surgical neck fracture—Presents in abduction. *Treatment: Splint in that position. One-part fracture requires sling and swath.*

Lunate dislocation—Piece of pie sign, spilled tea cup on lateral x-ray.

Lunate fracture—Most common serious carpal fracture.

Malgaigne's fracture—Fracture of ileum and a symphyseal dislocation.

Monteggia's—Proximal ulna with dislocation of radial head (usually anterior dislocation).

Nightstick fracture—*Treatment: For isolated ulnar nondisplaced transverse fracture apply splint.*

Nursemaid's—Subluxation of radial head.

Painful grip after playing tennis or golf—Suspect fracture of hook of hamate.

Perilunate dislocation—Lunate is ok, but capitate is dislocated.

Posterior fat pad sign (sail sign)—Abnormal. Fracture of radial head or distal humerus.

Reflex sympathetic dystrophy—Pain, restricted motion, and skin changes after trauma.

Scaphoid fracture—Most common carpal fracture. *Treatment: For nondisplaced fracture, apply thumb spica splint.*

Smith fracture—*Treatment: Closed reduction. If fails, patient needs ORIF.*

Snuff box tenderness—*Treatment: Thumb spica splint and orthopedic referral.*

Subungual hematoma:
- If hematoma covers <50% area beneath the nail—*Treatment: Simple trephination.*
- If hematoma covers >50% area—*Treatment: OK to do simple trephination.*
- If nail avulsion or distal phalanx fracture present—*Treatment: Nail removal, repair nail bed. Suture nail in place for protection and splinting.*

Volkmann's ischemic contracture—Muscle atrophy with disabling flexion contracture of wrist/hand. Complication of supracondylar fracture.

Wrist bone fracture—*Treatment: Apply splint and refer.*

▶ ORTHOPEDICS (LOWER EXTREMITY)

Achilles tendon rupture—Positive Thompson's test. "Weekend warrior." *Treatment: Posterior splint (equinus).*

ACL (anterior cruciate ligament) tear—Audible pop.

Ankle injury:
- Eversion—Transverse fracture of tip of tibia and oblique fracture of distal fibula. (Figure 3-80)
- Inversion—Transverse fracture of tip of fibula, and oblique fracture of distal tibia.

Anterior drawer sign—Checking for injury to anterior cruciate ligament.

Anterior drawer sign in ankle injury—Complete tear of anterior talofibular ligament.

Anterior hip dislocation—Externally rotated and abducted). Opposite of posterior dislocation: (**P**osterior: **I**nternal rotation and **A**dduction).

Anterior tibial compartment syndrome—Associated with tibial fracture. See Figure 3-76.

Avulsion type pelvic fracture:
- Forceful contraction of abdominal muscles—Iliac crest avulsion.
- Forceful contraction of hamstrings—Ischial tuberosity avulsion
- Forceful contraction of rectus femoris—Anterior inferior iliac spine avulsion.
- Forceful contraction of sartorius muscle—Anterior superior iliac crest avulsion

Calcaneal fracture—Associated with lumber fracture or disc prolapse and sometimes with cervical spine injury.

Deep peroneal nerve—Associated with proximal fibular fracture. Foot drop.

Femoral neck fracture—Leg shortened, abducted, and externally rotated (like anterior hip dislocation).

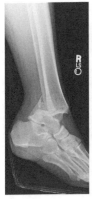
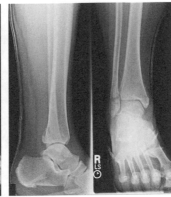

Figure 3-80: Distal tibial and fibular fractures. Pre and post reduction

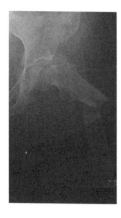

Femur fracture—May lose up to 1 liter blood before seen. (Figure 3-81)

Incomplete fracture—Buckle, Greenstick, and Torus.

Intertrochanteric fracture—Leg shortened and externally rotated.

Malgaigne fracture—Vertical shear fracture involving disruption of anterior and posterior elements of single hemipelvis.

MAST—For unstable comminuted pelvic fracture with hypotension. Not used much anymore since not readily available. Now stabilize with bed sheets, or external fixator.

Myositis ossificans—Painless formation of bone within muscles as a result of injury.

Figure 3-81: Left femur fracture S/P fall

Pelvic fracture, hip dislocation— Contraindications to femoral traction splints.

Pelvic fracture (KANE classification):
- Type I—Pelvic ring intact. Pain.
- Type II—Single break in pelvic ring. Pain.
- Type III—Double break in pelvic ring. Hemorrhage.
- Type IV—Acetabular fracture. Hip dislocation.

Posterior drawer sign—Checking for injury to posterior cruciate ligament.

Posterior hip dislocation—Associate with sciatic nerve injury. **P**osterior: **I**nternal rotation and **Ad**duction.

Thompson's test—Lay patient supine and squeeze calf. Positive test if no plantar flexion. Tests for achilles tendon rupture.

Valgus instability—Medial collateral ligament defect.

Varus instability—Lateral collateral ligament defect.

Vascular surgery—For gun shot wound (GSW) to thigh, with leg pale, cool, no pulse, and expanding hematoma.

▶ PREGNANCY

16 wks ~30 mL fetal blood volume—RhoGAM 300 µg/30 mL. >16 weeks do Kleihauer-Betke (KB) test. KB test is a blood test used to measure amount of fetal hemoglobin transferred to an Rh-negative mother's bloodstream. Mother's blood is taken to make a blood smear. Acid bath removes all maternal hemoglobin and on subsequent staining fetal hemoglobin appears rose-pink.

Abdominal x-ray of traumatic uterine rupture:
- Free intraperitoneal air.
- Extended fetal extremities.
- Abnormal fetal position.

Admission—If more than three contractions per hour, persistent uterine tenderness, vaginal bleeding, and abnormal fetal monitoring strip.

Carbon monoxide in pregnancy—Fetal CO level 10% to 15% > mother's. Elimination $T_{1/2}$ 3.5 × longer. Give 100% FiO_2.

Cardioversion—Safe in pregnancy.

Emergent c-section—If no signs of maternal life, perform a thoracotomy with open cardiac massage and C-section.

Hyperbaric—Not contraindicated in pregnancy.

Minor indirect trauma/pregnancy—Needs 4 hour observation > 20 weeks of gestation.

Rh sensitization—Needs 1 mL of fetal blood mixing for sensitization to occur. At 12 weeks of gestation, the fetus has approximately 4.2 mL of blood volume. *Treatment: 50 μg RhoGAM per 5 mL fetal blood.*

Supine hypotension syndrome—From inferior vena cava (IVC) pressure from uterus.

Tetanus toxoid and immunoglobulin diphtheria—Safe in pregnancy. Tetanus crosses placenta.

▶ ULTRASOUND

20/25—At 20-mm gestational sac, should see yolk sac. At 25-mm gestational sac, should see embryo.

AAA—Diameter > 3 cm, focal dilation, loss of normal distal tapering, and thrombosis present. Immediate surgery in patients with abdominal pain + hemodynamic instability. Elective in > 5.4 cm.

Acute cholecystitis—Wall > 3.5 mm, pericholecystic fluid, air in biliary tree, common bile duct (CBD) > 7 mm, and gallbladder (GB) transverse diameter > 4 to 5 cm. (Figure 3-82)

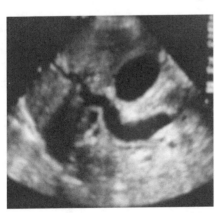

Figure 3-82: Transverse section of GB with dilated CBD

Aortic dissection—Look for presence of intimal flap.

Appendicitis—Immobile, tender, and noncompressible. Perforated: loculated fluid collection with circumferential loss of echogenic submucosal layer of appendix.

Beta-hCG level—Transvaginal detection of IUP at >1600 mIU/mL. Transabdominal detection >6500 mIU/mL.

Blighted ovum—Gestational sac >20 to 25 mm, but no yolk sac or embryo.

Cardiac arrest—No cardiac activity.

Cardiac shock—Marked global wall motion abnormality.

Cardiac tamponade—Dark circumferential area around heart. Diastolic collapse of right atrium and right ventricle.

Deep vein thrombosis (DVT)—Inability to compress vein walls.

Double-decidual sign—Intrauterine pregnancy (IUP). Hyperechoic surrounded by hypoechoic. Ectopic: see hyperechoic only.

Emergency ultrasound (US)—Goal is to expedite definitive treatment.

Hemothorax—Fluid above diaphragm.

Hyperdynamic myocardium in pulseless electrical activity (PEA)—Seen in hypovolemic patients.

Hypovolemia—Hyperkinetic heart with small right-sided collapse.

Moral pregnancy—Cystic placental tissue and no fetus.

Normal pregnancy (Table 3-21):
- Gestational sac initially, followed by yolk sac and then fetal pole.
- Cardiac activity if fetal pole present. Usually at 6 weeks by transvaginal US.
- Yolk sac: First reliable sign of IUP.

Pericardial fluid—Most reliable bedside ultrasound (US) finding in traumatic pericarditis.

Pulmonary embolism—Hyperkinetic heart with large hypodynamic right heart.

Table 3-21: Normal pregnancy

Ultrasound findings	Transvaginal	Transabdominal
Gestational sac	5 weeks	6 weeks
Yolk sac	5–6 weeks	6 weeks
See yolk sac if gestational sac	>10 mm	>20 mm
Fetal pole (embryo)	6 weeks	7 weeks
See fetal pole if gestational sac	>16 mm	>25 mm
Cardiac activity	6–7 weeks	6–7 weeks

Right upper quadrant (RUQ) abdomen hemoperitoneum—Fluid between diaphragm and liver or liver and kidney.

Sonographic Murphy's sign—Site of maximal tenderness corresponds to US location of gallbladder, and the patient's inspiration is inhibited by the probe at this location.

US to detect hydroureter—Study of choice in patient with flank pain, hematuria, and negative x-ray for stones.

Twin gestation—See Figure 3-83.

Wall dimension:

- Acute cholecystitis—Gallbladder wall > 3 mm.
- Pyloric stenosis—Pyloric muscle > 3 mm and canal > 1.2 cm elongated.
- Acute appendicitis—Appendix wall > 6 mm.

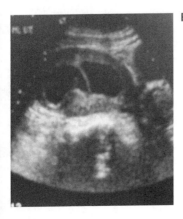

Figure 3-83: Twin gestation

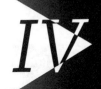

MC = most common

▶ ALLERGY and IMMUNOLOGY

Airway obstruction	MC cause of death in anaphylaxis.
"Chinese restaurant syndrome"	MC adverse food reaction (from direct histamine release).
Drugs	MC cause of serum sickness.
Epinephrine (110,000) intravenous	Most effective immediate treatment of anaphylactic shock.
Erythema nodosum	MC skin manifestation in sarcoidosis.
Fatigue	MC and most debilitating symptom in systemic lupus erythematosus.
Penicillin	MC cause and leading cause of fatal anaphylaxis. MC cause of drug reaction.
Phenolphthalein (over-the-counter laxatives)	MC cause of fixed drug eruption.
X-ray contrast media	MC anaphylactoid reaction.
Raynaud's disease	MC vasospastic disorder.
Serum sickness and urticaria	MC manifestations of penicillin allergy.
Urticaria	MC cause is never determined.

▶ CARDIOLOGY

3rd degree atrioventricular (AV) block	MC cause in AV dissociation.
Acute aortic insufficiency	MC causes are endocarditis, trauma, and dissection. MC symptom is dyspnea.
Aortic dissection	More common than ruptured abdominal aortic aneurysm (AAA). MC acute disease affecting aorta.
Aortic regurgitation	MC valvulopathy following blunt chest trauma.
Ascending aorta dissection	MC and most lethal type of aortic dissection.
Asthma or chronic obstructive pulmonary disease (COPD)	MC cause of pulsus paradoxus.
Atrial fibrillation	MC complication of mitral stenosis. MC sustained dysrhythmia.
Atrial tachycardia	MC dysrhythmia associated with Wolff-Parkinson-White (WPW) syndrome.
Bradycardia and atrial fibrillation	MC rhythm in hypothermia.
Chest pain	MC symptom in acute pericarditis. MC symptom associated with mitral valve prolapse.
Chest pain and dyspnea	MC presenting symptoms in pulmonary embolism.
Chest pain, dyspnea, and palpitation	MC symptoms reported by families of survivor of sudden cardiac death.
Chronic renal failure with missed dialysis in cardiac arrest	MC etiology of hyperkalemia.

Congenital bicuspid valve	MC cause of aortic stenosis in patients > 70 years of age.
Congenital heart disease	MC cause of congestive heart failure (CHF) in children.
Coronary artery disease	MC pathologic condition found in patients who die suddenly from ventricular fibrillation.
Coronary atherosclerosis	MC autopsy finding in sudden cardiac death patients.
Coxsackie virus	More frequent etiologic agent of acute myocarditis.
Dilated (congestive) cardiomyopathy	MC cardiomyopathy.
Dyspnea	MC complaint in atypical infarction, idiopathic hypertrophic subaortic stenosis (IHSS), aortic insufficiency, and esophageal perforation.
Dyspnea on exertion	MC presenting symptom of all valvular disease.
Dysrhythmia	MC cause of prehospital mortality in acute myocardial infarction.
Early defibrillation	Most important factor in surviving out-of-hospital arrest.
Embolism	MC source for acute mesenteric ischemia.
Esophageal perforation	MC cause in mediastinitis.
Heart	MC source of peripheral arterial occlusive disease caused by emboli.
Hyperkalemia	MC metabolic cause of cardiac arrest.
Hypertension	MC cause of chronic CHF. MC risk factor for aortic dissection.
Idiopathic	MC cause of dilated cardiomyopathy.
Idiopathic pericarditis	MC cause in restrictive pericarditis.

Infective endocarditis (IVDA)	MC organism is staphylococcus aureus. Affects tricuspid > aortic > mitral.
Ischemic damage to heart	MC cause of cardiogenic shock.
Ischemic heart disease	MC cause of left ventricular failure.
Left ventricular failure	MC cause of right ventricular failure.
Malaise and intermittent fever	MC complaints in subacute bacterial endocarditis.
Multifocal atrial tachycardia (MAT)	MC disease associated with COPD.
Myocardial infarction	Leading cause of death due to Kawasaki's disease.
Myxoma	MC tumor causing heart failure.
Oversensing	MC cause of failure to pace.
Pain	MC complaint in aortic dissection.
Papillary dysfunction and rupture	MC in inferior and posterior myocardial infarction.
Paroxysmal supraventricular tachycardia (PSVT) or premature ventricular contraction (PVC)	MC dysrhythmia in mitral valve prolapse (MVP).
PVCs	MC digoxin-induced rhythm disturbance with toxicity.
Rheumatic heart disease	MC cause of mitral stenosis and aortic regurgitation.
Ripping or tearing sudden chest pain	MC presentation of aortic dissection.
Shortness of breath	MC symptom of CHF.
Sinus tachycardia	MC finding on EKG in pericarditis.

Spread from distant site	MC mechanism for purulent pericarditis.
Stabbing chest pain	MC symptom of acute pericarditis.
Staphylococcus aureus	MC organism in right-sided endocarditis.
Streptococcus viridans	MC organism in left-sided endocarditis.
Sudden cardiac death	MC cause of out-of-hospital death in the United States.
Syncope	MC symptom in aortic stenosis or idiopathic hypertrophic subaortic stenosis (IHSS).
Transposition of great vessels	MC cause of death in first year of life.
Tuberculosis	MC cause of constrictive pericarditis in developed countries.
Viral	MC cause of myocarditis in the United States. Coxsackie virus B echovirus, influenza, parainfluenza, and Epstein-Barr virus (EBV).
Worsening of heart failure	MC precipitating cause of acute cardiogenic pulmonary edema.
Wolff-Parkinson-White (WPW) syndrome	MC type of preexcitation syndrome.

▶ DERMATOLOGY

Antibiotics	MC cause of drug eruptions.
Basal cell carcinoma	MC skin malignancy.
Clostridium perfringens	MC cause of gas gangrene.
Dermal injury	MC presenting complaint at mass gathering.
Diaper rash	MC skin disorder in infancy.
Drugs	MC cause of toxic epidermal necrolysis (TEN).
Erythematous or morbilliform rash	MC form of drug eruptions.

Herpes simplex virus (HSV)	MC cause of erythema multiforme.
Impetigo	MC skin infection in children.
Lyme disease	MC vector-borne disease in the United States.
Measles	MC cause of death worldwide that is preventable by vaccine.
Staphylococcus aureus	MC cause of cellulitis in adults.

▶ ENDOCRINE

Adrenal crisis	MC cause is abrupt cessation of long-term corticosteroids.
Alimentary hyperinsulinism	MC cause of postprandial hypoglycemia.
Diabetes mellitus (DM)	MC endocrine disease.
Diabetic medical treatment	MC cause of hypoglycemia treated in urban emergency department (ED).
Excess insulin administration	MC cause of coma in DM.
Exogenous glucocorticoid administration	MC cause of adrenal insufficiency.
Grave's disease	MC cause of hyperthyroidism and thyroid storm in adults.
Hashimoto's thyroiditis	MC cause of goitrous hypothyroidism in areas of adequate iodine.
Hypokalemia (severe)	Most life-threatening electrolyte complication from diabetic ketoacidosis (DKA) treatment.
Idiopathic	MC cause of primary chronic adrenal insufficiency.
Infection	MC cause of DKA and thyroid storm.

Lactic acidosis	MC metabolic acidosis.
Medications	MC cause of toxic epidermal necrolysis (TEN).
Post-radioablation treatment for Grave's disease or subtotal thyroidectomy	MC cause of primary hypothyroidism.
Pulmonary infection	MC precipitating cause for thyroid storm.
Sinus bradycardia	MC dysrhythmia in myxedema.

▶ ENVIRONMENTAL

Asymmetric multiplegias	MC presentation of arterial gas embolism (AGE).
Asystole	MC immediate cause of death in lightning strike.
Atrial fibrillation	MC dysrhythmia in hypothermia.
Aural barotrauma	MC type of barotrauma.
Barotitis media (middle ear squeeze)	MC form of barotraumas.
Carbon monoxide poisoning	MC cause of fire-related death. MC toxicologic cause of death in the United States.
Cataract	MC single eye complication following a lightning strike.
Coelenterates	MC of envenomations by marine animals.
Hands and skull	MC contact sites in electric injury.
Median nerve	MC peripheral nerve affected in electrical injury.
Pit vipers	MC (98%) of all venomous snakebites in the United States.
Sinus tachycardia	MC disturbance in electrical injury.
Skin	MC organ affected in radiation accident.

Stingray	Most commonly associated with human envenomation.
Ticks	Most frequent vector in tularemia (not rabbits).
Tympanic membrane	MC organ affected by blast injury or lightning.
Ventricular fibrillation	MC dysrhythmia in cardiac arrest from electrical injury. MC cause of death in electrical injury.
Yellow Jacket	Most potent sensitizer in Hymenoptera family.

▶ FLUIDS and ELECTROLYTES

Hyperkalemia	MC electrolyte abnormality in myoglobinuria.
Hypocalcemia	MC metabolic abnormality and occurs early in rhabdomyolysis.
Hyponatremia	MC clinical electrolyte abnormality.
Laboratory error	MC cause of hyperkalemia.
Lactic acidosis	MC cause of metabolic acidosis.
Magnesium containing antacids	MC cause of hypermagnesemia in renal failure patients.
Malignancies	MC cause of hypercalcemia.
Respiratory acidosis	MC acid–base disorder seen acutely in seizure patients.
Syndrome of inappropriate antidiuretic hormone (SIADH) secretion	MC cause of euvolemic hyponatremia in children.

▶ GASTROINTESTINAL

| Achalasia | MC motility disorder causing dysphagia. |
| Acute cholecystitis | MC cause of abdominal pain in individuals > 70 years of age.
MC surgical disease in elderly. |

Alcohol	MC cause of pancreatitis in urban hospitals.
Anal fissure	MC cause of painful rectal bleeding.
Calculus cholecystitis	MC cause of acute pancreatitis.
Campylobacter	MC bacterial cause of diarrhea in patients who seek medical care.
Carcinoma	MC cause of lower esophageal dysphagia. MC cause of large bowel obstruction (LBO). Diverticulitis is 2nd MC, and volvulus is 3rd MC cause of LBO.
Cerebrovascular accident	MC cause of neuromuscular swallowing dysfunction.
Cervical esophagus	MC site for foreign body impaction.
Cholecystitis	MC cause of abdominal pain and surgical emergency in the elderly. MC cause of extrahepatic jaundice in ED patients.
Cholesterol	MC type of gallstones.
Clostridium perfringens	MC cause of acute food poisoning in the United States.
Colovesical	MC fistula seen with diverticulitis.
Cryptosporidium and Isospora belli	MC cause of chronic diarrhea in acquired immunodeficiency syndrome (AIDS).
Cytomegalovirus (CMV) hepatitis	MC opportunistic viral infection in patients with liver transplant.
Diarrhea	MC gastrointestinal (GI) complaint in patients with AIDS.
Distal esophagus	MC site of esophageal rupture with Boerhaave's syndrome.
Diverticulosis	MC cause of painless significant lower GI bleed in adults.
Duodenal ulcer	MC cause of acute upper GI bleed.

Emboli from atherosclerotic cardiovascular disease (ASCVD)	MC cause of mesenteric ischemia.
Endoscopy	Most accurate diagnostic procedure for upper GI bleed evaluation.
Enterobius vermicularis (pinworm)	Most prevalent parasite in the United States.
Enterocolitis	MC cause of abdominal pain in AIDS patients.
Escherichia coli	MC cause of sterile bacterial peritonitis (SBP) in patients with cirrhosis and ascites.
Esophageal atresia	MC congenital obstruction of the esophagus.
Esophageal perforation	MC iatrogenic causation.
Esophagitis	MC cause of gastroesophageal (GE) reflux.
Ethanol-induced cirrhosis	MC cause of variceal bleeding.
Fecal impaction	MC cause of partial large bowel obstruction (LBO). Cancer is MC cause of complete LBO.
Femoral hernia	Most commonly found in women, but even in women, inguinal hernia is more common than femoral hernia.
Gastrointestinal bleeding	MC presentation of acute gastritis.
Giardia	MC cause of water-borne diarrhea outbreaks in the United States. MC intestinal protozoa.
Gilbert's syndrome	MC cause of mild unconjugated hyperbilirubinemia.
Hemorrhage	MC complication in ulcerative colitis.
Hemorrhoids	MC cause of rectal bleeding in adults.
Hernias and adhesions	MC cause of small bowel obstruction (SBO).

Hepatitis C virus	MC complication of intravenous drug abuse (IVDA). MC cause of intrahepatic jaundice in ED patients.
Indirect hernia	MC inguinal hernia in young men.
Inflammatory bowel disease	MC cause of lower GI bleed in young adults.
Inguinal hernia	MC type of hernia.
Intrinsic motility disorder (i.e., achalasia, spasm)	MC cause of lower esophagus dysphagia.
Intussusception	MC cause of LBO in children (seen at 5 to 10 months). Most often it is a combination of the large and small bowel that intussuscept.
Localized peritonitis or abscess formation	MC sequela of ruptured appendicitis.
Meckel's diverticulum	MC congenital abnormality of GI tract.
Medications	MC cause of nausea and vomiting in adults.
Melena	MC presentation of upper GI bleed in patients with peptic ulcer disease.
Monilia	MC organism for esophagitis.
Nasal trauma	MC cause of false-positive gastric aspirate result for blood.
Neuromuscular dysfunction (stroke)	MC cause of upper esophagus dysphagia.
Nonspecific abdominal pain	MC ED diagnosis given to patients who present with acute abdominal pain.
Norwalk virus	MC virus causing diarrhea in adults.
Pain	MC symptom in diverticulitis.
Pancreatitis	MC cause is alcohol in alcoholics. MC cause is gallbladder disease in nonalcoholics.
Perforation	MC complication in Crohn's disease.

Perianal abscess	MC anorectal abscess.
Polyps	MC overall cause of lower GI bleed in children.
Portal hypertension	MC cause of esophageal varices.
Pyogenic liver disease	MC after biliary tract obstruction.
Pyriform sinus (located in pharynx)	MC place of malplacement of nasotracheal tube.
Radionuclide imaging	Most useful for localizing lower GI bleed in stable patients.
Shigella	MC cause of bloody diarrhea.
Sigmoid colon	MC site for large bowel volvulus.
Staphylococcal food poisoning	MC cause of diarrhea involving preformed toxin.
Steatosis	MC variety of alcohol induced liver disease.
Toxic megacolon	MC complication seen in ulcerative colitis.
Ulcerative colitis	Most likely cause of massive lower GI bleed in young adults.
Ulcers	MC cause of visceral perforation.
Upper GI bleed	MC cause of apparent lower GI bleed.
Vibrio parahaemolyticus	MC cause of foodborne bacterial enteritis in Japan.
Viral gastroenteritis in children	MC cause of hypovolemic hyponatremia.
Viral illness	MC cause of acute diarrhea.

▶ GENITOURINARY

Acute tubular necrosis (ATN)	MC cause is ischemia (shocked kidney due to hypotension). MC cause of renal azotemia. MC tubulointerstitial cause of acute renal failure.

Benign prostatic hypertrophy (BPH)	MC cause of urinary retention in men > 50 years of age.
Chronic bacterial prostatitis	MC cause of recurrent urinary tract infection (UTI) in men.
Epididymitis	MC cause of acute painful scrotal swelling in > 18-year-old male adults.
Herpes simplex	MC cause of genital ulcers.
Hydrocele	MC cause of scrotal swelling.
Hypotension	MC complication during dialysis.
Hypovolemia	MC cause of prerenal azotemia.
Intradialytic hypotension	MC complication of hemodialysis from excessive ultrafiltration.
Ischemia	MC cause of acute tubular necrosis (ATN).
Periorbital edema	MC sign of glomerulonephritis.
Protein in urine	MC indicator of underlying renal disease.
Renal disease	MC cause of secondary hypertension.
Staphylococcus aureus	MC infection in hemodialysis patients.
Struvite (Mg-NH4-PO4) calculus	MC cause of staghorn calculi.
Testicular torsion	MC cause of acute painful scrotal swelling.
Trauma	MC cause of renal artery thrombosis.
Urethral prolapse	MC cause of "apparent vaginal bleeding" in premenarcheal girls.
Urethritis	MC urologic infection in men.

▶ HEAD, EYES, EARS, NOSE, and THROAT (HEENT)

Angle fracture	MC area of mandible fracture > condyle > body > ramus > symphysis.
Anterior displacement	MC direction of displacement in mandibular dislocation.

Anterior epistaxis	MC cause of epistaxis. Erosion of Kiesselbach's triangle vessels from trauma or dry air.
Cerumen impaction	MC cause of unilateral hearing loss in healthy patients.
Chlamydia trachomatis conjunctivitis	MC cause of preventable blindness worldwide.
Choanal atresia	MC congenital anomaly of the nose.
Coin	MC foreign body ingestion in children (peanuts and popcorn are second).
Dental caries	MC cause of pain of odontogenic origin.
Diplopia	MC finding after orbital floor fracture.
Fishbone, dentures, meat, and meat bone	MC foreign bodies in adults.
Group A Streptococcus	MC bacteria causing pharyngitis (viral > bacterial).
Haemophilus influenzae type B	MC cause of preseptal cellulitis. MC organism in epiglottitis.
Macular degeneration	MC cause of blindness in the United States.
Nasal bone	MC facial bone fracture.
Open angle glaucoma	MC type of glaucoma.
Otitis media and sinusitis	MC ear, nose, and throat (ENT) infections.
Peritonsillar abscess	MC deep-space infection of head and neck.
Poor tympanic membrane mobility on insufflation	MC sign of otitis media.
Pseudomonas aeruginosa	MC cause of chronic sinusitis.

Retropharyngeal abscess	MC ENT infection seen in children 1 to 5 years of age.
Rhinovirus and adenovirus	MC cause of pharyngitis.
Staphylococcus aureus	MC organism in orbital cellulitis.
Submandibular gland sialolithiasis	MC location of sialolithiasis.
Unilateral sensory loss	MC cause is viral neuronitis.

▸ HEMATOLOGY and ONCOLOGY

Acquired immunodeficiency syndrome (AIDS)	MC cause of death in hemophiliacs.
Acute lymphocytic leukemia (ALL)	MC leukemia in children < 15 years of age.
Bleeding	MC complication of massive transfusion.
Breast and lung	MC neoplasms causing pericardial tamponade or effusion.
Bronchogenic carcinoma	MC cause of obstruction of the superior vena cava (SVC).
Cancer	MC cause in SVC syndrome in adults.
Chronic lymphocytic leukemia (CLL)	MC type of leukemia in patients > 50 years of age.
Clerical error	MC reason for acute hemolytic reactions in transfusion.
Craniopharyngioma	MC hypothalamic–pituitary tumor in children.
Extreme anxiety, apprehension, and precordial oppressive feeling	MC symptoms in tamponade.

Fever	MC complication in blood transfusion (more common than allergic reaction).
Gram-negative bacteremia	MC cause of death in neutropenic cancer patients.
Hepatitis C virus	MC posttransfusion infection in the United States.
Hyperviscosity syndrome	MC cause of dysproteinemia. Waldenström's > multiple myeloma.
Hypercalcemia	MC life-threatening metabolic disorder associated with cancer. MC paraneoplastic syndrome.
Infection	MC cause of death in cancer. MC problem in peritoneal dialysis.
Iron deficiency anemia	MC anemia in women of childbearing age.
Lung cancer (small cell)	MC malignancy-related cause of syndrome of inappropriate antidiuretic hormone (SIADH) secretion.
Neuroblastoma	MC tumor in infants < 1 year of age. MC extracranial solid tumor in childhood.
Non-familial ichthyosis	MC malignant disease associated with Hodgkin's disease.
Osteochondroma	MC site is knee. MC benign bone tumor.
Osteosarcoma	MC primary malignant bone tumor in children.
Purpura	MC skin manifestation of leukemia.
Raynaud's disease	MC vasospastic disorder.
Retinoblastoma	MC primary malignant intraocular tumor of children.
Seizure	MC neurologic complication of cancer.
Teratoma	MC benign tumor of pericardium or mediastinum.

Thoracic back pain	MC initial presenting symptom (95%) in acute spinal cord compression.
Thrombosis	MC cause of death in polycythemia vera.
Vaso-occlusive crisis	MC cause of sickle cell crisis.
Von Willebrand's disease	MC inherited bleeding disorder.
Waldenström's macroglobulinemia	MC cause of hyperviscosity syndrome.

▶ INFECTIOUS DISEASE

Arbovirus	MC cause of endemic encephalitis in the United States.
Arthritis- dermatitis syndrome	MC presentation of disseminated gonorrhea.
Atrioventricular (AV) block	MC cardiac abnormality found in Lyme disease.
Candida albicans	MC cause of infectious pharyngitis in AIDS.
Cotton-wool spots	MC retinal pathology in AIDS due to microvascular lesions.
Cryptococcal meningitis	MC cause of AIDS meningitis.
Cytomegalovirus (CMV) retinitis	MC ocular disease in AIDS patients.
Escherichia coli	MC organism identified in gram-negative septicemia.
Gram-negative infections	MC infections in cancer patients.
Haemophilus influenzae type B	MC organism in epiglottitis in adults and children.
Heterosexual transmission	MC mode of human immunodeficiency virus (HIV) transmission worldwide.
Kaposi's sarcoma	MC cancer in patients with AIDS. MC cause of pneumothorax in patients with HIV.

Legionella	MC known bacterial etiology of rhabdomyolysis.
Lymphadenopathy	MC sign in tularemia: Adults: MC is inguinal lymphadenopathy; ulceration is 2nd MC sign in tularemia Children: MC is cervical lymphadenopathy; fever is 2nd MC sign in tularemia.
Lymphatic tissue	MC extrapulmonary site for tuberculosis.
Otitis media	MC complication of measles.
Otitis media and pneumonia	Two MC infections in adults caused by the pneumococci.
Paralysis of palatal muscles	MC initial neurological manifestation in diphtheria.
Paronychia	MC infection of the hand.
Peritonsillar abscess	MC abscess of head and neck.
Pneumocystis carinii pneumonia (PCP)	MC opportunistic infections of AIDS.
Pseudomonas	MC cause of osteomyelitis following a puncture wound (classically through the sole of a sneaker).
Rocky Mountain spotted fever	MC rickettsial disease in the United States.
Salmonella	MC cause of osteomyelitis in sickle cell patients.
Staphylococcus aureus	MC cause of osteomyelitis in all groups except neonates. MC cause of puncture wound infection (other than when the puncture is through a sneaker sole). MC organism associated with toxic shock syndrome (TSS).
Streptococcus pneumoniae	MC bacteria causing otitis media. MC cause of pneumonia in sickle cell disease.
Streptococcus pyogenes	MC cause of cellulites and lymphangitis.

Toxoplasmosis	MC cause of focal encephalitis in AIDS.
Trismus	MC presenting symptom in tetanus (>50%).
Urinary tract infection (UTI)	MC cause of hematuria in >20 years of age.
Viral conjunctivitis	MC type of conjunctivitis with concurrent upper respiratory infection (URI).

▶ NEUROLOGY

Central cord syndrome	MC incomplete spinal cord injury.
Headache and confusion	MC feature of central nervous system (CNS) involvement in lupus.
Lymphoma and multiple myeloma	MC tumors causing ischemic dysfunction of spinal cord.
Myasthenia gravis	MC disease of neuromuscular transmission.
Parkinson's disease	MC chronic neurodegenerative disease.
Ptosis and diplopia	MC symptom in myasthenia gravis.
Putamen	MC site of intracranial bleeding.
Trigeminal neuralgia	MC on right side of the face.
Uncal herniation	MC disease cause of unilateral dilated pupil. Mydriatic eye drops are MC nondisease cause of unilateral dilated pupil.

▶ OBSTETRICS and GYNECOLOGY

Abnormal development of zygote	MC cause of miscarriage.
Amniotic fluid embolism	MC cause of death in induced abortion.
Anatomic or functional abnormality of fallopian tube	Most important cause of ectopic pregnancy.

Appendicitis	MC surgical emergency in pregnancy.
Atrophic endometrium	MC cause of postmenopausal uterine bleeding.
Cerebral hemorrhage	MC cause of death in toxemia.
Chlamydia	MC cause of pelvic inflammatory disease (PID) in college students.
Dysmenorrhea	MC cause of cyclic pain in reproductive age women.
Esophagitis	MC cause of upper GI bleeding in pregnancy.
Gonorrhea	MC cause of PID in urban areas.
Hepatitis	MC cause of jaundice in pregnancy. Intrahepatic cholestasis of pregnancy is 2nd MC cause of jaundice in pregnancy.
Hormonal contraceptives	MC cause of abnormal vaginal bleeding in nonpregnant childbearing age women.
Malpresentation	MC cause of fetal dystocia.
Motor vehicle collision (MVC)	MC cause of blunt abdominal trauma in pregnant women.
Pain	MC presenting complaint of ectopic pregnancy.
Postpartum hemorrhage	< 24 hours—MC cause is uterine atony. >24 hours—MC cause is retained products of conception (POC).
Pyelonephritis (complicated urinary tract infection)	MC condition confused with appendicitis in pregnancy.
Refractory hemorrhagic shock (ectopic pregnancy)	MC cause of maternal death in first trimester.
Spontaneous abortion	MC cause of first trimester bleeding.

Thromboembolic disease	MC cause of death in pregnancy. Ectopic pregnancy is 2nd MC cause of death in pregnancy.
Unilateral adnexal tenderness	MC finding of ectopic pregnancy on pelvic examination.
Vaginal bleeding	MC gynecological complaints.
Von Willebrand's disease	MC hereditary disorder associated with menorrhagia.

▶ ORTHOPEDICS

▶ UPPER EXTREMITY

Anterior shoulder dislocation (sternoclavicular)	MC type of shoulder dislocation.
Axillary nerve	MC injured nerve after anterior shoulder dislocation.
Boxer's fracture (4th or 5th metacarpal neck fracture)	MC metacarpal fracture.
Clavicle	MC fractured bone in children. MC location is middle one-third.
Dislocation of proximal interphalangeal (PIP) joint	MC ligament injury of hand.
Fractured ribs	MC injury in blunt chest trauma.
Ganglion	MC synovial cyst arising from the metacarpophalangeal (MCP) joints.
Hand bones	MC fractured bones in the body.
Radial head fracture	MC fracture of the elbow.
Radial nerve	MC injury associated with humeral shaft fracture.
Scaphoid fracture	MC carpal bone fracture.

Scapholunate ligament injury	MC ligament injury of the wrist.
Subcoracoid	MC anterior shoulder dislocation.
Supraspinatus tear	MC rotator cuff injury.

▶ *LOWER EXTREMITY*

Ankle sprain	MC athletic injury seen in ED.
Anterior compartment	MC compartment syndrome.
Anterior cruciate ligament tear	MC cause of acute traumatic hemarthrosis of knee. MC serious ligament injury.
Anterior talofibular ligament	MC ankle ligament injury. Calcaneofibular ligament is 2nd MC. Posterior talofibular ligament is 3rd MC.
Calcaneus	MC fracture tarsal bone. Talus bone is 2nd MC.
Chondromalacia patella	MC cause of knee pain.
Compartment syndrome	MC after closed fracture of the tibia.
Fibular fracture	MC fracture of the leg.
Intertrochanteric fracture	MC hip fracture.
Inversion or plantar flexion	MC ankle injury.
Jones fracture	MC foot fracture (proximal 5th toe transverse fracture).
Knee	MC injured joint in the body.
Lateral dislocation	MC ankle dislocation.
Lateral patellar dislocation	MC patellar dislocation.
Ligamentous ankle injury	MC athletic injury.

Metatarsal stress fracture	MC stress fracture.
Navicular fracture	MC midfoot fracture.
Osteochondroma	MC benign tumor of the bone. MC site is the knee.
Posterior hip dislocation	MC type of hip dislocation.
Slipped capital femoral epiphysis	MC adolescent hip problem.
Stress fracture	MC occurs between 2nd and 3rd metatarsal bones.
Tibia fracture	MC long bone fracture. MC open fracture.

▶ PEDIATRICS

▶ CARDIAC

Bicuspid aortic valve	MC cause of significant aortic stenosis in infancy or childhood.
Congestive heart failure (CHF) in critically ill premature infant	MC cause is patent ductus arteriosus (PDA).
CHF in first few minutes after birth	MC causes are asphyxia, anemia, acidosis, hypoglycemia, or hypocalcemia.
Coarctation of aorta	MC cause of CHF in term infants in 2nd week of life.
Congenital heart disease	MC cause of CHF in children.
Feeding intolerance	Most reliable marker for exercise intolerance in infants.
Hemolytic-uremic syndrome (HUS)	MC systemic cause of hematochezia in patients < 3 years of age.
Hypoplastic left ventricle	MC cause of CHF in term infants in first week of life.

Idiopathic thrombocytopenic purpura (ITP)	MC cause of thrombocytopenic purpura of childhood.
Inguinal hernia repair	MC surgical procedure in children.
Kawasaki's disease	MC cause of acquired heart disease in children in the United States.
Myocarditis	MC cause of dilated cardiomyopathy in children.
Patent ductus arteriosus (PDA)	MC cause of CHF in premature infants.
Streptococcus and Staphylococcus	MC organisms to cause bacterial endocarditis in children.
Supraventricular tachycardia	MC symptomatic dysrhythmia in infants and children.
Tachypnea	MC first sign of CHF in infants followed by rales.
Tetralogy of Fallot (TOF)	MC cyanotic congenital heart disease in children > 1 year of age.
Transposition of great vessels	MC cyanotic congenital heart lesion appearing at first week of age.
Ventricular septal defect (VSD)	MC congenital cardiac defect.

▶ *CHILD ABUSE NONACCIDENTAL TRAUMA*

Abusers	MC are related caregivers.
Age	MC < 4 years of age.
Central nervous system (CNS) injury	MC cause of death related to child abuse.
Child abuse	MC cause of chronic subdural hematoma in infants.
Diaphyseal transverse and spiral fracture of long bones	MC fracture in child abuse.

Gonorrhea	MC infection in child sexual abuse.
Homicide	MC cause of death in children 6 to 12 years of age.

▶ ENDOCRINE

Adrenal cortical adenoma or carcinoma	MC noniatrogenic cause of Cushing's syndrome.
Dysgenesis of thyroid gland	MC cause of congenital hypothyroidism.
Lymphocytic thyroiditis	MC cause of acquired hypothyroidism in children.

▶ HEENT

Bacterial and viral conjunctivitis	MC cause of "red eye" in children.
Beads and nuts	MC nasal foreign bodies.
Chemical irritation	MC cause of neonatal conjunctivitis (no longer gonorrhea).
Chlamydial neonatal conjunctivitis	MC cause of neonatal conjunctivitis.
Conjunctivitis	MC ocular infection in childhood.
Cystic fibrosis or allergy	MC cause of nasal polyps in children.
Gingivostomatitis	MC type of herpes simplex virus (HSV) infection in children.
Group A beta-hemolytic streptococcal (GABHS) pharyngitis	MC treatable cause of pharyngitis in children.
Hearing loss	MC complication of otitis media with effusion (OME).
Laryngomalacia	MC cause of persistent inspiratory stridor in infants presenting in first month of life.

Parainfluenza	MC agent in laryngotracheobronchitis.
Periorbital cellulitis or orbital cellulitis	MC complication of sinusitis.
Peritonsillar abscess	MC deep infection of head and neck.
Retinal hemorrhage	MC physical sign of shaken baby syndrome.
Staphylococcus aureus	MC organism in bacterial tracheitis and cellulitis.
Staphylococcus aureus and GABHS	MC organism in retropharyngeal abscess.

▶ GASTROINTESTINAL

Anal fissure	MC anorectal disorder in children. Most common cause of rectal bleeding in infants.
Appendicitis	MC surgical condition in children.
Biliary atresia	MC indication for liver transplantation in pediatrics.
Campylobacter	MC cause of bacterial gastroenteritis in the United States.
Cystic fibrosis	MC cause of pancreatic insufficiency in childhood.
Dehydration from prolonged diarrhea	MC cause of metabolic acidosis.
Diarrhea	MC preceding illness in children with hemolytic uremic syndrome (HUS).
Duodenal atresia	MC cause of congenital small bowel obstruction.
Esophageal atresia with distal communication between trachea and esophagus	MC thoracic-esophageal fistula presentation.
Hirschsprung's disease	MC cause of partial or lower intestinal obstruction in early infancy.

Indirect inguinal hernia	MC type of hernia (also in adults).
Ileocolic	MC location of intussusception.
Intussusception	MC cause of intestinal obstruction < 2 years of age.
Isonatremic	MC form of dehydration in children.
Meckel's diverticulum	MC cause of significant lower GI bleed in children.
Mumps and trauma	MC cause of pancreatitis.
Pyloric stenosis	MC disorder requiring surgery in infancy.
Recurrent abdominal pain	MC symptom of constipation in school-age children.
Rotavirus	MC viral cause of acute diarrhea in infants. Adenovirus (enteric) is 2nd MC viral cause.
Shigella	MC bacterial cause of diarrhea in the United States.
Tracheoesophageal fistula	MC congenital esophageal lesions in infancy.
Upper GI bleed	MC causes are: Neonate—Idiopathic, gastritis, esophagitis, and swallowed maternal blood. 30 days to 1 year of age—Esophagitis, gastritis, and peptic ulcer disease. 1 to 12 years of age—Esophageal varices , and drug use. 13 to 19 years of age—Esophagitis and peptic ulcer disease.

▶ GENITOURINARY

Minimal-change disease	MC cause of nephrotic syndrome in children.
Neuroblastoma	MC extracranial solid tumor in childhood.
Wilms tumor	MC pediatric abdominal malignancy.

▶ INFECTION

Chlamydia pneumonia	MC cause of afebrile interstitial pneumonia in infants.
Chorioretinitis (inflammatory retinal lesion)	MC ophthalmic abnormality in congenital toxoplasmosis.
Escherichia coli	MC isolated organism in urinary tract infection (UTI).
Low birthweight	MC risk factor for sepsis in infants.
Neuritis with paralysis	MC neurologic complication of diphtheria.
Perianal pruritus	MC presentation of pinworm infection.
Salpingitis	MC complication of gonorrhea in adolescent female.
Vaginitis	MC manifestation of infection with gonorrhea in prepubertal girls.

▶ NEONATAL

GBS (group B streptococcus)	MC organism causing neonatal meningitis.
Hypoglycemia	MC metabolic abnormality in newborn.
Hypoxic-ischemic encephalopathy	MC cause of neonatal seizure.
Physiologic jaundice	MC cause of jaundice in unconjugated hyperbilirubinemia. Breast milk jaundice is 2nd MC cause.
Prematurity	MC predetermining factor in neonatal respiratory distress syndrome.

▶ NEUROLOGIC

Cerebral arteriovenous malformation (AVM)	MC cause of spontaneous intracerebral hemorrhage in children.

Shunt obstruction	MC cause of shunt malfunction.
Simple febrile seizure	MC seizure disorder in childhood.
Spastic	MC type of cerebral palsy.
Spikes over temporal lobes	MC characteristic electroencephalogram (EEG) finding in complex partial seizure.

▶ **ONCOLOGIC**

Abdominal mass	MC presenting sign of Wilms tumor.
Neuroblastoma	MC extracranial solid tumor in children.
Superficial painless (cervical) lymphadenopathy	MC presenting sign with Hodgkin's disease.
Wilms tumor	MC malignant tumor of genitourinary tract in children.

▶ **ORTHOPEDIC**

Hematogenous spread	MC mode of infection in septic joint.
Salter II fracture	MC growth plate injury.
Staphylococcus aureus	MC organism in septic joint and osteomyelitis.
Supracondylar fracture	MC occult elbow fracture in children.
Transient synovitis	MC cause of painful hip in children.

▶ **RESPIRATORY**

Airway obstruction and pneumonia	MC complication from bronchial trachitis.
Asthma	MC chronic disease of childhood.
Chlamydia pneumonia	MC afebrile pneumonia in 1- to 3-month old infants.
Dehydration	MC systemic complication of childhood pneumonia.

Group B streptococcus	MC cause of lower respiratory tract infection in newborn.
Group B streptococcus, escherichia coli, and listeria	MC cause of bacterial pneumonia in infants < 1 month old.
Hyperinflation	MC chest x-ray findings in bronchiolitis.
Laryngomalacia	MC cause of stridor in neonate.
Respiratory syncytial virus (RSV)	MC viral pathogen in bronchiolitis.
RSV and parainfluenza virus	MC cause of pneumonia in infants and small children.
Staphylococcus aureus and pseudomonas aeruginosa	MC bacterial pathogens in the lungs of patients with cystic fibrosis.
Streptococcus pneumoniae	MC cause of pneumonia in > 1 month of age. Hemophilus influenzae (H flu is 2nd MC cause.
Streptococcus pneumoniae and H flu	MC pathogens for acute otitis media.
Streptococcus pneumoniae and mycoplasma	MC cause of pneumonia in children > 5 years of age.
Sudden infant death syndrome (SIDS)	MC cause of post-neonatal death between 1 month and 1 year of age.
Tachypnea	Best single indicator of pneumonia (especially in children).
Upper respiratory infection (URI)	MC cause of acute asthma in children.
Wheezing	Most unreliable signs in evaluating degree of distress in asthma.

▶ *RESUSCITATION*

Asystole	MC pediatric arrest rhythm.
Hypoxemia	MC cause of pediatric cardiac arrest.
Tachycardia	Most sensitive and earliest sign of volume loss in pediatrics.

▶ *RHEUMATOLOGIC*

Hematogenous	MC origin of osteomyelitis in children.
Iridocyclitis	MC ophthalmologic complication in children with juvenile rheumatoid arthritis (JRA).
Juvenile rheumatoid arthritis (JRA)	MC rheumatoid disease of childhood.

▶ *TRAUMA*

Odontoid fracture	MC pediatric cervical spine fracture.
Spinal cord injury without x-ray abnormalities (SCIOWORA)	MC spinal injury in children < 8 years of age.

▶ PHARMACOLOGY

Azathioprine	MC cause of leukopenia in post-transplantation patients.
Dystonic reaction	MC adverse effect of neuroleptic agents.
Penicillin	MC cause of serum sickness in the United States. MC cause of drug-induced anaphylaxis.
Pericarditis	MC cardiac manifestation of lupus.

▶ PULMONARY

Bacterial pneumonia	MC cause of exudative plural effusion.
Bleb	MC predisposing factor for a spontaneous pneumothorax.

Chest pain	MC complaint of patients with suspected spontaneous pneumothorax.
Chronic obstructive pulmonary disease (COPD)	MC cause associated with secondary spontaneous pneumothorax.
Congestive heart failure	MC cause of pleural effusion. Bacterial pneumonia is 2nd MC cause.
Cryptococcus neoformans	MC fungus causing life-threatening infection in AIDS.
Deep veins in pelvis, thighs, and legs	MC source of thromboembolism leading to pulmonary embolism.
Dyspnea	MC symptom of left-sided congestive heart failure.
Dyspnea or tachypnea	MC sign and symptom associated with pulmonary embolism.
Elevated hemidiaphragm	MC sign in pulmonary embolism.
Emphysema	MC cause of secondary spontaneous pneumothorax.
Esophageal perforation	MC cause of mediastinitis.
Fever	MC symptom in tuberculosis.
Indirect immunofluorescence sputum stain	Most accurate method for diagnosing pneumocystis carinii.
Influenza pneumonia	MC cause of pneumonia in adults.
Klebsiella pneumoniae	MC gram-negative community-acquired pneumonia.
Malignancy	MC cause of chronic symptomatic effusion.
Parainfluenza virus	MC causative organism in croup.
Piriform sinus	MC malposition of nasotracheal tube (tip of the tube is seen as a bulge).

Pneumonia	MC cause of death from infectious disease. MC sequella in pulmonary contusion.
Pulmonary embolism	MC finding is normal EKG. MC abnormality is nonspecific ST-T changes. MC rhythm disturbance is sinus tachycardia.
Pulmonary tuberculosis	MC symptom is fever.
Respiratory complications	MC cause of mortality following suicidal hanging.
Right upper lobe lung	MC site for aspiration.
Sepsis	MC cause of noncardiogenic pulmonary edema. Shock is 2nd MC cause.
Streptococcus pneumoniae	MC cause of community acquired pneumonia.
Streptococcus pneumoniae and mycoplasma	MC cause of childhood pneumonia.
Tracheal intubation	MC complication of esophageal obturator airway.
Unexplained dyspnea	Most reliable symptom of significant pulmonary embolism.
Ventilation perfusion abnormality	MC respiratory function abnormality in bacterial pneumonia.

▶ RHEUMATOLOGY AND INFLAMMATORY

Back pain	MC cause of disability in people < 45 years of age.
Contiguous or direct spread	MC source of infection in osteomyelitis in adults.
Elevated erythrocyte sedimentation rate (ESR)	MC laboratory sign in osteomyelitis.

First metatarsophalangeal joint	MC site of gout (podagra).
Gonococcal arthritis	MC cause of septic arthritis in teenagers. MC septic arthritis seen in emergency medicine.
Group A beta-hemolytic streptococcus (GABHS)	MC cause of septic arthritis in neonate.
Hemophilus influenza (H flu) type b	MC cause of septic arthritis in children < 4 years of age.
Hepatitis	MC cause of polyarticular joint pain.
Olecranon bursitis	MC site of bursitis.
Osteoarthritis	MC cause of oligoarticular (few joints) pain and swelling.
Osteomyelitis	H flu type b—MC organism in pediatric osteomylitis. Pseudomonas and serratia marcescens—MC organisms in intravenous drug abuse (IVDA) patient osteomylitis. Salmonella—MC organism in sickle cell osteomyelitis. Staphylococcus aureus—MC organism in adult osteomylitis.
Pericarditis	MC cardiac manifestation of systemic lupus erythematosus (SLE). Seen in 30% patients with lupus.
Procainamide and hemodialysis	MC agents for drug induced SLE (reversible).
Pseudomonas	MC osteomyelitis in sneaker puncture wound, drug pushers, and prosthetics.
Reiter's syndrome	MC cause of inflammatory oligoarthropathy.

Seizure	MC central nervous system involvement in SLE.
SLE	MC collagen vascular disease with oral manifestations.
Staphylococcus aureus	MC cause of nongonococcal arthritis in healthy adults. MC organism in hematogenous osteomyelitis.

▶ TOXICOLOGY

Altered mental status (AMS)	MC complaint in patients in acute overdose of sympathomimetic agents.
Amanita mushrooms (cyclopeptides)	MC mushroom-related fatalities in the United States.
Arsenic	MC cause of acute heavy metal poisoning.
Carbon monoxide (CO)	MC cause of acute poisoning death. MC cause of fire-related deaths.
Cardiovascular depression	MC cause of early death in barbiturate toxicity.
Esophageal stricture	MC delayed complications of lye ingestions.
Lead	MC chronic heavy metal poisoning.
Liquefaction necrosis	MC severe injury in caustic ingestion.
Pyloric stricture	MC delayed complications of acid ingestion.

▶ TRANSPLANTATION

Acute rejection	MC type of graft rejection in renal transplantation.
Cytomegalovirus (CMV)	MC cause of infection in liver transplant patients. MC pathogen in interstitial pneumonitis in transplant patients.

▶ TRAUMA

▶ GENERAL

Children	Motor vehicle collision (MVC)—MC cause of death in children > 1 year of age. Suffocation—MC cause of death in children < 1 year of age.
Elderly	Falls—MC accidental injury in individuals > 75 years of age. Head injury—MC cause of mortality in elderly trauma. MVC—MC mechanism for fatal incidents in elderly. Type II odontoid fracture—MC cervical spine fracture in elderly.
Injury (trauma)	MC cause of death before age 45.
Mass gathering	Dermal injury—MC trauma injury at mass gathering. Headache—MC medical complaint at mass gathering.

▶ CARDIAC

Aortic valve	MC valve rupture in blunt cardiac trauma.
Deceleration injury	MC mechanism of injury associated with aortic transaction.
Esophagus pushed to right by 1 to 2 cm	MC reliable x-ray sign of traumatic aortic rupture.
Hemorrhagic shock	MC etiology of hypotension in trauma.
Interscapular pain	MC symptom present with traumatic aortic disruption (25%).
Isthmus of aorta	MC vessel for blunt traumatic injury (90%).
Penetrating trauma to chest or upper abdomen	MC cause of traumatic pericardial tamponade.

Right atrium	MC site of perforation from catheter placement.
Right ventricle	MC part of the heart affected in cardiac contusion.
Rupture of aortic valve	MC valve lesion. Papillary muscle rupture is second MC.
Sinus tachycardia	MC sign of myocardial contusion on initial presentation.
Widening mediastinum	MC x-ray finding in traumatic aorta rupture.

▶ *GASTROINTESTINAL*

Diaphragmatic hernia	MC on left side. MC secondary to blunt<penetrating trauma.
Duodenal hematoma	MC associated with handlebar injury.
Endoscopy	MC cause of iatrogenic esophageal perforation.
Esophageal injuries	MC missed injury in the neck.
Esophageal perforation	MC cause is iatrogenic.
Liver	MC solid organ injured in penetrating trauma.
Penetrating trauma	MC mechanism in diaphragmatic injury.
Spleen	MC solid organ injured in blunt trauma.

▶ *NEUROLOGIC*

Cerebellar hemorrhage	MC treatable intracranial hemorrhage.
Diffuse axonal injury	MC cause of coma in head injury.
Subarachnoid hemorrhage	MC type of intracranial hemorrhage in trauma.

▶ OBSTETRIC AND GYNECOLOGIC

Fetal death	MC causes are maternal death and maternal shock.
Trauma	MC nonobstetric cause of maternal death during pregnancy.
Uterine contractions	MC obstetric problem caused by trauma (90% self-limiting).

▶ ORTHOPEDIC

Anterior lower leg	MC site for compartment syndrome.
C_1–C_2	MC site of "true misses" fractures of cervical spine.
C_7–T_1	MC site of missed fractures due to inadequate films.
C_6–T_1	MC cause of morbidity resulting in medical litigation from failure to visualize.
Lisfranc fracture	MC mid-foot fracture.
Mandibular dislocation	MC cause is blow to the open jaw.
Motor vehicle collison (MVC)	MC cause of facial trauma.
Water's view	Most valuable x-ray study in evaluation of mid-face trauma.

▶ PULMONARY

Fractured ribs	MC injury in blunt chest trauma.
Pulmonary complications	MC cause of in-hospital death in near-hanging.
Pulmonary contusion	Most significant factor in respiratory insufficiency in flail chest.

▶ VASCULAR

Blunt trauma	MC cause of cervical vascular injury (penetrating rare).

Common carotid artery	MC injured artery in the neck.
Exsanguination from vascular injuries	MC cause of immediate death after penetrating neck trauma.
Forceful hyperextension and lateral rotation of neck	MC mechanism of blunt internal carotid artery injury.
Jugular vein	MC injured vessel in the neck.
Subclavian artery injury	MC sign of injury is absence of radial pulse on affected side.

▶ VASCULAR

Atherosclerosis	MC cause of thoracic and abdominal aortic aneurysms.
Brachial artery	MC site of an embolus in upper extremity.
Deep calf veins	MC site of thrombophebitis origin.
Femoral artery	MC site of posttraumatic infected aneurysm.
Heart	MC source of emboli causing acute occlusion of lower extremities.
Intravenous drug abuse	Arterial injury is MC in upper extremity. Pseudoaneurysm is MC in lower extremity.
Popliteal aneurysm	MC peripheral aneurysm (>60% bilateral).
Thromboembolic events	MC serious complication of prosthetic valve.

Practice Questions

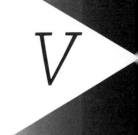

▶ QUESTIONS

1. A 73-year-old man presents with left flank pain. He has been complaining of backache for several weeks and states he has had spinal stenosis for years. This morning, the pain became very sharp, and he had an episode of dizziness. His wife states that he looked like he had passed out. He takes aldomet for hypertension.

   Vital Signs: BP 120/70 mmHg, P 110 beats/min, R 18 breaths/min, T 37°C, O_2 sat 90%.

   Physical examination is unremarkable, except that the patient appears very uncomfortable.

   What is the likely diagnosis?

   A. Renal colic
   B. Cardiac dysrhythmia
   C. Pulmonary embolus
   D. Abdominal aortic aneurysm

2. A 28-year-old man is involved in a motor vehicle crash and sustains multiple long-bone injuries, several broken ribs, but no head or spinal injury. After open reduction-internal fixation of a right tibial fracture, he is 3 days post surgery. He had noted left chest pain since the accident (the site of the rib fractures), but today he begins to complain of pain in the right abdomen.

   Vital Signs: BP 130/70 mmHg, P 110 beats/min, R 18 breaths/min, T 37°C, O_2 sat 96%.

   On physical examination, he has marked tenderness and guarding in the right upper quadrant; marked tenderness over the left lower chest, and no signs of edema, redness, or purulence of the operative site. Chest: diminished breath sounds bilaterally. Heart: no murmurs or rubs and regular rhythm. Abdomen: diminished bowel sounds and no masses or tenderness.

What is the diagnosis that should be investigated?

A. Atelectasis of the right lower lobe
B. Pulmonary embolus
C. Delayed splenic rupture
D. Acalculous cholecystitis

3. A 55-year-old woman enters the ED with a chief complaint of pain in the right eye. She states she felt well until she walked into a dark living room that had the curtains drawn, from her sunlit kitchen. On physical examination, the right eye is reddened, has a dilated pupil that does not react to light, and has a cloudy cornea.

The diagnostic test that will yield the correct answer is:

A. Doppler carotid ultrasound
B. X-ray study of the orbit
C. Ocular tonometry
D. Dilated retinopathy

4. A 60-year-old woman states that she believes she is having a stroke. She noticed that her face was distorted when she looked into a mirror to comb her hair.

On physical examination, she has an inability to close the right eye completely, cannot wrinkle the right side of the forehead, has decreased hearing in the right ear, has an unsteady gait, falls to the right, and has flattening of the right side of her face.

What pathology should be sought?

A. A left middle cerebral thrombosis
B. A right facial nerve palsy (Bell's palsy)
C. A left carotid dissection
D. A right cerebropontine-angle neuroma

5. A 68-year-old woman complains of severe substernal chest pain that radiates to the back. She has a 5-year history of hypertension. The pain started while she was at rest, but has

become progressively more severe, feeling like something tearing, and has caused her to become very restless. An EKG is obtained (see Figure 5-1).

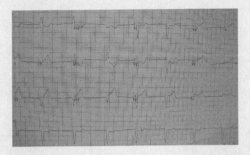

Figure 5-1

The most likely diagnosis is:

A. Third-degree heart block
B. Left bundle-branch block
C. Inferior wall myocardial infarction
D. Ascending aortic dissection

6. A 70-year-old man is brought to the ED by his wife complaining of chest pain. He has noticed some dizziness while bending over to play with his dog, and then an onset of substernal fullness. This was yesterday, and the pain has come and gone now for more than 24 hours. While he is being placed in a room, an EKG is obtained (Figure 5-2):

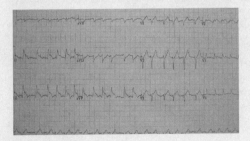

Figure 5-2

As the EKG is being obtained, he becomes very dizzy.

Vital Signs: BP 80/60 mmHg, P 180 beats/min and irregular, R 20 breaths/min, T 37°C, O_2 sat 90%.

The next steps taken should be:

A. Complete the history from the wife, perform a physical examination, and administer verapamil 10 mg. Give nasal oxygen via nose clip at 4 L/min.

B. Complete the history from the wife, perform a physical examination, and administer adenosine 4 mg IV. Give nasal oxygen via nose clip at 4 L/min.

C. Immediately obtain the cardiac catheter laboratory. Give heparin 5000 U IV. Give oxygen by nonrebreathing face mask at 100%.

D. Give versed 3 mg IV. Cardiovert at 200 wsecs. Prepare for rapid sequence intubation.

7. A 6-year-old boy is brought to the ED by his father. He has a very loud barking cough and sounds like a seal. His father states he was well until the evening prior when he began to run a fever. This evening, his temperature was 39.5°C taken by the mother orally. The father brought the child in because there are three other children at home, who while well, are all younger than this boy.

Vital Signs: BP 110/70 mmHg, P 120 beats/min, R 20 breaths/min, T 40°C, O_2 sat 96%.

Most likely the management will be:

A. Epinephrine, steroids, humidified air, and discharge to home

B. Imaging of the neck, antibiotics, visualization of the epiglottis, intubation

C. Humidified air, steroids, antibiotics, and admission to ICU

D. Bronchoscopy, antibiotics, and admission to ICU

8. A 75-year-old woman presents with confusion, weakness, and increasing inability to care for herself. She lives with her daughter, who states that her mother was alert and self-sustaining until about the last couple of weeks.

Vital Signs: BP 140/90 mmHg, P 90 beats/min and irregular, R 14 breaths/min, T 37°C, O_2 sat 94%.

A commonly overlooked diagnosis in this age group is:

A. Urinary tract infection
B. Diabetes
C. Alzheimer's disease
D. Hyperthyroidism

9. An 18-year-old man is involved in a motor vehicle crash. He was not wearing a seat belt, seemed repetitive and irritable at the scene, and was thought to be unconscious by some bystanders, although he was awake when the paramedics arrived. He has a bruise on his forehead, and the right tympanic membrane appears to be somewhat more purple than the left.

What imaging study will suggest an explanation of the patient's problem?

A. Skull x-ray study
B. Sinus film study
C. Panorex mandible study
D. Lateral cervical spine study

10. A 50-year-old man presents with a complaint of chest pain. He reports that he had become intoxicated at a dinner party the night before and had vomited copiously. Some hours later when he awakened after passing out, he felt like there was pain in his chest.

Vital Signs: BP 150/100 mmHg, P 120 beats/min, R 20 breaths/min, T 38°C, O_2 sat 95%.

A noticeable physical finding is a grating sound with each heartbeat.

To make the diagnosis in this patient, which of the following tests would be most useful?

A. A nasogastric aspirate for hemoccult blood
B. A serum iron level
C. A chest CT scan with contrast
D. A direct fiber-optic esophagoscopy

11. A 50-year-old man presents with chest pain, frequent urination at night, some fatigue, and increased hunger.

    Vital Signs: BP 140/90 mmHg, P 110 beats/min, R 24 breaths/min, T 37°C, O_2 sat 96%. An EKG shows nonspecific ST-T wave changes; no change from a recent prior tracing.

    Which test is most likely to yield a diagnosis in the ED?

    A. Echocardiogram
    B. Chest CT scan
    C. Rectal examination
    D. Fingerstick glucose

12. An 80-year-old woman presents with weakness and an episode of syncope.

    Vital Signs: BP 100/60 mmHg, P 120 beats/min, R 16 breaths/min, T 37°C, O_2 sat 96%.

    Which physical examination finding is most likely to lead to a diagnosis?

    A. Chest auscultation
    B. Abdominal palpation
    C. Neurologic examination
    D. Rectal examination

13. A 23-year-old women presents with joint pain in both knees. Physical examination reveals tender and swollen knee joints bilaterally. In addition, there are several blisters on her right index finger, and the proximal interphalangeal joint is tender. Additional history reveals that the patient has been taking penicillin throat lozenges for a sore throat, given to her by her boyfriend. She has been sexually active.

    What diagnosis is probable?

    A. Penicillin allergy
    B. Acute rheumatoid arthritis
    C. Degenerative arthritis
    D. Disseminated gonorrhea

14. A 25-year-old women is brought to the ED by her boyfriend, who states she has been raped and demands an examination, for which he insists upon being present.

She has had multiple visits to the ED, as well as many primary care offices for a number of fractures, bruises, and lacerations, all of which she states came from her women's soccer matches. The woman privately tells the nurse while she is undressing that she has not been raped, but that her boyfriend is jealous and believes she has been sleeping with another man. On physical examination, the physician notes circumferential bruising around the woman's neck.

What is the best strategy for the workup of this patient?

A. Complete hematologic workup to find a bleeding diathesis
B. A pregnancy test and a rape examination without the boyfriend
C. A bone density study to look for osteoporosis
D. A social service consultation and admission

15. A 1½-year-old boy is brought to the ED because he won't eat or drink. On examination, there is a red mark at the left corner of the mouth, and no sign of bleeding or bruising. The mother states he was with a babysitter this afternoon and was normal until then. The sitter stated he had been crawling around the living room, when she heard him crying and found him sitting, bawling holding a lamp cord.

What complication is of great concern in this scenario?

A. Nonaccidental trauma
B. Fifth disease
C. Electric burn hemorrhage
D. Hand, foot, and mouth disease

16. A 20-year-old man is a passenger in a motor vehicle crash that T-boned the vehicle from the driver's side. He was not wearing a seat belt; he hit his head on the right window and doesn't remember the crash or anything afterwards until he was in the ambulance on the way to the hospital. He is complaining of severe pain in his right ear. At the ED his vital signs are: BP 130/85 mmHg, P 92 beats/min, R 16 breaths/min, T 37.4°C, O₂ sat 99%. He is alert, although somewhat repetitive, and there are no significant physical findings. He repeatedly complains of severe pain in his right ear, but there is no hemotympanum, no Battle's sign, and no tenderness over the zygoma or mandible.

Which of the following imaging studies is most likely to reveal the significant pathology?

A. Panorex mandible film
B. CT scan of the cervical spine
C. CT scan of the head
D. Water's view of the facial bones

17. A 25-year-old man enters the ED complaining of pain in the right scrotum. He is sexually active. He states the pain has come on over the prior 36 hours and is now unbearable. He says it even hurts to urinate. On physical examination the vital signs are normal with no fever. The genitourinary examination reveals a very tender right scrotum that appears red and inflamed. The testicle is very tender and feels somewhat boggy.

Which of the following is the best management?

A. Urologic consult to take the patient to the operating room
B. Urinalysis, culture, and prescription for ciprofloxacin and pyridium
C. Urinalysis, ice to the scrotum, antibiotics, and lidocaine block of the spermatic cord
D. Doppler ultrasound of the scrotum, analgesics, and emergent urologic consultation

18. A 24-year-old man presents to the ED with a painful finger. He states that he pricked his finger with a wood splinter the day before. He removed the entire splinter but now has a painful index finger. The distal digit is red and tender, but there is no fluctuance or purulence observed. The fingernail is normal. The patient has no history of cold sores.

Correct management includes which of the following?

A. Antiviral therapy with acyclovir, splinting the finger, and follow-up with primary care physician
B. Incision and drainage of the finger, antibiotics, and follow-up with hand surgeon

   C. Antibiotics, analgesics, and incision and drainage for purulence or fluctuance

   D. Xerox-ray for wooden foreign body, follow-up with hand surgeon

19. A 57-year-old man enters the ED complaining of severe pain in his scrotum. He is a type 2 diabetic and states that he takes glyburide to control his blood sugar. He doesn't measure the levels of blood glucose. He has had some problems in initiating his urinary stream and states he gets up every few hours at night to void. He wants something for pain because he cannot stand the pain in his right groin.

Vital Signs: BP 150/100 mmHg, P 110 beats/min, R 16 breaths/min, T 38°C, O_2 sat 97%. On physical examination, there is no swelling in the right groin or scrotum. The testicle is tender but not enlarged, and the spermatic cord feels normal. There are no indirect or direct inguinal hernias present. On rectal examination, the prostate is enlarged x 2 without any nodules and is somewhat tender.

What diagnosis is suggested by this presentation?

   A. Inguinal sliding hernia that has reduced spontaneously

   B. Testicular torsion

   C. Fournier's gangrene

   D. Acute bacterial prostatitis

20. An 18-year-old woman is brought to the ED by her friends. They state she had been at a frat party, did a lot of drinking, and passed out. They watched her for about an hour, but when they couldn't arouse her, they decided to bring her to the ED.

Vital Signs: BP 120/70 mmHg, P 100 beats/min, R 12 breaths/min, T 37°C, O_2 sat 96%.

She has no focal neurologic findings. She is lightly comatose, responding to pain but not verbal or light touch stimulation. She does not appear to have a gag reflex and does not struggle when the oral cavity is examined. The emergency physician decides to intubate her and does so without incident. About 30 minutes after intubation, she is observed to be struggling against the endotracheal tube, and appears to be awake.

Management of this patient should include which of the following?

A. Urine and serum toxicology screens
B. Rape examination
C. Admission to the ICU
D. Extubation and discharge when fully awake

21. An 8-year-old girl is brought to the ED at the request of her chiropractor. The mother states the girl has had a mild upper respiratory infection for about 10 days prior and some muscle stiffness, so she took her to the chiropractor for a manipulation. The mother is divorced from a chiropractor, and her father was also one, so she is adamant that the manipulation is all the child really needs. The chiropractor sends a note that says: This child will not benefit from manipulation; her tissues feel very doughy to me. The mother tells me her urine is dark and that she has no appetite.

What diagnostic test would you wish to order?

A. Urinalysis
B. Cervical spine x-ray study
C. Chest x-ray study
D. Blood culture

22. A 23-year-old women complains of abdominal pain and that her eyes are yellow. She reports that she has had some lower abdominal pain and discharge as well. Social history reveals that she is sexually active and has several partners. On physical examination the vital signs are: BP 120/80 mmHg, P 110 beats/min, R 16 breaths/min, T 38.5°C, O_2 sat 98%. She appears uncomfortable. The sclerae are yellow. The abdomen is tender, especially in the right upper quadrant. Bowel sounds are minimal.

Workup should include which of the following?

A. CBC, chest x-ray, blood cultures, and urine cultures
B. Pelvic examination, vaginal cultures, metabolic panel, and urine hCG test
C. RUQ ultrasound, hepatic enzymes, lipase, and bilirubin level
D. Abdominal CT scan, CT scan of the abdomen, abdominal paracentesis, and culture

23. A 25-year-old man presents with weakness. He states that he has had a flu syndrome for about a week prior to entrance to the ED. He noticed some cough, some pharyngeal discomfort, and some muscle aching. He states he just got back from a business trip, and a lot of people on the plane were coughing. He has noticed over the past 24 hours that his legs were "tired," and he felt like he was using a great effort just to walk. He came to the ED because he was having trouble breathing: "It feels like I don't have the strength to get air in." No past history of asthma, pneumonia, familiar weaknesses, thyroid disease, or other serious illnesses. All childhood immunizations are up to date. Vital signs are: BP 130/70 mmHg, P 100 beats/min, R 20 breaths/min, T 38°C, O$_2$ sat 93%. On physical examination, the chest is clear to percussion with a few crackles but no wheezes on auscultation. The cardiac examination is normal. The abdomen is nontender. The neurologic examination reveals that the legs are bilaterally weak, and the patient cannot hold them up off the examination table. The deep tendon reflexes are diminished with absent knee jerks bilaterally. The Babinski's examination is nonresponsive to plantar stroking. The arms are of normal strength with good biceps and triceps reflexes. There are no sensory deficits.

What diagnostic and therapeutic measures does the patient need?

A. A lumbar puncture and external respirator
B. A metabolic panel and potassium therapy
C. A lumbar puncture and endotracheal intubation
D. A chest x-ray study and albuterol breathing treatment

24. A 64-year-old woman is a tourist traveling to Yellowstone Park. She and her husband are on vacation with their church group and have traveled by bus from their home in Green Bay, Wisconsin. They have just stayed overnight in Jackson Hole, Wyoming (altitude 6200 feet). She did not sleep well in the motel the prior night and felt like she was having trouble breathing. Today, on the bus, as they crossed the continental divide (8400 feet), she became aware of even more difficulty breathing so has come to the clinic at Yellowstone Lake (altitude 7000 feet). She is feeling a little better now but is still having trouble getting enough air. She has a past history of mild congestive heart failure from hypertension, which has

been successfully treated with Lasix. She stopped taking the Lasix during the trip, because it was so difficult to urinate on the bus.

Vital Signs: BP 150/100 mmHg, P 110 beats/min, R 22 breaths/min, T 37.2°C, O_2 sat 90%.

What is this patient likely to need?

A. Endotracheal intubation; helicopter transport to the nearest ICU; and urgent blood pressure lowering

B. Oxygen therapy, mild diuresis, and descent to sea level

C. Nitrate therapy, IV lasix, and serial cardiac enzymes

D. Antibiotics, endotracheal intubation, ventilation

25. A 48-year-old man presents with pain in his left lower chest. He describes the pain as a mild ache that has persisted for about a week in the back of the left chest, where he cannot visualize the area. The ache has turned into a burning sensation, and he states that he is quite uncomfortable. It seems to him that the pain, while worsening, is now crossing to the right side of his back and chest, but at the same level as the original pain on the left. On questioning about the past history, he states that he is HIV positive, with a CD4 count of 100 several months ago. He has not been sexually active for several months. He remembers having chicken pox as a child.

Vital Signs: BP 130/80 mmHg, P 90 beats/min, R 14 breaths/min, T 37.4°C, O_2 sat 98%. On physical examination, there is an erythematous rash with some clear blisters that extends from the left sixth posterior midscapular line to the right midscapular line. The patient states that this is where he feels the pain, but there is no direct tenderness in the area.

What is the appropriate management for this patient?

A. Tell him he has Herpes zoster, give him adequate vicodin, and have him follow with his primary care physician.

B. Offer him analgesia, oral acyclovir, start him on tegretol, and have him follow up with a neurologist.

C. Start him on topical steroids, tell him he has pityriasis rosea, and have him follow up with dermatology.

   D. Check the current CD4 level, admit him to the hospital, and start him on IV acyclovir.

26. A 57-year-old man gets his hand caught in a taco-making press; he wraps the hand in a rag and comes to the ED. On physical examination, the digits are crushed, dirty, and blue, and hanging by the flexor tendons. See Figure 5-3.

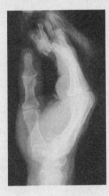

Figure 5-3

Which of the following plans for management is correct?

   A. Antibiotics, cooling of the fingers, and reimplantation with microvascular surgery

   B. Antibiotics, repair of fingers, and referral to hand surgeon

   C. Antibiotics, amputation of the digits by emergency physician, and follow up with primary care physician

   D. Antibiotics, splint fingers, and amputation by hand surgeon at a time of his choice

27. A 26-year-old man comes to the ED from his brother's birthday party because of pain in the right groin. He states he has had painful swelling in his right groin for about a month. Initially, he became aware of a lump there and went to see a physician who treated him for epididymitis, but the lump stayed the same, and he became aware of his leg swelling and becoming tender. The day before, he went to an ED for the discomfort and swelling, and they did an ultrasound study of the leg that was normal. He was advised to be admitted for workup but wanted to attend the birthday party. At the party, he felt uncomfortable but had acute pain when he had a toast to his brother. On physical examination, the vital signs are normal. The circumference of the right thigh is 4 inches greater than that of the left. There is no swelling or reddening. There is a mass of matted lymph nodes in the right groin. There is no hernia or hydrocele, and the right spermatic cord feels a little boggy and is larger than the left, but is nontender.

Which diagnostic study is likely to reveal the pathology?

A. Repeat Doppler ultrasound of the right calf and thigh
B. Urinalysis, rectal examination, and urethral swab for culture and Gram's stain
C. Pelvic CT scan with contrast
D. Right leg venography with IV contrast

28. A 64-year-old man enters the ED complaining of cough. His wife who accompanies him says his eyes look funny. She can't say exactly why. She also says that he has had the cough for years, and she made him come because it seems worse at night, and she is having trouble sleeping because of it. The patient reports that he has smoked more than two packs of cigarettes per day for as long as he can remember. The vital signs are normal. On physical examination, the pupils are unequal, the left being 2 mm greater than the right. Moreover, the right eyelid appears droopy. The patient can wrinkle both sides of the forehead, and extraocular eye movements appear normal. It is a hot and humid day, and the patient appears to be sweating, mostly on the left side of his face. The chest examination is normal except for some bilateral rhonchi.

What diagnostic test is likely to give the answer?

A. Sputum for Gram's stain, culture, and acid-fast study
B. Right carotid Doppler ultrasound study
C. Chest x-ray study
D. Bronchography with contrast

29. A 5-year-old girl is brought to the ED by her mother because she is "bruising easily." The child has had a mild cold for about 5 days. Today the mother noted that the child's shins were purple

and became concerned about leukemia. The child has been complaining of pain in her ankles and knees as well as a stomach ache. Prior to all of this, she had been normal with only a couple of ear infections in the past. All immunizations are up to date.

Vital Signs: BP 110/70 mmHg, P 110 beats/min, R 12 breaths/min, T 37.4°C, O_2 sat 99%. The child appears alert but seems to be uncomfortable. She sits with her arms around her mother, and she does not want to be examined. HEENT: the nose is crusted; the pharynx appears slightly reddened with no exudate. There is some minor jugular digastric lymphadenopathy. The neck is supple. The tympanic membranes are clear, gray, and move well on insufflation. Back: there is one patch of ecchymosis over the left posterior chest. Chest is normal to auscultation and percussion. Cardiac: no murmurs or rubs. Abdomen: diffusely tender in midepigastrium with no masses, splinting, or rebound; the bowel sounds are normal. Extremities: there are purple ecchymoses over the shins.

Neurologic: normal

Which of the following is probable?

A. This is early leukemia. Clotting studies and a bone marrow will be necessary.

B. This is Henoch-Schönlein purpura. No imaging studies will be necessary, but the child should be admitted.

C. This is nonaccidental trauma. Not only should a skeletal survey be performed, but a serum lipase should be obtained to look for traumatic pancreatitis.

D. This is meningococcemia. The child will need blood cultures, isolation, and a lumbar puncture. Start steroids because of adrenal hemorrhage.

30. A 68-year-old woman presents complaining of weakness. She states that she isn't sure when she started feeling poorly, perhaps some months ago, but comes in because she just can't take care of herself any longer, because she lives alone. She believes she is gaining weight but doesn't weigh herself. She has noticed her hair falling out, and her friends tell her that her voice is getting "full of gravel." She states she is thinking of moving south because she is cold all the time.

Vital Signs are normal. The patient appears in no distress. HEENT: the face looks somewhat diffusely swollen. The neck has no masses. The arteries in the neck have no bruits. Chest: the lungs are clear and the heart has no murmurs. Abdomen: soft, nontender, and no masses. Extremities: the ankles are swollen, but there is no pitting edema. Neurologic: there are no focal findings. The deep tendon reflexes seem very slow.

Which strategy would you choose to evaluate this patient?

A. Basic metabolic panel, urinalysis, EKG, and social service consult for placement if all are normal.

B. Cardiac enzymes, EKG, chest x-ray study, and admit for observation and an early treadmill study.

C. Complete metabolic panel including thyroid studies and admission for commencement of thyroxin therapy.

D. Cortisol level, and admit for adrenocorticotropic hormone (ACTH)–stimulation study. Commence steroid replacement therapy.

31. A 53-year-old man presents to the ED complaining of shoulder pain. He states he was well until he went to sleep the night before and awoke with pain in his shoulder. He can barely move his arm. He leads a sedentary life and has no physical hobbies. He has not lifted anything heavy at work or at home. On physical examination, he cannot elevate the involved left shoulder. He cannot flex the left shoulder, abduct it, or reach behind his trunk to his wallet pocket. There is no swelling, bruising, or deformity. The shoulder is diffusely tender to touch. The only other positive physical finding is a bite mark on the left buccal mucosa. He states he doesn't remember biting his cheek.

What diagnostic imaging study would you wish to see?

A. Plain shoulder x-ray series

B. Left shoulder x-ray with and without weights

C. Left shoulder arthrogram or left shoulder CT scan

D. Head CT scan with and without contrast

32. A 28-year-old Laotian woman is brought to the ED in status epilepticus. The paramedics state that she lives alone, and that the neighbor who heard her scream and found her seizing doesn't know much about her. She thought the patient was getting a divorce and knows that she goes to a medical clinic, but is not sure why, but thought she had tuberculosis. Despite receiving multiple doses of versed, valium, dilantin, and phenobarbital, the patient continues to seize.

What step should be taken next to stop the seizures?

A. Perform a rapid sequence intubation and give curare

B. Repeat dilantin and valium and stop the oxygen

C. Give another dose of versed and prepare for general anesthesia

D. Obtain as much pyridoxine as your pharmacy has and start it as an IV infusion

33. A 1-year-old infant is brought to the ED because the mother reports he awakened screaming in the middle of the night. She was unable to console him, but then he had a bowel movement and stopped crying. He has never been ill before, and the mother had a full-term vaginal delivery after an uneventful gestation.

    Physical examination reveals a quiet, sleeping infant, who periodically sucks on a pacifier.

    Vital Signs: BP not taken, no cuff small enough in your ED, 130 beats/min, R 14 breaths/min, T 37.4°C rectally, O_2 sat 98%. On physical examination, the child appears to be completely normal. A rectal examination reveals no stool. The mother did not save the diaper that appeared to relieve him, but she thought it had a funny dark purple color.

    Your plan for the child is which of the following:

    A. Don't disturb the child with blood tests, but have the child follow the next day with the pediatrician

    B. Call in the pediatric surgeon to take the child to the operating room for exploration

    C. Obtain a barium or air-contrast enema

    D. Obtain an ultrasound study of the abdomen

34. A 49-year-old alcoholic man is found down and brought to the ED. The paramedics found his fingerstick glucose to be 60 mg/dL and administered an ampule of 50% dextrose.

Vital Signs: BP 150/100 mmHg, P 120 beats/min, R 24 breaths/min, T 36°C, O_2 sat 96%.

What is your initial management of this patient while you define the metabolic abnormalities?

A. IV normal saline heparin lock, metabolic panel, arterial blood gases, and blood alcohol level.

B. IV 5% dextrose with normal saline with an ampoule of multivitamins, thiamine 100 mg, and observe in the ED for appropriate alcohol metabolism.

C. Rapid-sequence intubation, head CT scan, and immediate neurosurgical consultation.

D. CT scan of head, chest, and abdomen, and immediate trauma surgery consultation.

35. An 8-year-old African American boy limps into the ED complaining of a painful right knee. He denies trauma, but he is an active child and runs around with his friends constantly. On physical examination, the knee is not swollen and is not tender; however, there is a limited range of motion of the right leg.

What diagnostic studies would you order from the following choices?

A. Sickle cell preparation, complete blood count, and reticulocyte count

B. Right knee x-ray series

C. Right hip x-ray series

D. All of the above

36. An 18-year-old woman enters the ED complaining of severe odynophagia, fever, and feeling very tired. She is living in a dormitory and is in her first year of college. Student health service saw her yesterday and started her on amoxicillin for a "strep throat." Today, her throat is worse. She can't eat or drink anything, has a new-onset rash on her trunk, face, and back, and has new abdominal pain. She feels weak and a little dizzy.

Vital Signs: BP 100/60 mmHg, P 110 beats/min, R 14 breaths/min, T 38.4°C, O_2 sat 98%.

She appears to be fatigued, somewhat anxious, and has dry mucous membranes. There is an erythematous rash on her face and anterior and posterior trunk. The throat has severe erythematous and purulent ulcerations over both tonsils. There is marked tender lymphadenopathy of the cervical nodes, inguinal nodes, and both elbow epitrochlear nodes. The thorax examination is normal, but the abdominal examination shows enlargement of both liver and spleen. The extremities are normal. The neurologic examination is normal.

What diagnostic and therapeutic steps would you choose from the following?

A. Monospot, abdominal ultrasound, IV fluids, stop ampicillin, analgesics, and admission

B. Abdominal CT scan, benadryl, steroids, H_2 blocker, epinephrine, and stop ampicillin

C. CT scan of the chest, add clindamycin, IV fluids, and discharge to dormitory

D. Admit for bone marrow and lymph node biopsy, ENT consult for tracheotomy, and lupus erythematosus panel

37. An 8-year-old boy is brought to the ED by his mother because he has a painful swollen face. He has been sick with low grade fever, runny nose, and sore throat for several days. Today his fever was better, but he complains of pain in his left jaw, and the mother thinks his face is swollen. He is up to date on his immunizations, the mother thinks, but she forgot to bring the shot card with her. On physical examination, the throat is reddened without ulceration or exudate. There is a tender swelling above the mandible on the left side of the boy's face. Compression over the swelling does not produce any pus in the mouth. There are some tender jugular digastric lymph nodes and some firm but nontender cervical nodes. The neck is supple. The tympanic membranes are normal.

The extremities show some long scratches. (The mother states there is a new kitten at home with which the boy has been playing.)

The most likely diagnosis is which of the following?

A. Submaxillary gland stone

B. Cat scratch fever

C. Infectious mononucleosis

D. Mumps

38. A 29-year-old woman is driving to her prenatal appointment when she is involved in a minor car crash. She is in the third trimester of her first pregnancy. Although she has no complaints, she wants her baby checked out. There is no obstetric service at this hospital to which she has come.

Vital Signs: BP 100/60 mmHg, P 90 beats/min, R 12 breaths/min, T 37.4°C, O_2 sat 99%. On physical examination, she has some slight tenderness in the lower abdomen. She was not wearing a seat belt. There is no vaginal discharge externally, and there is no blood in the vagina. There are fetal heart tones at 130 beats/min in the right lower quadrant of the abdomen.

Which of the following is your management plan?

A. Reassure the mother that she and her baby are all right, and have her continue on her way for her prenatal check

B. Transfer her to your sister hospital where there are obstetric services for fetal monitoring and obstetric consultation

C. Ask one of your staff gynecologic surgeons to evaluate the patient for emergent cesarean section

D. Admit the patient to the trauma service for observation, and request that her obstetrician come and consult

39. A 40-year-old alcoholic woman comes to the ED complaining of leg pain. She states that she can't stand the pain in her leg and wants you to give her some pain medicine. She has been drinking, her speech is slurred, and she is well known to your ED for her multiple visits, usually for extreme intoxication. In addition, she has a history of diabetes mellitus, which is usually poorly controlled, since she is often too intoxicated to take insulin on a regular basis. She states that the pain began several days prior. She thinks she may have been kicked in the leg but can't really remember because "I have been on a binge."

Vital Signs: BP 150/100 mmHg, P 110 beats/min, R 16 breaths/min, T 37.9°C, O_2 sat 96%. The skin shows multiple generations of bruises, and the newest ones are not on the painful right leg. The head and neck are clear, and the chest reveals some diffuse basilar rhonchi. The cardiac examination is normal. The abdomen is soft and nontender, and the liver is enlarged 4 cm below the right costal border. The left leg is normal, but the right leg is extremely tender, although there is no reddening or swelling. The neurologic examination has no focal neurologic deficits, other than that the patient is clearly intoxicated.

A fingerstick glucose is 300 mg/dL. The blood alcohol is 220 mg%.

What is your preferable management strategy among the following?

A. A yellow IV (D5%NS plus multivitamins and thiamine), analgesia, 2 units of regular insulin, and repeat finger stick glucose (FSG) every 1 hour; and observation until the patient is functionally sober, and the blood sugar < 200 mg/dL.

B. X-ray study of the right leg, analgesia, and if the x-ray is negative, observe until functionally sober and discharge.

C. Ultrasound study of the right leg, yellow IV, analgesia, antibiotics, and surgical consultation.

D. Yellow IV, analgesia, valium as the patient sobers, and then discharge.

40. A 40-year-old woman is picking up her son from hockey practice at the local skating rink, but she slips on the wet floor and strikes her chest on the railing around the rink. The next day, she has increasing pain in her chest that worsens with trying to lie flat. She took some motrin, but with no relief. Her prior medical history is positive only for one pregnancy, the usual childhood diseases, and an appendectomy at age 19. She has been in good health and takes no medications. She is not pregnant and is still having regular menses.

Vital Signs: BP 130/80 mmHg, P 92 beats/min, R 18 breaths/min, T 37.4°C, O_2 sat 96%. The pertinent physical finding is that she has a mitral click (which she says she has had for several years, and a rubbing sound that accompanies diastole.

The chest x-ray study is normal with no rib fractures, normal sized cardiac silhouette, and no hemopneumothorax, no sternal fracture, and no pleural effusion.

The EKG shows a sinus tachycardia; normal intervals, and some nonspecific ST-T wave changes in the left precordium. She has never had a prior tracing.

There is no ST depression. The PR interval is normal, and there is no PR depression.

Prudent management strategy includes which of the following:

A. Serial troponin levels, serial EKGs, hospital admission, and early treadmill test in the morning.

B. Start therapy with indocin after a dose of IV toradol, repeat EKG over the next few days, and follow with primary care physician.

C. Start steroids with prednisone taper, add nonsteroidal anti-inflammatory drugs (NSAIDs), and follow with cardiology.

D. Obtain a CT angiography (CTA), give a dose of lovenox while waiting for the study, and admit to the hospital if the CTA is positive.

41. A 55-year-old alcoholic man enters the ED complaining of nausea, vomiting, feeling flushed, chest pain, and weakness. He was just discharged from a detoxification program and was given a new medication.

Vital Signs: BP 80/60 mmHg, P 120 beats/min, R 20 breaths/min, T 37°C, O_2 sat 92%.

The skin is red and flushed, although there are no urticaria to be found. The chest has distant heart sounds with a sinus tachycardia and no murmurs, and some diffuse rhonchi. The abdomen is soft and nontender. The extremities have some old bruising. The neurologic examination is nonfocal.

What is the most likely explanation from the choices below?

A. Alcohol/antabuse reaction
B. Acute coronary syndrome
C. Acute anaphylaxis
D. Acute withdrawal syndrome

42. A 48-year-old women is brought in by the paramedics in a coma. A friend called 911 when she went to visit and found the woman down and unarousable. The paramedics state there was a suicide note, and that, according to the friend, the patient has been depressed over a divorce. There was an empty pill bottle without label at the house. The friend did not know any of the medical details of the patient's history but stated that she had been complaining of insomnia.

Vital Signs: BP 100/80 mmHg, P 110 beats/min, R 8 breaths/min, O_2 sat 84%.

There are multiple bullae over the patients back. The HEENT are atraumatic. There is no jugular venous distention. The neck is supple. The pupils are midrange and reactive. The fundi are normal. The chest is clear to percussion, but there are diffuse rales throughout. The heart reveals a regular tachycardia. There are no murmurs, rubs, or gallops. The abdomen is soft, scaphoid, and nontender with no organomegaly. The pelvic examination was not done. The extremities were not edematous. The neurologic examination revealed no focal findings, but very depressed deep tendon reflexes at +1 everywhere tested. The patient reacted only with withdrawal to very deep pain. A fingerstick glucose had been 90 mg/dL in the field. The patient had not reacted to Narcan in the field.

Management strategies include which of the following:

A. Physostigmine, charcoal per nasogastric tube, toxicology screen, and admit to ICU

B. Rapid-sequence intubation, bicarbonate drip, and hemodialysis

C. Rapid-sequence intubation, ICU admission, and IV fluid maintenance

D. Hyperbaric chamber, cyanide kit, and prophylactic tympanoplasties

43. An 82-year-old woman is brought to the ED by EMS, who have called her in as a stroke. They have intubated her in the field. They also gave her an ampoule of 50% dextrose because their glucometer was broken, and the husband gave a history of insulin-dependent diabetes mellitus.

Vital Signs: BP 150/100 mmHg, P 100 beats/min, R 12 breaths/min, T 37°C, O_2 sat 92%.

The HEENT is atraumatic, with supple neck. The back is normal. The chest is clear to percussion and auscultation. The heart is not enlarged; there is a regular tachycardia; and there are no extra beats, murmurs, or rubs. The abdomen is soft and nontender. The extremities show no edema. The neurologic examination shows constricted pupils and the eyes deviated to the left. The deep tendon reflexes are brisk on the right side but absent on the left. The left arm and leg are straight and do not respond to pinprick, whereas the right side moves in response to pain. The rectal examination shows normal tone. The toes are upgoing to plantar stroking on the left and withdraw on the right.

The husband appears and offers the following history: The patient was eating dinner and became unresponsive. This was about 3 hours ago. Neither had talked much during the meal, but that was customary. The patient took her usual dose of 20 units NPH insulin that morning before breakfast, as was customary. She had eaten lunch. She was in good health and was taking aldomet for longstanding hypertension that was well controlled, although he didn't know her usual blood pressure. She had a history of some kind of eye problem and had just that week been given a new set of eyedrops; he didn't know the name but seemed to recognize atenolol.

What is your next step (of the following) in managing this patient?

A. Obtain a noncontrast CT scan, and summon the stroke team to give TPA

B. Obtain a noncontrast CT scan and an MRI to follow, and admit to the ICU

C. Give another ampoule of 50% dextrose, and prepare to extubate the patient

D. Obtain a PET scan, and admit the patient for comfort care

44. A 24-year-old woman is brought to the ED by her mother, with whom she lives. They had been having an argument about the need for the patient to go to work, when the young woman fell to the ground. She did not lose consciousness but said she could feel nothing in her legs, and could not stand up, bear weight, or walk. She was carried to the car by two brothers. They said they did not call an ambulance because they couldn't afford the bill.

Vital signs are normal. The rectal examination is normal. All the extremity pulsations are normal. The neurologic examination reveals no sensation from the mid-thigh down to the toes. There is no response to pain in either leg, including deep pinprick. There is no response to vibration, temperature, hot or cold, or light touch with a cotton-tipped swab. When the leg is passively elevated, it is held upright, without falling to the gurney, but the patient cannot lift the heel of her foot off the bed. In addition, she can neither abduct or adduct the hip. The deep tendon reflexes are normal. On stroking the sole of the feet, the toes do not move. The patient appears unconcerned about her condition and requests a food tray.

Select the appropriate management from the following:

A. Neurosurgical consultation, MRI of the back, and place on fluid and food restriction in the event that surgery is needed.

B. Vascular surgical consultation, Doppler ultrasound of the pelvis, and administer lovenox 1 mg/kg.

C. High-dose steroids 5 mg/kg followed by 1 mg/kg infusion, orthopedic spine consultation, and CT scan of the spine.

D. Reassure the patient that she will get well and obtain a psychiatric consultation.

45. A 53-year-old alcoholic man was brought in by EMS because they found him wandering in the middle of the street with cars whizzing past him. They could obtain no coherent history from him. Although he was shouting gibberish at the cars, he had no odor of alcoholic beverages on him.

Vital Signs: BP 150/100 mmHg, P 110 beats/min, R 18 breaths/min, T 37.9°C, O_2 sat 94%.

The patient is disheveled, dirty, but answers questions, although the answers are convoluted and nonresponsive. HEENT reveals a nystagmus that is horizontal, with the eyes not moving well to the left. The pupils are midrange and equal. The fundi are not visualized because of the nystagmus and the patient's inability to cooperate. The neck is supple. The chest examination reveals bilateral coarse rhonchi. The heart is not enlarged or tachycardic, and there are no murmurs, rubs, or gallops. The abdomen is soft, and the liver is enlarged 4 cm below the right costal border. The bowel sounds are normal. The extremities have multiple-generation bruises, in that some look fresh and some old. The neurologic examination shows brisk 3+ deep tendon reflexes that are symmetric. There are no focal deficits. The patient confabulates upon questioning. When asked to draw a clock face with the time of 2:30, he states he is no artist. Following additional requests, he tries but cannot place the clock hands within the clock and has no idea of where 2:30 would be. He has a coarse tremor in both hands and arms.

Your best management strategy of the following would be which option?

A. A yellow IV (5% dextrose with normal saline with an ampoule of multivitamins and thiamine 100 mg) fingerstick glucose, valium IV, admission to the ICU, and neurologic consultation.

B. Noncontrast CT scan, lumbar puncture, IV antibiotics, and admission to the ICU.

C. IV D5W keep open, MRI ordered, dilantin bolus, and admission to medical unit.

D. Psychiatric consult, social worker consult for placement, haldol 2 mg orally, and admission to nonmedical detoxification unit.

46. A 68-year-old man has a syncopal episode in the bathroom at his home. EMS is called and transports to your ED. Vital signs in the field: BP 70/palpated mmHg, P 120 beats/min, R 16 breaths/min, O_2 sat 92%. In the ED, the patient is awake and complains of pain in the back, which he states has been bothering him for a few weeks, but was more severe this morning. He states he was hospitalized for an upper gastrointestinal bleed 4 months ago, but the source was not found. This was in another city. He has moved here to live with his daughter. Past history includes a myocardial infarction (MI) 2 years ago that was treated with an angioplasty. He no longer takes plavix but does take an aspirin every day. He had a transient ischemic attack after the MI, but he has never had a stroke. He smoked heavily for many years but quit after the MI. He has had type 2 diabetes for 15 years, but he does not test blood sugars because he says he is well controlled with glyburide.

Vital signs in the ED: BP 102/60 mmHg, P 110 beats/min, T 37°C, O_2 sat 90%. On physical examination, he has a bilateral arcus senilis. The neck is supple. There is a grade 3 bruit in the right carotid artery. The chest is clear to percussion and auscultation. The heart is enlarged to the left anterior axillary line. There is a grade 3/6 systolic murmur heard best over the left sternal border in the sixth intercostal space. The rate is regular but rapid. The abdomen is diffusely tender but no masses are palpated. The rectal examination shows no blood or occult positive stool, but the prostate is enlarged times two, with no nodules. The groin shows no herniae. The extremities have very faint femoral pulses and absent popliteal, dorsalis pedis, and posterior tibial pulses. The legs are somewhat wasted and hairless.

Which of the following is your selected management?

A. EKG, type and cross 4 units packed red blood cells (PRBCs), metabolic panel, CBC, focused abdominal sonography for trauma (FAST) examination of the abdomen, NG tube insertion, foley catheter insertion, emergency vascular consultation, and alert the OR that the patient is coming.

B. NG tube insertion, abdominal CT scan, alert interventional radiology that the patient needs embolization, CBC, and metabolic panel.

C. NG tube insertion, type and cross 2 units PRBCs; alert GI the patient needs endoscopy; CBC, and metabolic panel.

D. EKG, cardiac enzymes, aspirin administration, propranolol administration, and notify the catheter laboratory the patient needs percutaneous angioplasty.

47. A 72-year-old man enters the ED complaining of chest pain. He states it is typical of angina that he has not experienced for 20 years. It radiates to the left elbow. He states it started 3 days earlier as he was riding a bicycle into a cold wind. He reports that 25 years ago, he had an MI that was treated with bedrest. He had severe angina for about a year, usually when walking into a cold wind. After a number of years of therapy with calcium channel blockers, he felt fine and had no more chest pain. Three years prior he had an episode of pulmonary edema, but it was thought due to steroid-induced edema. At that time, he had a stress test that was normal. He was taking the steroids for a severe asthmatic bronchitis. Two days ago, he again experienced angina when he was walking up a hill. He was planning to see his physician during the week, but this evening, he was merely sitting in his living room and had an episode of angina. He had bought some nitroglycerin the day before, and this time the nitrates didn't relieve the chest pain, so he thought he should be seen. He had not experienced any weight gain, shortness of breath, or ankle edema. He had no cough. He had not noticed any irregular heart beat. Past history was noteworthy for type 2 diabetes mellitus, controlled with metformin. He also had a history of hypertension, well-controlled with cozaar. He neither smoked nor drank. He also had a history of degenerative arthritis, for which he took NSAIDs, and gout, for which he took allopurinol. He was taking digoxin and occasional lasix for weight gain.

Vital Signs: BP 140/90 mmHg, P 82 beats/min, R 12 breaths/min, T 37°C, O_2 sat 99%. The physical examination was unremarkable. The chest was clear; the heart was a regular rhythm, with no murmurs, rubs, or gallops. The abdomen was soft and the liver not enlarged.

An EKG was obtained at triage that showed ST nonspecific changes with some ST depression in the left precordium. The patient stated that it looked like his past EKGs. He was also given an aspirin at triage.

A metabolic panel was obtained that was normal. A serum troponin was 0.09 ng/mL, the upper limit of normal.

What is your preferred management of the following choices?

A. Give the patient another nitroglycerin and, if he is pain free, have him follow-up with cardiology.

B. Admit the patient for serial troponins, and administer heparin and TPA.

C. Give the patient a dose of lasix, obtain another EKG, and admit the patient for overnight observation.

D. Obtain another troponin, repeat the EKG, give heparin, give integrilin, and if the troponin level rises, admit for cardiac catheterization.

48. A 38-year-old man enters the ED complaining of fever and fatigue. He states that he felt hot about 2 days ago, but he didn't check his temperature. The day before he had had a shaking chill and couldn't get warm. A friend told him that he felt like he had a fever, but he still didn't check his temperature because he did not have a thermometer. He also noted that he had lost his appetite and felt very drained. He has been taking motrin for the fever. Today, he felt cold again and decided to come to the ED.

His past history is unremarkable except for an appendectomy at age 18. No history of any medical disease other than a couple of ear infections as a child.

Social History: the patient works as a carpenter. He reports on questioning that he occasionally takes crystal methamphetamines because he has to work many hours of overtime. He also reports that he occasionally uses IV heroin when he can't sleep after the crystal methamphetamine. He also says that he has noted a sensation of "bugs" crawling under his skin.

Vital Signs: BP 150/100 mmHg, P 120 beats/min, R 16 breaths/min T 39.4°C, O_2 sat 98%.

The patient is thin, somewhat anxious in appearance, and looks drawn and ill.

HEENT are unremarkable. There are no enlarged lymph nodes. The neck is supple. Chest examination reveals some diffuse, but mainly basilar rales. The heart is not enlarged, but there is a 2/6 blowing diastolic murmur at the right sternal border in the 5th intercostal space. The rate is regular and rapid. There are no friction rubs or gallops. The abdomen is tender in the right upper quadrant, and the liver is enlarged 3 cm below the right costal margin. Bowel sounds are normal. The extremities appear somewhat wasted. There are several subungual hematomas, which are vertical and linear. (The patient states he is always hitting his hands with a hammer doing his carpentry.) There is no edema. The neurologic examination reveals no focal findings.

Which management strategy would you select for of this patient from the following?

A. Obtain chest x-ray, CBC, urinalysis (UA), and basic metabolic panel. If all are normal, discharge the patient to follow with primary care physician (PCP) for a viral syndrome.

B. Obtain an EKG, give the patient some IV toradol; if the fever comes down, treat the patient with NSAIDs, and have him follow with a PCP for the pericarditis.

    C.   Obtain blood cultures, chest x-ray, complete blood count, urinalysis and culture, echocardiogram, IV fluids, and start the patient on IV antibiotics, including vancomycin. Admit to ICU.

    D.   Obtain an EKG, HIV test, CD4 count; start the patient on bactrim and have him follow in AIDS clinic.

49. A 35-year-old man enters the ED with a rapid heartbeat and dizziness. He works as a head waiter in a local bar and grill, and states that he drinks pretty heavily every night during cleanup. Tonight, there were many St. Patrick's Day parties going on at the bar. He started drinking with the customers. About an hour into the cleanup, he noticed that his heart was pounding in his chest, and he felt that it was beating very irregularly. He felt very dizzy, like he was going to pass out. He thinks he had about six drinks, but he did not feel intoxicated. He smokes a pack of cigarettes per day. He denies recreational drug use. He has never had any problems in the past. He takes no medications.

Vital Signs: BP 100/70 mmHg, P 250 beats/min, R 20 breaths/min, O_2 sat 92%.

The monitor shows an atrial fibrillation at a rapid rate. The patient is now complaining of anterior chest pain.

Which of the following is the strategy you would choose to manage the patient?

    A.   Give the patient a yellow IV (5% dextrose with NS with thiamin 100 mg, and multivitamins), start heparin; give the patient some valium; admit to cardiology for elective cardioversion.

    B.   Same, but instead of admission, give the patient some calcium channel blockade, and watch in the ED observation unit.

    C.   Start as above, but in addition to some nifedipine, prepare the patient for conscious sedation with versed, etomidate, and cardiovert at 75 watt/sec. Admit the patient for cardiac observation.

    D.   Same as B, but give the patient some quinidine, and some digitalis, to slow the atrial fibrillation. When he is more comfortable, admit to medical floor for observation.

50. A 59-year-old man develops a chest sensation of fluttering, along with some dizziness and a feeling that he might pass out. He was riding home from the movies with his wife, and because they were right in front of the hospital, he had her stop at the ED. He has had a high cholesterol, but no chest pain, no heart attack, and no failure. He has been somewhat overweight (height, 5'9"; weight, 200 lbs), but he does not smoke. He has not had diabetes, drinks socially, and does not use recreational chemicals.

Vital Signs: BP 100/60 mmHg, P 160 beats/min, R 18 breaths/min, T 37°C, O_2 sat 93%.

He is now complaining of chest pain that radiates to the left arm.

An EKG is immediately obtained, and it shows a wide complex tachycardia at a rate of 160 bpm. (Figure 5-4)

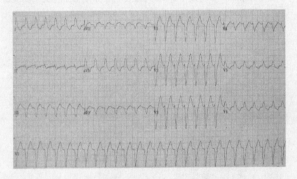

Figure 5-4: Wide complex tachycardia

Physical examination shows a normal HEENT with no jugular venous distention. Chest has some basilar crackles, but no rales or effusion. The heart is enlarged to percussion to the anterior axillary line. There are no murmurs, rubs, or gallops. The heart tones are faint. The abdomen is scaphoid and nontender. The liver is not palpated. The extremities show no edema. The neurologic examination has no focal findings. The patient is anxious but can respond to questions.

What strategy would you pursue for this patient from the following?

A. Give adenosine 12 mg IV push followed by 10 mL of NS push; give IV toradol 30 mg for analgesia; admit the patient for observation.

B. Give lidocaine 1 mg/kg IV, followed by pronestyl 100 mg IV slow push if there is no change with the lidocaine; admit to the critical care unit (CCU).

C. Prepare for conscious sedation, give versed, rapid-sequence intubation; cardiovert the patient at 200 watt/sec; admit to the CCU if the postconversion EKG does not show signs of ischemia that require catheterization.

D. Give amiodarone 100 mg, nitroglycerin, aspirin, propranolol, and heparin; and notify the catheter laboratory that the patient needs an emergency catheterization.

51. A 32-year-old man falls from a stepladder while hanging a picture. He has immediate pain in his shoulder. At the ED, his shoulders are unequal, with the left one, the painful one, being depressed. The clinical diagnosis is anterior dislocation. X-ray studies were obtained (Figures 5-5 and 5-6).

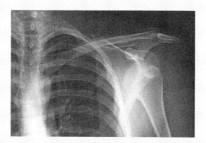

Figure 5-5: Initial x-ray: shoulder dislocation

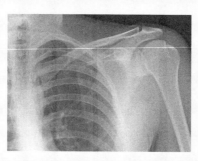

Figure 5-6: Post-reduction shoulder

Following the post-reduction x-ray, the patient complains of new chest pain, shortness of breath, and feeling dizzy.

Vital Signs: BP 100/60 mmHg, P 110 beats/min, R 22 breaths/min, T 37°C, O_2 sat 90%.

The patient's shoulder looks now to have the same contour as the right, but there are some eggshell sensations over the left deltoid.

What problem do you suspect from looking again at the x-ray studies?

A. Chronic anterior dislocation, deformity of the humeral head, and vasovagal reaction to pain

B. Acute pulmonary embolus; absence of vascular markings in left upper lobe

C. Early pulmonary edema; acute ischemic coronary syndrome

D. Left pneumothorax, absent vascular markings, and subcutaneous emphysema

52. A 48-year-old alcoholic man falls from a bar stool, landing on his shoulder. Witnesses state he made no effort to break the fall. He is driven by a friend to the ED, where he complains of left shoulder pain. He has slurred speech, but is cooperative and coherent. The left clavicle has a hump deformity. An x-ray study is obtained (Figure 5-7).

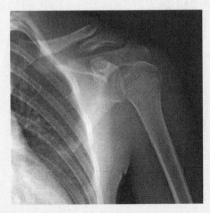

Figure 5-7: Left clavicular fracture

On physical examination, the patient has some numbness over the left deltoid muscle. He also has a loud bruit over the clavicle that seems to end at the left sternal border. He also has a large bruise over the left anterior chest and around the clavicle.

Which of the following options would you elect?

A. Place the patient in a figure-of-eight bandage; give adequate analgesia, and have the patient follow with his primary care physician.

B. Obtain an ultrasound study of the clavicular fracture; consult with vascular surgery.

C. Obtain clotting studies, give the patient valium, and observe until the patient is functionally sober.

D. Refer the patient to orthopedics for elective repair of the clavicle; obtain neurosurgical consultation for the peripheral nerve injury.

53. A 68-year-old man trips in his home and has a fall on his outstretched left hand. He is brought to the ED by his son.

An x-ray study is obtained (Figure 5-8).

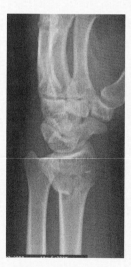

Figure 5-8: Left wrist x-ray

Which of the following postreduction management strategies would you choose?

A. Long-arm cast from above the elbow to the distal palmar crease with the wrist in extension and in ulnar deviation

B. Short-arm case from below the elbow to the distal palmar crease with the wrist neutral but in ulnar deviation

C. Sugar-tong splint from wrist to just above the elbow, with the elbow and wrist in neutral position

D. Radial gutter splint with slight ulnar deviation and the wrist neutral

54. A 70-year-old man presents to the ED because of abdominal pain, no bowel movement, and nausea and vomiting. He reports that he has been ill for 2 days, and that he felt worse today and couldn't eat or drink anything. He states that he has had a "rupture" for many years, for which he wears a truss, but that the abdominal pain, nausea, and vomiting are new.

His past history is unremarkable.

Vital Signs: BP 150/100 mmHg, P 110 beats/min, R 16 breaths/min, T 37°C, O_2 sat 92%.

Physical examination of the abdomen reveals diffuse tenderness and a very large inguinal hernia, the size of a large grapefruit. It cannot be easily reduced. It appears to originate above the inguinal ligament. The internal ring is palpable and seems to be separate from the hernia. There are increased bowel sounds over the hernia. There is no guarding or rebound tenderness. The rectal examination is Hemoccult negative. An abdominal CT scan is obtained (Figures 5-9 and 5-10).

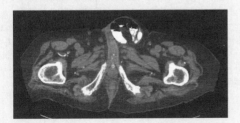

Figure 5-9: CT pelvis: scrotal hernia

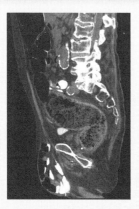

Figure 5-10: CT abdomen/pelvis: scrotal hernia

Which of the following management strategies would you select for this patient?

A. Sedation, reduction of the hernia, and follow-up with surgeon.
B. Enemas to clean out the fecal impaction; ignore the hernia; follow-up with primary care physician.
C. Emergency vascular surgery consult for immediate laparotomy for a leaking abdominal aortic aneurysm.
D. IV antibiotics for gram-negative and anaerobic bacteria, nasogastric tube, foley catheter, and surgical consultation for herniorrhaphy and possible bowel resection.

55. A 47-year-old house painter falls from a scaffold while painting a house. He is transferred to your ED from a rural clinic. He complains of having passed out while painting. This has never happened to him before, and he has never had episodes of dizziness while working on the scaffold. He did not experience any shortness of breath, and he does not remember any dizziness before falling. He denies any chest pain prior to falling. Now he has severe pain in the left leg, in the left arm, and in the back. He thinks he blacked out before he fell, but he cannot remember anything until he was in the ambulance on the way to the hospital ED. He remembers no chest pain, shortness of breath, or palpitations. He takes aldomet intermittently for hypertension but states he has had no recent problems. He has not had surgery. He takes no medications at present other than the intermittent aldomet. He smokes one pack of cigarettes per day and drinks about two six packs of beer each week. He does not drink on the job and had no alcohol the day of the fall. The paramedics state they gave him some demerol on the way to the ED after immobilizing him at the clinic. The clinic is staffed by a nurse practitioner.

Vital signs in the ED: BP 130/90 mmHg, P 110 beats/min, R 16 breaths/min, T 37°C, O$_2$ sat 92%.

The patient is in some distress from pain, but alert and able to answer questions. HEENT: atraumatic. The neck is supple and nontender. Back is tender in midline. Chest compresses without pain. Normal breath sounds bilaterally. Heart is not enlarged. Regular rhythm; tachycardic; no murmurs or rubs; has loud first heart sound (S$_1$).

Abdomen: soft and nontender. Pelvis compresses without tenderness. Extremities: left midshaft leg is swollen, tender, and deformed. Left elbow is swollen, tender, and deformed. Neurologic: the patient is alert and oriented, and answering questions lucidly. There are no sensory deformities. The deep tendon reflexes are equal and 2+ but are not tested in left leg or left arm because of pain and deformity. The Glasgow coma scale score is 15. Rectal: good sphincter tone and no hemoccult blood.

Initial x-ray study is shown in Figure 5-11.

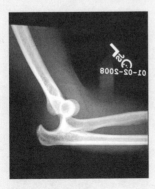

Figure 5-11: Initial x-ray

What is the next diagnostic study this patient needs from the following?

A. CT scan of the head
B. Cervical spine series
C. FAST ultrasound series
D. EKG

▶ ANSWERS

1. D	**20.** D	**39.** C
2. D	**21.** A	**40.** B
3. C	**22.** B	**41.** A
4. D	**23.** C	**42.** C
5. D	**24.** B	**43.** C
6. D	**25.** D	**44.** D
7. C	**26.** D	**45.** A
8. D	**27.** C	**46.** A
9. D	**28.** C	**47.** D
10. C	**29.** B	**48.** C
11. D	**30.** C	**49.** C
12. D	**31.** D	**50.** C
13. D	**32.** D	**51.** D
14. D	**33.** C	**52.** B
15. C	**34.** B	**53.** D
16. C	**35.** D	**54.** C
17. C	**36.** A	**55.** D
18. B	**37.** D	
19. C	**38.** B	

▶ EXPLANATIONS

1. The best choice is **D**. Explanation:

   A. Flank pain and renal colic are commonly seen in adults. While the pain of colic is often excruciating, it is vacillating in intensity and does not produce syncope.

   B. Cardiac dysrhythmia is a common problem in the elderly and certainly can produce syncope. There should be some evidence of heart block or dysrhythmia on the electrocardiogram (EKG), and it does not produce flank pain.

   C. Pulmonary embolus can of course produce syncope but does not produce flank pain. There should be some evidence of thrombophlebitis or a predisposing injury or condition.

   D. The patient's back pain may have not been related to his degenerative arthritis, but instead to the expanding aneurysm. It is often not possible to palpate a mass with an abdominal aortic aneurysm (AAA), since the swelling of the aorta is filled with very soft grumous material of atheroma. Any patient with syncope, back pain, and hypotension must be considered immediately for the possibility of leaking or ruptured AAA. The BP of 120/70 mm Hg should be alarming because this is not normal for the patient's age, and with a history of hypertension.

2. The best choice is **D**. Explanation:

   A. Atelectasis should have occurred earlier, should have been accompanied by a high fever, and should have been on the left, the side of the rib fractures.

   B. A pulmonary embolus (PE) is always possible with long-bone fractures, but more often presents with chest symptoms or signs of thrombophlebitis. The patient has no new chest pain, has tenderness over the rib fractures, and has significant abdominal tenderness.

   C. Delayed splenic rupture is certainly a consideration but should produce pain in the left abdomen, the left chest, or left shoulder. It is very unlikely to produce pain in the right upper quadrant.

   D. Acalculous cholecystitis is commonly described in patients with diabetes, patients with long-bone fractures, or those with serious burns. Although the patient is young, and would not be a likely candidate for cholelithiasis, acalculous cholecystitis is often not considered until the patient spontaneously perforates the gallbladder.

3. The best choice is **C**. Explanation:

    A. A retinal artery occlusion should not result in a dilated pupil or a steamy cornea. A transient ischemic attack (TIA) might come on suddenly, but the clue here is the sudden dilation of the pupil upon entering the dark room, suggesting a narrow-angle glaucoma.

    B. An ocular foreign body might yield a dilated pupil, sudden onset of pain, and a red eye, but there should be some kind of history of ocular trauma, such as from hammering metal on metal.

    C. Tonometry should immediately reveal the high chamber pressure.

    D. A retinal detachment can come on suddenly but should not dilate the pupil or result in a red eye, and is not triggered by walking into a dark room.

4. The best choice is **D**. Explanation:

    A. The patient has a peripheral facial nerve deficit on the right; she has decreased eighth nerve function on the right; she had right cerebellar dysfunction. These cannot be accounted for by a central right cortical lesion.

    B. The patient has a right peripheral facial nerve lesion, but this would not cause the eighth nerve dysfunction, nor the cerebellar dysfunction.

    C. A carotid dissection should cause pain in the left neck and cerebrocortical dysfunction of the left brain, not lesions of the right peripheral seventh and eighth nerves, and not a cerebellar lesion.

    D. With the combination of peripheral nerve and cerebellar lesions, look for a tumor compressing the cerebropontine angle, the most common being a neuroma.

5. The best choice is **D**. Explanation:

   A. There is a first-degree heart block, along with a left bundle-branch block (LBBB) and a sinus bradycardia, but there is no failure of the p wave to transmit.

   B. There is an LBBB, but there is much more ST elevation in the direction concordant with the main QRS complex, especially in V_3, V_4, and V_5. Although there is definitely more ST elevation in II, III, and aVF than would be expected with an LBBB, the elevation is discordant to the main QRS. This suggests perhaps reciprocal involvement with the left coronary artery, where the ST segment is concordant.

C. and D. Given the LBBB and the signs of an acute myocardial infarction (MI), along with the history of chest and back pain, and a tearing sensation, it would be imperative to rule out an ascending aortic dissection that is retrograde with involvement of the left coronary artery.

6. The best choice is **D**. Explanation:

   A. Although the patient appears to be having an inferior wall myocardial infarction, he clinically suggests recurrent ventricular tachycardia. A calcium channel blocker might be useful if you knew this was his first episode of atrial fibrillation (AF), but this clinical presentation suggests ventricular tachycardia (VT) more than AF. Moreover the low blood pressure would argue against using the calcium channel blocker.

   B. Even if you are sure this is paroxysmal atrial tachycardia (PAT), you have to explain the ST elevations in leads II, III, and aVF, and the episodes of dizziness and low blood pressure. It is safer to assume the patient is not in a supraventricular block.

   C. There is no harm in anticoagulating this patient, but with symptoms present for more than 24 hours, he is not a candidate for the catheter laboratory and needs immediate treatment for his shock.

   D. For the reasons discussed previously, this is a patient who is in a symptomatic tachycardia. This needs treatment, and afterwards, one can define the best management for his probable myocardial infarction.

7. The best choice is **C**. Explanation:

   A. It would be reasonable to start with epinephrine and steroids, but the child is old for croup and has a very high fever. This makes it more likely that one is dealing with bacterial tracheitis, and, therefore, the child needs antibiotics and admission.

   B. This does not sound like epiglottitis, but there would be no harm in obtaining an image of the epiglottis and the trachea while the child is being treated. He may be capable of being managed without intubation, however.

   C. This is the safest approach for this sick child, who as explained in A, probably has bacterial tracheitis.

   D. There is no indication of a foreign body in this child. There is nothing wrong with obtaining a chest x-ray imaging study, but there is no need for bronchoscopy in this child, unless his condition worsens and he cannot handle the secretions from the bacterial tracheitis.

8. The best choice is **D**. Explanation:

   A. Although this is the most common cause for an acute organic brain syndrome, it rarely occurs in the absence of some suggestion of sepsis.

   B. Diabetes certainly can cause acute confusion, but it is less likely to cause problems over a few weeks. It is always prudent to check a fingerstick glucose, however, because sometimes patients are given hypoglycemic medications incorrectly.

   C. The most common error is to assume the confusion is due to aging rather than to an acute organic brain syndrome caused by an acute and treatable disease. It is very useful to listen to a relative's account of the patient's status before she became ill.

   D. Hyperthyroidism in the elderly, often called apathetic, can present only with the cardiac dysrhythmia of atrial fibrillation, with the lowered cardiac output leading to an acute organic syndrome.

9. The best choice is **D**. Explanation:

   A. Skull plain film studies are almost never valuable any more unless looking for a foreign body. They do not give a good view of the basal skull.

    B. Sinus films do not usually show the base of the skull, and although useful for detection of anterior facial fractures, they really do not give a good view of the sphenoid sinus.

    C. The Panorex is an excellent study for the mandible, but not for the skull below.

    D. A true lateral of the cervical spine will often reveal an air–fluid level in the sphenoid sinus and thus confirm the presence of a basilar skull fracture. This can be very helpful because sometimes early after a trauma, it is difficult to see a hemotympanum.

10. The best choice is **C**. Explanation:

    A. There may not have been much bleeding with the esophageal tear. The history is typical for a Boerhaave's syndrome, first described in a Dutch Admiral who had consumed too much wine and duckling. Boerhaave was the physician. If the hemoccult test were positive, the patient might have a Mallory-Weiss tear, which usually leads to a self-contained minor upper gastrointestinal bleed. This is more often seen in young bulimic women, and the erosion of the front teeth enamel may give a clue to its presence. The Hammond's crunch described suggests a mediastinitis from the esophageal tear.

    B. Patients with chronic minor GI bleeds, especially often seen in older women, develop severe microcytic anemia. More useful than an iron level may be a red blood cell isotope study to detect the longevity of the red blood cell and the presence of a bleed.

    C. A CT scan with contrast will reveal the tear, as well as the mediastinal spill. This will lead to an early decision for surgery, and the earlier the repair, the better the outcome.

    D. Direct esophagoscopy can totally miss the tear, and will not reveal the mediastinitis as well, so the imaging study is preferable.

11. The best choice is **D**. Explanation:

    A. The patient might still have an ischemic coronary syndrome, but that will not be shown by a cardiac echocardiogram, but rather serial troponin levels, because the patient does not have ST elevation changes on the EKG.

    B. A chest CT scan is unlikely to show any chest pathology that lies outside of the heart. The increased respiratory rate is more likely due to disordered acid–base metabolism than to pneumonia or congestive heart failure.

    C. A rectal examination might show an enlarged prostate, but benign prostatic hypertrophy should not alter the breathing pattern, produce chest pain, nor cause fatigue and increased appetite.

    D. This clinical presentation is typical of mild diabetic ketoacidosis (DKA). A blood sugar level would be expected to be elevated (ascertain first that the patient has not just eaten), and the urine should also be checked for sugar and ketones. A blood gas will also show acidosis. Do not ignore the chest pain, because 25% of new-onset DKA will occur in conjunction with an acute myocardial infarction.

12. The best choice is **D**. Explanation:

    A. Although the physician might hear a murmur of aortic stenosis, this would not explain the tachycardia. It is improbable to hear a pleural friction rub from an early pulmonary embolus.

    B. Women are less likely than men to have an abdominal aortic aneurysm, and fewer than 20% of these are palpable, especially if the patient is at all obese.

    C. Despite the episode of syncope, the neurologic examination is likely to be normal unless the patient complains of acute neurologic dysfunction.

    D. Painless colonic bleeding is often observed by the patient, but there can be significant bleeding without expulsion of blood. Rectal examination is most likely to reveal the bleeding and lead one to search for diverticulosis or an upper gastrointestinal bleed.

13. The best choice is **D**. Explanation:

    A. Although penicillin allergy can produce an acute arthritis, it is unlikely to be the earliest manifestation of the allergy. The finger blisters are not characteristic of a penicillin skin rash, which is much more likely to be a diffuse truncal erythematous measles-type rash.

B. Acute rheumatoid arthritis can occur in this age group but will not come on acutely and will not produce the finger rash.

C. Degenerative arthritis is uncommon in this age group, without a history of trauma, and is more likely to be monoarticular. It also will not produce the finger rash.

D. Although the penicillin consumption can lead the physician astray, the finger rash and the sexual history are important. The blisters may not culture positive for gonococcus but are worth looking at, along with a pelvic examination and culture. The finger blisters are an important clue not to overlook.

14. The best choice is **D**. Explanation:

A. Frequent bruising may well be the sign of a bleeding diathesis or a blood dyscrasia but should not produce fractures.

B. While it is important to respect the possibility of rape, this should not be done against the wishes of the patient.

C. Congenital bone disorders are unlikely to present in young adulthood, and the bruising suggests a different kind of trauma, as does the suspicious behavior of the boyfriend.

D. The presence of strangulation bruises is an extremely serious presentation of domestic violence. These women have a high mortality facing them if they cannot be removed from the person inflicting the violence. All efforts should be made to obtain the proper kind of help and to admit the patient to attempt to prevent these deaths.

15. The best choice is **C**. Explanation:

A. Although child abuse is always of concern, the clinical scenario is plausible, and there are no physical findings that are suggestive of child abuse.

B. Fifth disease, also known as the slapped face syndrome, produces an exanthem that is more diffuse, often across the child's cheeks. It should be accompanied by fever and more signs suggestive of a viral illness; for example, runny nose, cough.

C. Children in this age group explore the world through their mouths. Unfortunately, we don't know if the cord was plugged in when the child was playing with it, although it probably was, because this sounds like a mouth burn. The problem with these electric burns is that they often look more innocuous than they will evolve to be. Necrosis of the burn area is common and can lead to necrosis of the labial arteries with a significant hemorrhage.

D. Hand, foot, and mouth is a viral disease that is often causative of painful ulcerations of the tongue and palate, as well as in producing an exanthem involving the palms and soles of the hands and feet. It often causes the child to stop eating and drinking but should not involve the corners of the mouth.

16. The best choice is **C**. Explanation:

A. Even if the patient has a coronoid process fracture of the mandible, the neurologic confusion, as well as the history of unconsciousness with amnesia for a period of time, suggests that the most urgent imaging need is to look at the brain for an extra-axial hemorrhage.

B. Even if the patient cannot have the cervical spine cleared without an imaging study, because of the possible concomitant head injury, a cervical fracture will not cause pain in the ear.

C. The CT scan of the head is critical; ear pain may well reflect temporal bone fracture, and this patient fits the clinical picture of a potential epidural hematoma. He lost consciousness, and although he is now alert, he still betrays some confusion with repetitive questioning, With the amnesia for the events of the crash, he has had a significant concussion. Waiting for him to develop focal neurologic findings prior to identification of the intracranial bleed may lose the window of opportunity to decompress the brain.

D. Although this view may show facial bone fractures, blood in the antrum, and the frontal views of the mandible that might reveal a mandible fracture, none of these injuries should take precedence in searching for intracranial pathology.

17. The best choice is **C**. Explanation:

A. The patient might have a torsion, but it is improbable with this history and with these scrotal findings. There is nothing wrong with obtaining a urologic consultation after workup, but the workup should occur first.

B. Although this management includes some of the data that are reasonable to obtain, this is probably not a simple urinary tract infection, but more probably an epididymitis, for which anti-neisserial and chlamydial antibiotics would be more logical.

C. A urinalysis may help in the identification of epididymitis, the ice pack will help relieve the swelling, and spermatic cord block is not used often enough to provide pain relief while the diagnosis is confirmed. As indicated previously, antibiotics for sexually transmitted disease will be indicated.

D. There is nothing wrong with obtaining a Doppler ultrasound study to ensure there is blood flow to the testicle, and there is nothing wrong with giving adequate analgesia. If the patient has the data to confirm the diagnosis, it is appropriate to have the patient follow up with a urologist, but this is hardly necessary on an emergent basis.

18. The best choice is **B**. Explanation:

A. This is not the appearance of a viral paronychia, also known as herpetic whitlow. Therefore, while splinting the finger is a good idea, the patient has a felon, and this needs immediate antibacterial management and surgical therapy.

B. If one awaits the appearance of purulence or fluctuance for this infection in a tight closed space, the distal digit will become necrotic and may well be lost. A felon is one of two infections (the other being a bacterial infection of the parotid gland), where the fascial compartments of the infected space will not permit fluctuance to develop until the entire space is necrotic.

C. Antibiotics alone are inadequate for the management of a felon. The patient requires surgical relief of the digit space that is under pressure. See also the explanation for B.

D. Although it is possible that the patient did not completely remove all of the splinter, xerox-ray is not readily available. The patient needs the digit space incised and drained, and a foreign body could be looked for at that time. Ultrasound imaging can also reveal wooden foreign bodies, so this could be done in the ED while setting up for the incision and drainage.

19. The best choice is **C**. Explanation:

   A. Hernias can be painful while extruding but are unlikely to be so when reduced spontaneously. Although a sliding hernia can still be incarcerated (it represents one wall of the hernia sac being bowel wall), this is seen only after a forced reduction, not after a spontaneous one.

   B. Torsion in this age group is possible but extremely unlikely. Moreover, neither the spermatic cord nor the testicle would be normal.

   C. A patient with diabetes who has signs of early sepsis and pain out of proportion to any physical findings must be considered to have an anaerobic infection of the groin until it can be disproved. Fournier's gangrene can appear innocuous before the sepsis begins to spread and must be aggressively managed to save the patient's life.

   D. Acute bacterial prostatitis is improbable in this age group. It is certainly likely that the patient has a benign prostatic hypertrophy, and this obstruction certainly may have caused a urinary tract infection that has involved the prostate, but acute bacterial prostatitis is so painful as to prevent a satisfactory evaluation of the size of the prostate, and this should lead the physician to consider Fournier's gangrene. Also see answer C.

20. The best choice is **D**. Explanation:

   A. The most likely diagnosis is gamma-hydroxybutyrate (GHB) ingestion. This won't show up on a toxicology screen, and it is not necessary to prove because no other drug overdose will produce this picture of coma that reverses spontaneously.

   B. Although it is certainly possible that the woman has had sexual intercourse without her permission, nothing suggests this, although certainly the friends who brought her should be quizzed about the possibility. There is nothing wrong with doing such an examination, but it is most probably not necessary.

C. There is no need to admit to the ICU, or even to a floor bed, once the patient awakens and no longer needs intubation. Obviously, if the patient doesn't awaken, another source of the coma needs investigation, with ICU admission for persistent coma.

D. The patient's struggling against the ET tube, and her quick arousal, essentially clinch the diagnosis of GHB intoxication. Once the patient is fully awake, able to communicate, and able to protect her own airway, there is total logic to extubating her, and discharging her to someone competent to watch her. This is unlikely to be the friends who brought her in themselves instead of calling an ambulance for her and might need to be a parent, or a competent school counselor, depending on the social circumstances.

21. The best choice is **A**. Explanation:

A. The child appears edematous. The dark urine may have been bloody. The child had a URI, which was probably a streptococcal infection, and most likely has acute glomerulonephritis. One would also like to see the protein content of the urine and whether there are red cell casts.

B. Despite the manipulations, there do not appear to be any neurologic disorders. Cervical spine fractures have been reported after chiropractic manipulation, but this chiropractor seems a good deal more sensible than the mother.

C. Despite the history of the prior upper respiratory infection, this clinical presentation doesn't sound like pneumonia or congestive heart failure. It might well be worthwhile to obtain a chest x-ray study, but this can be done as the child is being admitted.

D. This doesn't sound like sepsis. It would certainly be worthwhile to obtain a basic metabolic panel, but the best initial test is still the urinalysis.

22. The best choice is **B**. Explanation:

A. While the patient has an unknown febrile illness, the source is unlikely to be in the chest. It is true that sometimes a right lower lobe pneumonia will imitate acute cholecystitis but should not produce jaundice, certainly will not produce lower abdominal pain, and will never produce vaginal discharge.

B. The diagnosis that would tie all together is pelvic inflammatory disease, with perihepatitis; that is, the Fitz-Hugh-Curtis syndrome. If the physician doesn't consider this, it is unlikely that a pelvic examination will be performed, and thus it would be easy to miss the pelvic infection. Even if one considers this entity, it is always prudent to ensure that there is no pregnancy, although pelvic inflammatory disease is almost never seen during pregnancy.

C. Given the patient's history, it would be easy to focus upon the right upper quadrant (RUQ) for the source of disease, but acute cholecystitis should have more tenderness along with a palpable mass in the RUQ, in addition to a positive Murphy's sign, a lower degree of fever, and no pelvic complaints. There is nothing wrong with looking at the gallbladder with an ultrasound, but the tendency is to stop looking for an alternative diagnosis when cholecystitis is being considered, even in the face of a normal ultrasound examination. The lipase can be elevated in pelvic inflammatory disease as well as pancreatitis, so that if the pelvic examination is omitted, one might conclude the patient has gallstone pancreatitis, even if no stones are visualized in the gallbladder.

D. With no alcoholic history, no history of cirrhosis, whether secondary to alcoholism or primary biliary cirrhosis, it would be very unlikely to have primary peritonitis. Other causes of peritonitis, such as a perforated appendix, or a perforated peptic ulcer, shouldn't produce jaundice, although the pelvic examination can easily look like pelvic inflammatory disease.

23. The best choice is **C**. Explanation:

A. The patient does have the appearance of poliomyelitis, but given that he had normal immunizations, this is unlikely to be polio. He does appear to be having difficulty with ventilation, and although one might think of myasthenia gravis, this is less likely in a man; the weakness is not diffuse throughout the entire body, but started in the legs before the breathing difficulties were noted. An external respirator is not likely to be available given the absence of polio for so many years.

B. The patient has no family history of weakness. Moreover, his weakness appears to be localized first to the legs and then to the chest, but is not present in the upper extremities. Even if this is the first onset of hypokalemic intermittent paralysis, it should not affect only parts of the body. This is similarly true for thyroid disorders that can accompany hyperthyroidism. Moreover, the patient has no neck mass, no eye changes, and only a mild tachycardia.

C. The lumbar puncture may help with the diagnosis if there is elevated protein and some cells. The patient needs intubation; has a decreased oxygen saturation; with the history of ascending weakness, and the absent deep tendon reflexes in the legs, but normal in the arms, this should suggest an ascending paralysis, or Guillain-Barré syndrome. These patients tend to die of ventilatory failure before it is recognized that their weakness has risen to the level of the intercostal muscles and diaphragm.

D. Although a chest x-ray study is certainly worth obtaining to be sure there is no intrinsic lung pathology or mediastinal tumor, the crackles in the chest represent hypoventilation from chest wall paralysis rather than bronchospasm or pulmonary secretions. The lungs should clear with artificial ventilation after intubation.

24. The best choice is **B**. Explanation:

A. Although the patient has a low SaO_2, she is at unaccustomed altitude and probably is beginning to decompensate her compensated failure.

B. Oxygen will certainly improve her general condition. It will raise her oxygen saturation, and when combined with mild diuresis, such as with Diamox, along with descent to sea level, the patient should recompensate and do well. If the bus is to descend to sea level the next day, the patient can probably be managed without ending her vacation trip with her group, but if the plan is to stay at altitude, the patient should stop traveling with the group and return home.

C. The patient does not have high resistance congestive heart failure with acute pulmonary edema. It is very unlikely that she is having an acute coronary ischemic syndrome, but more probable that she has a mild high altitude pulmonary edema. This was probably induced by the change in the oxygen saturation, the failure to continue diuresis, and a borderline cardiac compensation. She doesn't need the kind of aggressive therapy that one would use for acute high resistance pulmonary edema. Mild diuresis, as suggested with diamox, will do. Diamox is a carbonic anhydrase inhibitor and will produce a mild respiratory acidosis that will cause the patient to hyperventilate, especially helpful during sleep. Combined with some external oxygen, this will allow the patient to recover compensation, descend from altitude, and return home safely.

D. It is very unlikely the patient has pneumonia. There are no fever, no chills, and no cough, and though she is in close contact with her fellow passengers, the clinical presentation does not appear to be sepsis.

25. The best choice is **D**. Explanation:

A. Herpes zoster is the most likely diagnosis, and the recommendations for therapy would be adequate if the patient was not HIV positive, and if the patient did not already appear immunocompromised: CD4 count of oral acyclovir has not been shown to shorten the course of herpes zoster, and Tegretol should be reserved for patients who have a chronic pain syndrome. There is nothing wrong with asking a neurologist to see the patient in consultation, but this should not be just to follow up with one.

B. Although pityriasis rosea can resemble herpes zoster, the blisters are not in a single dermatome; the heraldic patch is usually an erythematous clump away from the Christmas tree patterns of blisters, and it is not a painful rash.

C. and D. The prior CD4 count was already low, and that was before this acute infection. Therefore, it is likely the patient is already immunosuppressed. Moreover, the rash crosses the midline, thereby involving more than one dermatome. This means that the virus is disseminating, and one can anticipate this patient becoming much more ill. Hopefully IV acyclovir and more aggressive antiviral HIV medications can check the spread of this reactivated virus and prevent widespread dissemination.

(When the patient knows his childhood illnesses, there is almost always a childhood history of chicken pox. Why the virus lies dormant for many years before reactivation is unknown. Perhaps there is a more recent exposure to the acute virus, or perhaps it is triggered by other stimuli, since the herpes zoster can often appear after surgery or some other intercurrent illness.) Given that this is an HIV-positive patient, the onset of zoster may be the AIDS-defining illness.

26. The best choice is **D**. Explanation:

   A. This is clearly a crush, contaminating, and severe distal amputation. The level of the amputation probably precludes any microvascular reimplantation, but the fact that the wound is dirty, and crushed, makes reimplantation moot. The decision can be left to the hand surgeon, but there is no rush to have a hand surgeon see this injury.

   B. It is probably not incorrect to sew the fingers back in place to make splinting and bandaging of the hand easier, especially if the hand surgeon is not available or in the same institution as the ED, but these fingers are not going to be salvageable.

   C. For the reasons given in B, the emergency physician could complete the amputation, but if uncomfortable with doing this, there is no reason to undertake this procedure. For psychologic reasons, it is preferable to have the hand surgeon see this patient the same day.

   D. This is probably the best choice in most EDs, although as indicated in C, it is only prudent to have the hand surgeon see the patient in the ED and let him decide when and where to amputate.

27. The best choice is **C**. Explanation:

   A. Although it would be nice to see the study from the other hospital, this may be impractical logistically; it might not even be possible to talk to the prior treating physicians and radiologists. The leg does not have the appearance of deep venous thrombosis; the appearance is more compatible with lymphatic obstruction.

   B. Although this is a young man, who (by history) is sexually active, the swelling of the leg suggests more than the lymph node enlargement related to sexually transmitted disease such as lymphogranuloma venereum. Certainly gonorrhea would neither produce the lymphadenopathy nor the leg swelling, and lymphogranuloma should not cause the leg to enlarge.

C. What this patient most likely has is an obstruction of the vena cava, and a CT scan should show why the leg is swollen and perhaps also show a mass contiguous with the inguinal mass. This most probably will be lymphoma, and it certainly will require a full workup, but the most likely imaging study that will give initial information is the CT scan. This will also help with disposition if the patient comes from a different city and would prefer hospitalization near his home.

D. There is no reason to further compromise venous flow in this extremity with a venogram, 25% of which will actually cause a venous thrombosis. The reasoning is the same as in A, but if there is a lymphoma causing this swelling, fear of an increased risk for thrombosis would be justified.

28. The best choice is **C**. Explanation:

A. Although tuberculosis is becoming more common and certainly is always a source for concern with a worsening cough, this is a disease that is unlikely to produce the neurologic findings described.

B. Certainly a carotid dissection can produce neurologic disease that is not always anatomically focal; however, these particular findings might occur after carotid surgery, but not before.

C. The findings are the triad that suggest a Pancoast syndrome: meiosis, anhydrosis, and ptosis. This is not a facial nerve palsy, since the patient can wiggle his forehead, and since the patient has lost sweating ability on the right side, the same side as the ptosis. The cervical sympathetic chain has probably been invaded by a pulmonary carcinoma. This is often accompanied by palpable cervical lymphadenopathy, but sometimes even palpation of the supraclavicular fossa doesn't reveal the lymphadenopathy.

D. Bronchiectasis is certainly a strong possibility for cough that is worsening at night, but which is always present, especially in a long-time cigarette smoker. It is well demonstrated with bronchography. This study, however, should not proceed until an explanation has been discovered for the neurologic findings that would not be explicable by bronchiectasis.

29. The best choice is **B**. Explanation:

A. Just because the mother fears blood dyscrasia, it does not mean that the physician must as well. There is certainly every reason to do a complete blood count in this child, but any elevation of the white blood cells will be consistent with B, and not with early leukemia.

B. With the joint pain, abdominal pain, and the purpura, this child clearly fits the picture of Henoch-Schönlein purpura. Admission is for pain control, and some would advise early steroid therapy.

C. Certainly this is always a prudent consideration, especially if one thinks purpura are contusions. The child's unwillingness to be examined is normal behavior, and not fear from being abused, because she looks to the mother for comfort. Surely other sites of tenderness and evidence for typical nonaccidental trauma must be sought, but it is unlikely to present with this constellation of findings.

D. Meningococcemia petechiae are easy to confuse with Henoch-Schönlein purpura, although the mistake is usually to think the sepsis is Henoch-Schönlein, rather than the meningococcemia. The petechiae can precede much of the other signs of meningococcemia, but there is usually high fever, alteration in level of mental awareness, and headache if there is a meningitis component. When there is not, the child is usually older and should not have the joint and abdominal pain. Certainly if one cannot distinguish the two, the safest plan is to aggressively search for the meningococcus with pancultures, start antibiotic therapy, and perform a lumbar puncture if there are any signs of meningitis present.

30. The best choice is **C**. Explanation:

A. Simply because the easy workup is normal, and the patient is elderly, it is premature to consider the disposition before you have an explanation of why she is in the ED. Remember that patients with metabolic disease often have complaints that don't match the seriousness of their disease, because there are often such dissimilar symptoms with which metabolic disease presents.

B. Fatigue rather than chest pain is certainly common in elderly patients, especially women, but the patient will probably have a normal EKG, or nonspecific ST-T wave changes on the EKG. Few patients with hypothyroidism have actual low voltage. The enzymes will be normal, and the stress test will fail because the patient won't have enough muscle strength to perform it.

C. The patient actually has a clinical picture that suggests the metabolic failure of thyroid disease: cold intolerance, muscle fatigue, and weight gain with a sensation of edema. Remember that hyperthyroidism can present with very similar symptoms, especially in the elderly, but should include a tachycardia, or atrial fibrillation. These patients should have brisk reflexes even when presenting with primarily cardiac dysfunction. The hypothyroid patient will have a slowing of metabolism. The deep tendon reflexes are slow, especially with a prolongation of the relaxation phase. The patients are edematous, but it doesn't pit: the classical myxedema. The gravelly voice is very common, as is a dry sense of humor, often described as myxedema wit.

D. Adrenal insufficiency is most commonly secondary rather than primary. That is, the patient has stopped taking a recommended steroid therapy, often seen in moderate to bad asthma, which has improved with long-term steroid therapy. Weakness and fatigue are common complaints, and there is often fluid retention from the steroid therapy. Diabetes, if present, will worsen, and sometimes that causes the patient to stop the steroids. Typically the metabolic panel will show hyponatremia and hyperkalemia. Increased pigmentation is hard to detect in many patients, and not often observed by the patient, relatives, or others. The patient may also have psychiatric complaints, and primary depression can also resemble hypothyroid-depressed metabolism.

31. The best choice is **D**. Explanation:

   A.   The patient has the physical findings of a rotator cuff tear. A plain shoulder series is unlikely to show any abnormalities.

   B.   The patient has no history of trauma, no fall onto the shoulder, and no physical deformity. There is no tenderness over the acromioclavicular joint. Therefore, there is little chance here of an acromioclavicular separation, and the imaging study to demonstrate one is not needed.

   C.   Given the fact that the patient has a rotator cuff tear, this will not be well demonstrated on a CT scan. The arthrogram will give the extent of the tear, which is often used to help decide the need for surgery.

   D.   There is no way that a patient goes to sleep well and awakens with a complete rotator cuff tear without significant trauma. The patient can give no such history, but he does have a buccal bite mark. Ninety percent of patients who have a grand mal seizure will have such a mark. It would also be useful to ask the patient if he had wet the bed on the prior night. (He had, but was ashamed to describe it, because he had never experienced this before.) He, therefore, most probably has had a grand mal seizure and should have a workup for new-onset first-time seizure. (In this particular case, the patient proved to have a meningioma that was benign and successfully resected. His rotator cuff was also repaired.)

32. The best choice is **D**. Explanation:

   A.   Although the patient would benefit from paralysis and intubation, as long as seizures continue, neither succinylcholine nor longer-acting agents such as curare or pavulon will stop the seizures. If long-term paralysis is used, the patient must have continuous EEG monitoring as therapy to break the seizures.

   B.   If a maximum dose of an antiseizure agent has been used, there is no point in giving higher doses. This will merely lead to the consequences of overdose, and all antiseizure medications can cause seizures in overdose. It is true that oxygen administration can perpetuate seizures, and sometimes just lowering oxygen levels is enough to break the cycle, but in a patient in status, it is unlikely to work because the status itself will have produced hypoxia before the patient was intubated and artificially ventilated.

C. General anesthesia has been effective in stopping status epilepticus and certainly should be considered in patients who have been maxed out with other antiseizure medications. There is no point in giving more versed, if this method of therapy is chosen. Although this may be a reasonable strategy in any given case of prolonged status epilepticus, see D for why that answer's suggested therapy should be tried first.

D. The patient might have tuberculosis. Although no empty pill bottle has been found containing the prescription for isoniazid, the diagnosis should be considered because the patient has not stopped seizing with use of conventional treatment methods. The neighbor's report that she is getting a divorce suggests that she might have been depressed and taken an overdose of isoniazid. The reversing agent is vitamin B6, pyridoxine, and it requires large amounts, because one must use almost the milligram equivalent of the ingested isoniazid. Most toxicology laboratories cannot test for isoniazid levels, and most hospital pharmacies don't carry much pyridoxine, so it may be necessary to use the drug empirically and obtain supplies from nearby institutions.

33. The best choice is **C**. Explanation:

A. Although the child looks and acts normally, one cannot be sure that an intussusception is not still present without an imaging study. Blood tests won't help, so there is little reason to torment the child with them, but the imaging study is imperative.

B. If you don't have a good pediatric radiologist who can help you elucidate whether the child needs surgery, you may have little choice but to attempt laparotomy. However, if you don't have pediatric radiology, you probably don't have pediatric surgery, and you may have to transfer the child to obtain either or both. It is hard to convince people in the middle of the night to accept transfers when the child appears well, but intussusception is a dangerous enough diagnosis that you must persist in getting the help the child needs before necrosis of the bowel occurs.

C.   Barium or air contrast, if well performed, is diagnostic and often therapeutic. The advantage of barium is that you can see if there is good flow into the terminal ileum, after the column of enema material has reduced the intussusception. The disadvantage is the difficulty in passing the barium that sometimes can cause a recurrence of the intussusception.

D.   The ability to diagnose intussusception with ultrasound is not as good as with barium or air-contrast enema, and, furthermore, it cannot produce a reduction of the intussusception. Therefore, it is usually a waste of time to obtain this study, even if it can be read correctly, and may eliminate the time left before the bowel undergoes necrosis.

34. The best choice is **B**. Explanation:

A.   The patient is not fluid overloaded as is often suggested in alcohol intoxication. He most likely is ketotic and acidotic. As opposed to diabetic ketoacidosis, which has been defined as starvation in the midst of plenty, alcoholic ketoacidosis is starvation in the midst of starvation. If the patient is well known to your institution, he may not need much workup, and only observation to be sure he is metabolizing the alcohol load appropriately. The blood gas is useful, but unnecessary if you help the patient reverse the ketoacidosis. The blood alcohol is useful for suggesting the duration of observation, but not necessary, because what you are trying to determine is functional sobriety as opposed to chemical sobriety. You may find the blood alcohol level rises, because the patient may not have finished absorbing the alcohol in his gastrointestinal tract.

B.   If the patient is a chronic user of your ED, he may not need the thiamine and multivitamins, because he probably received them on one of the recent prior visits. If, on the other hand, he is unknown, it is always safe to administer these. He did receive a glucose bolus in the field, and while there is a theoretic danger of inducing a Wernicke's encephalopathy, it won't happen if the thiamine is given in reasonable proximity to the administration of glucose. The patient will reverse the metabolic abnormalities with the administration of normal saline and glucose. Alcoholic ketoacidosis, as alluded to in the answer to A, is starvation induced. The alcoholic patient has no glycogen reserve in the liver, so gluconeogenesis cannot occur. Fat and protein must, therefore, catabolize. The patient develops hypoglycemia and ketosis. The reversal is by administration of glucose, which enables glycogen to be built up and to restore the glucose aerobic metabolism. The patient should be observed in the ED until functional sobriety has been reached. This often takes between 6 and 8 hours. The chronic alcoholic patient cannot metabolize alcohol any faster than a nonchronic drinker; the rate is approximately 25 mg/dL per hour. What is true is that the chronic drinker can function well at an alcohol level that would put the amateur drinker into a coma. When the alcoholic patient can walk, talk, and give a history of what is bothering him, it is safe to institute an appropriate workup or discharge the patient. If he fails to become less intoxicated, or if he develops neurologic deficits, then the workup can begin to search for an extra-axial bleed.

C. There is no need to obtain an immediate CT scan of the head on every intoxicated patient. If there are obvious signs of trauma, if the patient is failing to lighten the level of coma, or if the patient develops focal neurologic signs, the head CT scan is appropriate. Not every alcoholic requires endotracheal intubation, but if observed appropriately while lying on a side, the patient will be protected from silent aspiration.

D. Simply because a patient is comatose from alcohol does not mean that he or she is a major trauma victim. Obviously, if there is a history of trauma, for example, a motor vehicle collision, or if there are physical findings of trauma, then a trauma evaluation can be undertaken. This, however, is not necessary for most of these patients.

35. The best choice is **D**. Explanation:

A. Children with sickle cell disease, but sometimes even with only sickle cell trait, develop painful ankles and wrists with and without swelling. Although most patients with sickle cell disease have been recognized by age 8, there are some patients with sickle cell trait who may not have been diagnosed. They are unlikely to be anemic but can sometimes have similar hemolytic crises if exposed to the right stimulus, and if they are glucose-6-phosphate deficient.

B. Pain in the knee even without local tenderness may represent growth deformity; for example, tibial epicondylitis known as Osgood-Schlatter's disease, although this patient is a little young, given that most cases present during adolescence. There are sometimes hidden stress fractures in young active boys, so it is worthwhile to look for tibial plateau deformities.

C. With a limp, it is always worth looking at a hip for a source of referred pain. Children with sickle cell disease have a higher than normal incidence of septic arthritis and may have congenital hip deformity or the growth deformity of the hip known as Legg-Calvé-Perthes disease. This child is too young for slipped capital femoral epiphysis, but he could be an outlier, and, therefore, a hip series is worth ordering.

D. Therefore, it would be best to entertain all the possibilities for this problem, and thus this is the correct answer.

36. The best choice is **A**. Explanation:

A. There is almost no disease that enlarges the lymph nodes just above the elbow other than mononucleosis or lymphoma. The odds are high this is mononucleosis, even if the Monospot is not yet positive. The young woman is a student, has all the clinical symptoms of infectious mononucleosis, and has many of the signs. The terrible looking throat is not a streptococcal overgrowth, but the normal, if scary, appearance of the viral pharyngitis produced in this disease. The diffuse lymphadenopathy helps clinch the diagnosis, along with the enlargement of the liver and the spleen. The rash is most probably not due to a penicillin allergy but is the rash that is produced in patients with mononucleosis who are given ampicillin. The patient clearly needs some fluid rehydration, because she is not able to eat or drink. Because the spleen is enlarged, and the patient has abnormal vital signs, the ultrasound is prudent to ensure that spontaneous rupture of the spleen has not occurred. The indications for admission are to get her out of her dormitory, watch the spleen, and ensure that the patient is rehydrated and able to eat and drink before sending her out.

B. As already explained, this is not a penicillin allergy, and there is no reason to treat the patient for anaphylaxis.

C. The patient's diffuse lymphadenopathy might be a cause for concern about lymphoma except that the clinical picture looks so much like infectious mononucleosis. Therefore, at this point in time, it is premature to look at the chest for a primary lymphoma. The clindamycin is not necessary, looking for Vincent's angina of the mouth that has spread to the neck and chest. The terrible looking oral ulcers over the tonsils are typical of mononucleosis.

D. The rash is not that of lupus erythematosus, which more typically is a fixed malar rash that does not come on suddenly. The picture is not that of acute lupus, which usually presents without fever, but with joint swelling and tenderness, or acute renal problems such as changes in renal function, red blood cell casts, or hematuria.

37. The best choice is **D**. Explanation:

A. Despite the jugular digastric lymphadenopathy with some tenderness, the clinical picture is more of a viral illness with fever, sore throat, and runny nose. Submaxillary stone produces a painful swelling that is unilateral but is also submandibular.

B. Despite the scratches, cat scratch fever usually produces a painful lymphadenopathy of a single set of lymph nodes. This can be within the substance of the parotid gland, but usually comes some days to weeks after the exposure to the cat, usually doesn't produce much fever, despite the name of the disease, and usually does not have systemic symptoms.

C. Infectious mononucleosis can produce this picture but usually is accompanied by more fatigue, worse fever, oral ulcerations with exudate, and is more frequent in older patients.

D. With the advent of mumps immunization, the disease is so much rarer that many emergency physicians have never seen a case. The involvement of the parotid glands is often unilateral in mild cases, and, in any event, usually involves one side before the other. The fever and viral flu type symptoms often precede the swelling. The disease should be considered when the swelling is above the mandible, there is a viral syndrome, or the swelling is bilateral. The virus can also attack the pancreas and the testicles, but this is more common in adults than in children with the disease. A parotid duct stone is also possible but should not be associated with any fever or viral flu symptoms. Bacterial parotid abscess is almost never seen in children unless they are immunosuppressed and, when present, can often produce pus in Stenson's duct with compression of the gland. Remember that fluctuance of the parotid gland is a very late finding, as with a felon, because of the very firm fascial stroma that supports the gland.

38. The best choice is **B**. Explanation:

   A. This option would be correct if the mother were in the first trimester of pregnancy, and most probably in the second. The baby is hydraulically protected during this period, although more vulnerable in the second than the first trimester, in which the amniotic fluid protects the fetus from even high pressure blunt blows, such as a punch or a kick. In the third trimester, however, the fetus is very vulnerable to even minor trauma, and the patient must be observed for several hours before concluding that an abruption has not occurred.

   B. Because of the reasoning in A, it is most prudent to transfer the patient for fetal monitoring, fibrinogen monitoring, and the ability to perform emergent caesarean section should the patient show signs of abruption. Although a pelvic ultrasound study can be helpful in looking for abruption, one shouldn't waste time trying to obtain this study prior to transfer to the facility that can manage the pregnancy.

   C. This might be your only option if you are working in a rural community that does no obstetrics, and if the patient is showing signs of abruption, namely, abdominal pain, decreasing fibrinogen, rising pulse, and vaginal bleeding. Sometimes a general surgeon has had enough gynecologic experience to be able to perform a cesarean section, but in most cases, you will be better served by transferring the patient to the institution that can care for both the mother and the child.

   D.   This is an unlikely option, since any hospital that has a
            trauma surgeon is likely to have an obstetrician, but if that
            is the staffing pattern of your institution, you may be forced
            into this decision. You will probably find that the obstetrician
            would prefer the patient to be transferred to his or her
            institution where the patient can be monitored on the labor
            deck, and this is a preferable option unless the mother is
            already having an abruption. A cesarean section may then be
            life-saving for both mother and child.

39. The best choice is **C**. Explanation:

   A.   This is fine as far as the management of her usual
            intoxication goes, but the leg pain out of proportion to what
            is observed on physical examination is worrisome. Moreover,
            the patient has a low-grade fever. Therefore, it is unlikely that
            it will be safe to discharge the patient even if she becomes
            functionally sober. Furthermore, it is unlikely that the
            diabetes will slip into control easily because of the possibility
            of serious infection.

   B.   There is nothing wrong with obtaining a plain film study of the
            leg. Alcoholic patients are notorious for walking about with
            serious bone trauma pathology, and the patient could easily
            have a fracture from the distantly remembered altercation.
            Nevertheless, if the plain film is negative, there still remains
            the need to explain the patient's extreme pain. The reasoning
            is the same as for A.

   C.   The ultrasound may give you an indication of air or fluid
            in the tissues that would signify necrotizing fasciitis. The
            patient needs emergency surgical consultation because
            aggressive debridement will be necessary to save her life.
            These are always difficult patients to manage because they
            are a great deal sicker than they look, and it is always a
            challenge to convince your consultants that the patient needs
            an operation. The ultrasound study has been more helpful
            than plain film in revealing early fasciitis.

   D.   If the patient didn't have the signs of sepsis already alluded
            to, it would be prudent to think about preventing withdrawal
            symptoms as the patient sobered, but as already discussed,
            this should not be a concern until your investigation and

management of the probable necrotizing fasciitis is well under way.

40. The best choice is **B**. Explanation:

    A.   Although the exact rise in troponins after trauma is poorly understood, there clearly can be a rise. The patient may well have a rise in troponin from a myocardial contusion, but this does not mean that all chest pain has to be an ischemic coronary syndrome. The early EKG changes in pericarditis are nonspecific, and it may well be a matter of some hours to days before the classic changes of pericarditis are seen.

    B.   This is a prudent strategy, although it may fail because of a lack of pain control. It is sometimes necessary to add steroids to control a traumatic or a viral pericarditis, but there is no need to start them before determining if pain can be adequately controlled with NSAIDs. Given that the patient has a normal-sized heart on chest x-ray study, there is no need to obtain a cardiac echocardiogram to look for a pericardial effusion, and that is the principle indication for admission with pericarditis.

    C.   There is no need to start therapy with steroids, and they may not always be free of complication in the trauma patient; fluid retention, electrolyte disturbance, and impaired glucose metabolism are all seen, although infrequently. There is nothing wrong with a cardiology follow-up, but it is probably unnecessary, since virtually all primary care physicians are capable of following pericarditis.

    D.   This is not the clinical picture of pulmonary embolus, and it is preferable not to start anticoagulation on a trauma patient; since if the patient does develop a pericardial effusion, it would be far preferable for it not to contain blood. Certainly pulmonary embolus can take place after almost any trauma, but the patient has not been bedridden, is not taking hormones, is not pregnant, and does not have a history of prior disease.

41. The best choice is **A**. Explanation:

A. and B. The patient has the appearance of an alcohol/aldehyde reaction seen when drinking after taking antabuse. It can also be seen after drinking alcohol when taking flagyl. Patients often test the effects of antabuse when they first start taking it, or else they simply cannot avoid returning to alcohol consumption. The reaction can be extremely severe, and although the patient's chest pain is probably not coronary ischemia, if he has severe underlying arteriosclerosis, the drop in blood pressure can certainly induce a myocardial ischemia. The treatment for the alcohol/antabuse reaction is IV fluids and observation. While doing this, it would be prudent to obtain an EKG and some cardiac enzymes, and to ensure the patient has not induced an ischemic syndrome.

C. True anaphylactic reactions to antabuse are rare. It can be difficult to distinguish anaphylaxis from the alcohol/antabuse reaction, but there are no hives or angioedema, and the patient should not have the flushed erythema of the alcohol/aldehyde interaction.

D. Alcohol withdrawal can be life-threatening but should not produce flushing. The blood pressure is usually elevated rather than below normal. Severe withdrawal is often heralded by tachycardia, shakiness, and jitteriness, and may begin with a grand mal seizure.

42. The best choice is **C**. Explanation:

A. Although a toxicology screen might be useful, there is no point in giving charcoal to someone who is comatose from an overdose, because it will cause a severe charcoal aspiration. Physostigmine is unlikely to reverse drugs that cause coma.

B. and C. The intubation is a good idea, but not the hemodialysis, until one identifies the agent. Given the bullae, the signs of noncardiogenic pulmonary edema (normal-sized heart, no jugular venous distention, diffuse rales, and tachycardia), and the history of insomnia and depression, this is likely a barbiturate overdose, and supportive care is what the patient needs, rather than aggressive intervention to attempt to remove the barbiturates.

   D. There is no reason to believe this is carbon monoxide
   poisoning, although that could easily be verified. There is also
   no reason to believe that this is cyanide poisoning, since the
   bottle that was empty was for pills and not liquids. Because
   the patient doesn't need a hyperbaric treatment, she doesn't
   need to have the tympanic membrane decompression.

43. The best choice is **C**. Explanation:

   A. The patient would appear to have a brainstem stroke,
   probably a hemorrhage, according to the neurologic findings.
   Therefore, she is very unlikely to be a candidate for TPA.
   There is nothing wrong with involving the stroke team, if you
   have one in your institution, but more thought is required
   for this patient, and she should not be cared for only by the
   stroke team. Moreover, she is 3 hours out from the onset
   of her symptoms, so even with thrombosis as the etiology
   of the stroke, combined with the hypertension, she is not a
   good candidate for reperfusion.

   B. The same reasoning applies as in A. The patient, if she has
   had a stroke, has had a major brainstem hemorrhage. There
   is, therefore, no reason to obtain an MRI, and if the patient
   has a large brainstem hemorrhage, there is little reason to
   take up an ICU bed while she completes the act of dying.

   C. β-Blockers can themselves produce hypoglycemia and
   prevent the adrenergic gluconeogenesis from anything that
   causes blood sugar to fall, such as the peak effect of an
   NPH insulin dose. Ophthalmologists sometimes don't find
   out that patients are diabetic and, therefore, prescribe
   β-blockers for the treatment of glaucoma. Remember that
   eyedrops are absorbed systemically, so that the body
   reacts as to an oral or parenteral medication. These facts
   together suggest that despite the administration of 50%
   dextrose in the field, the patient is still hypoglycemic.
   There of course is nothing wrong with checking another
   fingerstick glucose prior to administering more glucose. The
   patient will awaken and doesn't need further artificial
   airway management, so she can be safely extubated. She
   will need admission and observation to be sure she doesn't
   develop further hypoglycemia, and for safety, she should

have a glucose drip throughout the night, probably with 10% glucose. The diabetes can be controlled with regular insulin until it is safe to restart the long-acting insulin. The key to this case, in addition to the interaction of β-blockers with insulin, is to recall that hypoglycemia can produce not only seizure activity but any focal neurologic deficit that can be imagined. Prolonged hypoglycemia obviously will produce brain death, but despite the focal neurologic deficits, early glucose administration will reverse the focal findings.

D. Giving up on the patient and calling the clinical picture one of brain death before confirming what has been the cause is premature, and, in this case, a self-fulfilling prophecy, because aggressive management will prevent the brain death.

44. The best choice is **D**. Explanation:

A. The patient's neurologic examination does not fit any anatomic localization. Although an epidural abscess can sometimes give a confusing picture, this patient has lost sensation from no known dermatome. She can hold the leg in the air but cannot raise it from the table. She has normal deep tendon reflexes. She cannot move either hip, although the sensory deficit is from the mid-thigh. She, therefore, does not have an acute spinal cord syndrome.

B. Although acute paralysis of both legs is possible from acute thrombosis of the aorta, this is never a pain-free event. Bilateral thrombosis of the aorta and the inferior vena cava is theoretically possible but has not been described. Moreover, if this were phlegmasia cerulea dolens, the patient would have pain, swelling, and blue discoloration of the legs, and the cutoff would probably be at the inguinal ligament rather than at the mid-thigh. If this were phlegmasia alba dolens, suggesting clotting of the aorta, there would still be severe pain in the legs, and the pulsations below the aorta would not be normal.

C. Even if you are convinced that spinal cord injury does benefit from high-dose steroids, there is no evidence here for a spinal cord injury. There is no pain, there is no sign of trauma, there is no history of trauma, and even if you postulate a herniated disk that suddenly ruptured when the patient twisted during the argument, the patient should have pain, muscle spasm, urinary incontinence, abnormal deep tendon reflexes, and involvement of one side greater than the other.

D. The patient has a clear conversion reaction. She exhibits the classical "belle indifference," would appear to have a clear secondary gain to win the argument with the mother about going to work, and has neurologic deficits that fit no anatomic pattern. The best treatment for these patients is reassurance that she will get better. Don't feed her until she improves, and this can also be suggested. Finally, this patient may well benefit from psychiatric counseling.

45. The best choice is **A**. Explanation:

A. The patient has an acute delirium, an organic brain syndrome. Moreover he has nystagmus and perhaps a paralysis of the lateral rectus eye muscle. He is confabulating and cannot perform coordinated mental activity. Together these suggest an acute Wernicke's encephalopathy. This is caused by an acute thiamine deficiency; and the patient, therefore, definitely needs thiamine administration. He probably has some alcohol withdrawal component to his presentation and, therefore, needs to have a glycogen substrate, namely glucose. This won't worsen the encephalopathy. He needs a fingerstick glucose to see if he needs a bolus of 50% dextrose for an acute hypoglycemia that might also be contributing to the encephalopathy.

B. There would certainly be every reason to obtain a head CT scan for this patient, because alcoholic patients are notorious for having extraaxial subdural bleeds that might well be contributing to the delirium. There is no need to obtain a lumbar puncture at this time, because the patient does not appear septic, but if the fever spikes higher, this would also be a reasonable diagnostic test, along with a chest x-ray study, and a urinalysis, to seek a source for the sepsis. He is in no need of antibiotics but certainly would be prudently placed in an ICU bed.

C. Even if the patient had sustained an observed seizure, or had a history of alcohol withdrawal seizures, dilantin is not effective to prevent or treat alcohol withdrawal seizures. Benzodiazepines are much more effective and are also useful for treating some of the symptoms and signs of alcohol withdrawal. Neither agent is useful for the treatment of Wernicke's encephalopathy, which requires thiamine. There is nothing wrong with admitting the patient to the medical unit, but an ICU bed is indicated as is a neurology consultation.

D. This man's behavior is organic, not psychotic. There is no reason to involve psychiatry. At this stage of management, it is premature to involve social services, because his disposition clearly must be in-patient. Haldol is not needed to control the agitation, but rather treatment of the organic brain syndrome as described previously. Furthermore, if there is a question of the patient having had a seizure, or a history of alcohol withdrawal seizures, it is safer to withhold haldol, because it can induce or enhance seizures. This patient is entirely too ill for nonmedical detoxification.

46. The best choice is **A**. Explanation:

A. The scenario presented is of a vasculopath who has already had disease in both cerebral and cardiac circulations. With a syncopal episode and back pain, and with the signs of hypovolemic shock, the most likely diagnosis is a leaking or ruptured abdominal aortic aneurysm (AAA). This could certainly trigger another heart attack, or stroke, but before concluding the patient is in pump failure, he ought to be investigated for AAA. The FAST examination may not be helpful, or may actually show the aneurysm, but will not show the leakage. A CT scan with contrast might well do so, but he is too unstable for the scanner. With the history of an UGI bleed 4 months ago, it is reasonable to conclude that was a heraldic bleed that was caused by the aneurysm eroding into the third portion of the duodenum. The fact that you cannot palpate an aneurysm is not helpful. This is very common, and the only useful data would be if you felt one. Absence of positive proof is not proof of absence. The patient needs an immediate operation if he is to be salvaged.

   B. To go down the pathway of a recurrent UGI bleed is to move in the wrong direction. Even if the patient has blood in the NG tube, the most probable diagnosis is AAA. The prior bleed as already mentioned was probably due to the aneurysm eroding the wall of the duodenum. The interventional radiologist cannot help with this pathology.

   C. This is another variation on the thinking in B. The gastroenterologist cannot help you with the bleeding from an eroded duodenum. First of all, it is most likely in the third portion, which is well below where endoscopy can be achieved, and secondly this does not represent duodenal ulcer, or *Helicobacter pylori* infection, but rather pressure necrosis on the bowel.

   D. A syncopal episode can of course be seen with pulmonary embolus, acute myocardial infarction, and transient cerebral ischemia, but that still leaves the hypotension, tachycardia, and back pain to be explained, as well as the prior UGI bleed. The patient may well have another MI postoperative, and a stroke as well, but you have no choice but to focus on the AAA and attempt to control this immediate threat to the patient's life.

47. The best choice is **D**. Explanation:

   A. The fact that the patient had angina on exertion in and of itself is not especially significant, because the pain resulted from significant isometric exercise, although it certainly needed investigation given that the patient has not had angina in so many years. There did not seem to be a failure trigger, because the patient had no symptoms, and he had not experienced any weight gain. Moreover, the second episode the next day suggests that perhaps the patient had ruptured a plaque with the bike ride, and when he had a third episode, especially since it was at rest and was unrelieved by nitroglycerin, this can only represent accelerating unstable angina and needs urgent investigation. Even if the patient is now pain free, he needs serial troponin levels, repeat EKG, and assessment by cardiology to take the patient to the catheter laboratory.

   B. There is no value of reperfusion of non-ST-elevated MI or for accelerated angina. The patient's repeat troponin was 0.10

and 0.20, 2 and 4 hours later. The patient has probably had a small infarction and will benefit from catheterization and perhaps angioplasty or coronary artery bypass grafting.

C. There is no need for lasix if the studies are not showing any failure. The new onset of failure can trigger angina, but in this case, it would appear to be the exercise that was the trigger, and it is more likely that this represents a ruptured plaque. There is still some blood flow, even with the bump in enzymes, because there is no ST elevation.

D. This strategy was the one chosen. The patient's troponins did rise, although without change in the EKG. He was taken to the catheter laboratory the next day and found to have a fresh hemorrhage around a 99% occlusion of the right main coronary artery—the dominant artery in this patient, with a 95% occlusion of the circumflex artery, which in this patient came from the right main. There was disease in the left, but not much narrowing. The two narrowed vessels were stented successfully, because the patient did not wish to have CABG. The negative stress test 3 years prior raised the interesting dilemma of first, how much reliance one can place on a negative stress test, and two, for how long a stress test is reliable. In answer to one, it is safest to assume that the only meaningful stress test is a positive one. A negative one is not proof of absence of coronary artery disease. In answer to two, when Philip Bleiberg died (he was the South African dentist who received the first heart transplant), his autopsy showed quadruple-vessel severe narrowing. He survived for one and one half years, and at autopsy, he had not died of rejection. However, in one and one half years, the healthy heart, taken from an 18-year-old, showed severe atheromatous disease. One should conclude that negative evidence is thus not useful for more than about a year.

48. The best choice is **C**. Explanation:

A. The patient must be assumed to have a bacterial infection. He has a high fever, he has had shaking chills, he has a new heart murmur, and last but not least, he has reported IV drug abuse. There is no safe way to conclude the patient has a viral syndrome, no matter how many of the above tests are normal. He needs an echocardiogram to examine the heart valve, as well as an investigation of his sepsis.

B. This is not the picture of pericarditis, although it might be the picture of a bacterial pericarditis. This would require an echocardiogram to look for a pericardial effusion and would require aspiration and culture of the effusion. The patient might also require a surgical drainage of the pericardium. In any event, this patient is too ill to send home.

C. This is the only prudent approach. One can assume the patient has a staphylococcal endocarditis, and that it may well involve the tricuspid valve, because he has been an IV drug abuser. He may well have a community-acquired methicillin resistant *Staphylococcus aureus* (MRSA) infection, since one can never predict his source for needles and any sterile technique. He is a very sick patient and may well require acute valve replacement.

D. Certainly one should worry about AIDS in an IV drug-abusing patient. This is not the picture of *Pneumocystis carinii* pneumonia, however. There would be nothing wrong with checking the HIV status as an inpatient, but the patient is looking more like an acute bacterial endocarditis and needs admission and workup for that entity while the HIV status is being investigated.

49. The best choice is **C**. Explanation:

A. The controversy over the wisdom of immediate conversion of atrial fibrillation (AF) does not truly apply to the patient with new-onset AF from binge drinking, known as "holiday heart." The natural history of this form of AF is that it is self-limited, and if the patient ceases alcohol consumption, it will convert on its own. The process of conversion need not occur in the hospital, especially if the patient is tolerating the dysrhythmia. If this is true, than save the admission and watch the patient in the ED.

B. This would be a good strategy in general for holiday heart, but for the fact that the patient has developed an almost maximum AF rate and is not tolerating the decrease in cardiac output. He has developed chest pain, and likely his blood pressure has decreased. The SaO_2 is low, and the heart rate is almost 300. Therefore, even with calcium channel blockade, which is usually very effective in the conversion of holiday heart, the patient needs more aggressive management of the dysrhythmia.

C. The more aggressive management option is immediate cardioversion. This can be done with or without the use of conscious sedation. If the patient is not failing rapidly, you can give a single dose of calcium channel blocker while you are preparing to sedate and intubate the patient. If he is failing rapidly, you can give a small dose of versed and proceed with cardioversion. The reason for admission of the patient, even after successful cardioversion, is because he was unstable and you wish to ensure that he does not lapse back into the dysrhythmia or develop necrosis because of the very rapid rate.

D. In the days prior to cardioversion, and prior to chemical agents such as calcium channel blockers, there was no choice but to try to convert the patient with AV nodal blockers including quinidine and digitalis. Today, with the ability to shock the patient into a regular rhythm, there is no need to use these agents. It is a mistake to give digitalis to any patient who is likely to need an electric jolt to the heart because it increases the risk for ventricular fibrillation. If you wish to augment the calcium channel blocker, 2 g IV magnesium are safe and may assist the cardioversion and the maintenance of sinus rhythm post conversion.

50. The best choice is **C**. Explanation:

A. The differentiation of supraventricular tachycardia from ventricular tachycardia is difficult, and often the choice is made in the wrong direction. To assume this is supraventricular tachycardia in a patient who is symptomatic with chest pain, low blood pressure, and rapid cardiac rate invites disaster. Even if one cannot find Ashman phenomenon, or rabbit ears that suggest ventricular tachycardia, it is safe to assume ventricular tachycardia is present and cardiovert the patient to a sinus rhythm, rather than attempt to convert with drugs known to work well for supraventricular tachycardia.

B. Although lidocaine and procainamide are both useful for conversion of VT, along with magnesium and amiodarone, as suggested in A, the patient is too symptomatic to attempt chemical conversion. You also have not determined if there is an underlying ischemic syndrome that has caused the dysrhythmia,

C. This is the most prudent approach. The patient is symptomatic and failing. Quit trying to sort out the origin of the dysrhythmia and concentrate on restoring a sinus rhythm and a better cardiac output. Once converted, the patient needs a workup to ascertain if the dysrhythmia was caused by an acute ischemic coronary syndrome. If this is not present, the patient can be admitted to the CCU.

D. This would not be a bad strategy if the patient were more stable, but with the chest pain, low BP, and acuteness of onset of the dysrhythmia with symptoms, this might cause the patient to deteriorate into ventricular fibrillation while you are waiting for the antidysrhythmic agents to work. The patient might well need the catheter laboratory (see C), but first he needs stabilization.

51. The best choice is **D**. Explanation:

A. The humerus does show the deformity suggestive of chronic or repeated dislocation, but there are other findings as well that would be more explanatory of the patient's sudden change in condition.

B. Pulmonary embolus might diminish vascular markings visibly in a young thin patient such as this man, but it should be more lobar, and not a rim of missing lung changes in the apex.

C. The lung does not look congested; there are no Kerley B lines, and the heart is normal sized.

D. The rim of pleura can be seen below the clavicle, there is no lung in this area, and there is a clear line of subcutaneous air along the shoulder. This is not seen in the pre-reduction film. The patient has a small pneumothorax; this could be confirmed with ultrasound or a CT scan. The patient could be given 100% O_2 with a nonrebreather mask and observed to see if the pneumothorax expands. He probably will not need a chest tube. The fall may well have fractured a rib, which is not always visible on the x-ray study.

52. The best choice is **B**. Explanation:

A. and B. For a simple clavicle fracture, A is correct; however, there are other issues of concern here. The patient should not have a bruit in the area; this suggests an injury to the subclavian vessels with an arteriovenous fistula; especially since the bruit disappears at the junction of the internal jugular vein with the right atrium. There is also much more bruising than one sees with most clavicular fractures. Therefore, the patient needs an investigation of the fistula possibility. An ultrasound Doppler study may well reveal the fistula, but the vascular surgeon might still desire angiography. In either event, a vascular surgeon should be consulted because the patient will probably need an operative repair.

C. Clotting and liver function studies would probably not be a bad idea in an alcoholic, nor would treatment with a yellow IV (5% dextrose NS with thiamine 100 mg, and an ampoule of multivitamins), nor would it be incorrect to give some valium to prevent seizures and other alcohol withdrawal symptoms. The disposition is premature, however, due to the considerations that must be addressed for the AV fistula.

D. Clavicular deformities are rarely in need of operative repair, either for cosmetics or for function, because the clavicle is not a weight-bearing bone. The widely disparate ends of the fracture will probably line up when the patient is placed in a figure-of-eight dressing. The deltoid numbness may represent a brachial plexus injury, but that will be more readily defined after the shoulder swelling abates and the patient is more sober. The possibility of the fistula should be addressed before the patient sobers.

53. The best choice is **D**. Explanation:

A. Long-arm casts are not advisable in elderly patients; the elbow becomes stiff too quickly, and, moreover, a long-arm cast hides the swelling that will occur in this very comminuted Colles' fracture. No fracture should have a circumferential cast in patients at any age until the swelling has diminished in 48 to 72 hours.

B. This short-arm cast will be a useful management cast for the patient, but not initially. If there will be trouble having the patient return, this cast could be placed and then immediately bivalved to avoid any possibility of a Volkmann's contracture.

C. A sugar-tong splint is not useful for this fracture, because it immobilizes anteriorly and posteriorly and gives no lateral stability.

D. A radial gutter splint will be very useful. It gives lateral stability; the ulnar deviation helps hold the fracture reduction. It allows for swelling at the fracture site and provides comfort to the patient.

54. The best choice is **C**. Explanation:

A. The hernia has been displaced for years. There is contrast in the small bowel in the hernia sac. Although hernias are best repaired electively, it is impossible to conclude from this presentation that it is the hernia that is the cause of the patient's signs and symptoms.

B. There is a large amount of stool in the colon and no contrast. Perhaps this is due to timing of the contrast, and that it was only given orally. There appears to be both large and small bowel in the hernia sac, and it is possible that this has produced a partial large bowel obstruction.

C. There is an ominous finding on the CT scan; the patient has about a 7-cm aortic aneurysm that is rimmed by calcification, except anteriorly, where it is adjacent to the duodenum. It is hard to see any leakage here, because it does not appear that any IV contrast was given. There is so much distention that an ultrasound would be difficult to interpret. The patient may need more cuts with contrast, but a safer strategy would be to have a combined general and vascular surgical approach to the patient through a laparotomy.

D. D is only half the answer, because one must also consider C; nevertheless, everything in suggested management for D should be initiated along with the investigation of the aorta.

55. The best choice is **D**. Explanation:

A. There is every reason to obtain a head CT scan in this patient. He did have a fall after a syncopal episode, but that is what must take priority.

B. Clinically, the patient has no cervical spine injury, but given the competing pain from the skeletal fractures, he needs to have the cervical spine cleared, but not immediately.

C. Given the fall, the competing pain from skeletal injuries, and the possibility of head injury, it wouldn't be unreasonable to obtain a FAST examination next, but one still needs to ask why this man fell?

D. An EKG might reveal the answer, and in fact it shows why the patient had a syncopal episode that led to the fall:

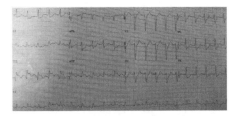

Figure 5-12: EKG: Inferior MI

Given that the patient is having an acute inferior myocardial infarction, with reciprocal lateral changes, right-sided ventricular leads should be obtained looking for a right ventricular infarction. The patient needs to go to the catheter laboratory, have the left elbow reduced, and have the CT scan, cervical spine x-ray studies, and FAST series.

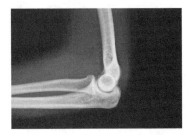

Figure 5-13: Left elbow post-reduction

At a tertiary care center, it would be possible to admit the patient and have cardiology consult and take the patient to the catheter laboratory. The leg can be splinted, the elbow reduced, and the other studies obtained. It would be hard to administer TPA to this patient given all the traumatic injury contraindications, and, in fact, he might not be a candidate for angioplasty and stent placement because of the need for antiplatelet activity post stent placement. It might be most prudent to have him receive a coronary artery bypass graft, along with open reduction-internal fixation of the leg and whatever care the abdomen needs. Given the neurologic examination, the patient will probably have a normal CT scan.

Appendix I: Signs

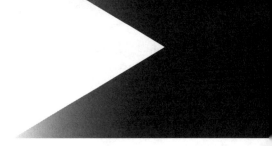

Anterior drawer sign—A test for anterior cruciate ligament injury. The patient lies supine with the hips and knees flexed. The examiner stabilizes the patient's feet and pulls the tibia forward. The test is positive if the tibia moves forward easily.

Battle's sign—Following blunt head traumas. A positive sign is bruising in the mastoid area. This indicates a basilar skull fracture.

Blue-dot sign—Seen with testicular pain, often of sudden onset. A bluish discoloration over the superior aspect of the testicle. This signifies torsion of the appendix epididymis.

Brudzinski's sign (a test for meningitis)—With the patient lying supine, when you flex patient's neck (chin toward sternum), the knees flex.

Chinese restaurant syndrome—This is seen as flushing, nausea, headache, and sometimes diarrhea and abdominal pain, and it is caused by a histamine release in response to monosodium glutamate (MSG).

Chvostek's sign—Facial nerve tapping causes ipsilateral facial muscles to go into spasm. This is classically seen in the tetany of hypocalcemia, but may also be seen with hypomagnesemia.

Coffee-bean sign—This is seen in an abdominal series, best on the upright films. It shows distended, air-filled and U-shaped bowel loops separated by an edematous bowel wall. This sign connotes a small bowel obstruction.

Colon cut-off sign—This is seen in an abdominal series. There is a dilated small bowel loop over pancreas that stops abruptly at the level of the pancreas. This connotes an acute pancreatitis.

Cortical ring sign—This is seen on the posterior-anterior (PA) view of the wrist series. In a scapholunate dislocation, the scaphoid bone appears shorter, with a dense ring appearance. This is also known as the signet-ring sign.

Courvoisier's sign—There is a palpable nontender mass and jaundice. The mass is the gallbladder. These findings suggest a pancreatic cancer obstructing the common bile duct.

Crescent sign—There is a blue-black discoloration around the ankle. It is caused by a hematoma formed from a ruptured baker's cyst (ganglion of the popliteal space).

Cullen's sign—There is a periumbilical ecchymosis. This is classically supposed to connote an acute hemorrhagic pancreatitis but may be seen with any intraperitoneal hemorrhage.

De Musset's sign—Bobbing of head in association with the heartbeat. This connotes severe aortic regurgitation.

Destot's sign—There is a hematoma along the inguinal ligament extending into the scrotum. This is seen post trauma and connotes a pelvic fracture.

Double bubble sign—There are two round circles within the fetus seen on an abdominal ultrasound study. This connotes duodenal atresia.

Double decidual sign—A hyperechoic area surrounded by a hypoechoic area, giving the appearance of a double echogenic ring seen on pelvic or abdominal ultrasound study, suggests an early pregnancy of 6 to 7 weeks.

Duroziez's sign—There is a bruit heard in conjunction with the heartbeat over the femoral arteries. This is another sign of severe aortic regurgitation.

Earle's sign—A palpable bony prominence or a large hematoma on rectal examination. Connotes a pelvic fracture.

Grey-Turner's sign—There are blue-black ecchymoses in the abdominal flank regions bilaterally. This classically connotes acute hemorrhagic pancreatitis but can be seen with peritonitis and intraperitoneal hemorrhage.

Groove sign—There is an inguinal lymphadenopathy above and below the inguinal ligament. This connotes lymphogranuloma venereum.

Halo or double ring sign—After blunt head trauma, if there is persistent nasal or otic bleeding, place a few drops of this fluid on litmus paper or a Kleenex. If the blood separates into two rings on the paper, this connotes the spinal fluid leak from rhinorrhea or otorrhea.

Hutchinson's sign—If there are blisters along the tip of the nose and next to the eye, this connotes herpes zoster involvement of CN V.

Kehr's sign—If the patient complains of shoulder or neck pain on palpation of the abdomen, after blunt abdominal trauma, this suggests an intraperitoneal hemorrhage, probably from splenic rupture.

Kernig's sign—This is another meningitis sign: When sitting, or with the leg flexed onto the abdomen, the leg cannot be extended because contraction of the hamstrings is accompanied by pain in the neck and back.

Kussmaul's sign—If the heart sounds are muffled, the cardiac silhouette is enlarged, and tachycardia and a pulsus paradoxus are present, the patient has a pericardial tamponade. Just prior to arrest, the patient will develop a bradycardia.

"Lead lines" —A blue-gray line at the junction of the tooth and the gum may be seen in lead poisoning.

Lhermitte's sign—The patient reports an "electric shock" radiating from the back to the arm and leg. This may be seen along with the neck in flexion. This sign connotes multiple sclerosis.

Lincoln-log sign—Also called H-shaped or "fish-mouth" vertebrae. This is seen on the lateral spine views in patients with sickle cell disease. There is central endplate depression with sparing of the anterior and posterior segments of the endplate.

Nikolsky's sign—When the skin is lightly rubbed, the epidermal layer of the skin slips free from the bottom layers or the skin.

Obturator sign—With the patient supine, raise the right leg with the knee flexed and rotate the hip internally. If right lower quadrant abdominal pain is elicited with this maneuver, the patient has acute appendicitis.

O.K. sign—If the patient can successfully make a ring between the thumb and index or any of the other fingers, the median and radial nerves are intact.

Posterior drawer sign—This tests the integrity of the posterior cruciate ligament. The patient lies supine with the hip and knees flexed. The examiner stabilizes the patient's feet and pushes the tibia posteriorly, holding the tibia just below the knee. The test is positive if the tibia moves backward easily.

Posterior fat pad sign (sail sign)—The posterior fat pad is not normally visible. If present on a lateral elbow view, it indicates a fracture of the radial head or the distal humerus due to a displacement of the fat pad from a joint effusion. The black density of the fat pad against the white bone looks like the spinnaker sail of a sailboat.

Psoas sign—With the patient in a left lateral decubitus position, extend the right leg at the hip. If this produces right lower quadrant pain, the patient has acute appendicitis.

Quincke's sign—There is visible capillary pulsation of the nail bed at rest. This is another sign of severe aortic regurgitation.

Raccoon's eyes—Bilateral periorbital ecchymoses, after blunt head trauma, connotes a basilar skull fracture.

Rovsing's sign—Palpation of the left lower quadrant of the patient's abdomen causes the patient to perceive pain in the right lower quadrant. This is another positive sign suggesting an acute appendicitis.

Sonographic Murphy's sign—When the ultrasound probe is pushed into the gallbladder image during an abdominal ultrasound examination, it tests the presence of cholecystitis. In the presence of this, the patient will experience pain and inhibition of inhalation due to pain of the inflamed gallbladder.

Steeple sign—In the soft tissue x-ray image of the neck or chest of a patient with croup, the subglottic area is narrowed, producing an inverted V shape or steeple shape.

String sign—In pyloric stenosis, barium contrast appears as a thin string when passing through the narrow pylorus during an upper gastrointestinal study.

Thumbprint sign—Epiglottis is enlarged and takes on the shape of a thumb in the epiglottitis compared to its normal pencil shape. Seen in the lateral neck x-ray imaging study.

Tracheal rock sign—In the presence of a retropharyngeal abscess, pain is elicited when moving the trachea and larynx from side-to-side.

Trousseau's sign—A blood pressure cuff on the upper extremity is inflated to greater than systolic pressure for 3 minutes. If the patient develops carpopedal spasm, it connotes hypocalcemia. It may also occur with hypomagnesemia.

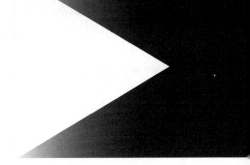

Appendix II: Syndromes

Acute chest syndrome—This is seen in a patient with sickle cell anemia, who presents with cough, chest pain, and an infiltrate on chest x-ray study.

Adult respiratory distress syndrome (ARDS)—The patient is in acute ventilatory and respiratory failure from trauma, sepsis, anaphylaxis, toxic overdose, altitude sickness, or barotraumas. The chest x-ray study shows diffuse infiltrates with a normal-sized heart.

Anterior cord syndrome—This is seen in a patient with spine trauma, who has absent motor function distal to the lesion, loss of pain and temperature sensation distal to the lesion, but who retains normal vibration and position sensation. This is seen after hyperflexion injury to the cervical spine.

Behçet's syndrome—Vasculitis. These patients demonstrate a triad that suggests vasculitis—oral ulcer, genital ulcers (epidermal or mucosal sloughing), and repeated involvement of the eye (iridocyclitis).

Boerhaave's syndrome—A full thickness tear of the esophagus from forceful vomiting.

Brown-Sequard syndrome—After penetrating trauma of the spinal column, there are ipsilateral loss of motor function and vibratory sensation below the lesion. There is a contralateral loss of pain and temperature sensations distal to the lesions.

Brugada syndrome—This lesion is either congenital or a fresh mutation of dysfunction of the cardiac sodium channels. There are ST elevations in V_1-V_3 along with a right bundle-branch block, and T-wave inversions. These patients are prone to cardiac arrest.

Carcinoid syndrome—The patient exhibits vomiting, diarrhea, and hypotension. It is induced by an endocrine tumor that can arise anywhere in the gastrointestinal tract, but occurs only if hepatic metastases are present. The patient has elevated excretion of 5-hydroxy-indoleacetic acid.

Cauda equina syndrome—An acute cord syndrome manifested by both motor and sensory losses in the legs, bowel and bladder dysfunction, and saddle anesthesia. It is most commonly seen after a herniated central intervertebral disc.

Central cord syndrome—This is a cervical spine injury induced by trauma that causes forced hyperextension of the neck. The patient exhibits an upper extremity motor weakness that is much greater than that of the lower extremities. There is also some loss of pain and temperature in the upper extremities greater than in the lower.

Compartment syndrome—Because of an increased intracompartmental pressure from trauma or repetitive physical activity, the patient develops ischemic necrosis of the muscles within the compartment. The patient has severe and constant pain in the extremity and exhibits the "5 P's": pain, pallor, paresthesias, paralysis, and pulselessness. Pain on passive extension of the digits is a sign of increased compartment pressure.

Cushing's syndrome—Hyperadrenocorticism: The patient exhibits weight gain, truncal obesity, striae, fatigue, and hypertension. The patient will be hypokalemic.

Down's syndrome—The congenital anomaly of trisomy 21. Physical features include a single transverse palmar crease, an epicanthic fold of the eyelid, short limbs, and a protruding tongue. Accompanying congenital anomalies include duodenal atresia, congenital heart disease, atlantoaxial instability, and ovarian agenesis (Turner's syndrome).

Dressler's syndrome—The patient presents with chest pain, fever, and a pleural effusion 2 to 6 weeks after myocardial infarction. This is caused by pleuropericarditis, thought to be an autoimmune reaction to the necrotic muscle cells.

Felty's syndrome—An autoimmune disease presenting with the triad of rheumatoid arthritis, neutropenia, and splenomegaly.

Fitz-Hugh-Curtis syndrome—The patient has gonorrhea, but in addition to pelvic inflammatory disease, she also has right upper quadrant abdominal tenderness and jaundice.

Goodpasture's syndrome—The patient has the signs of glomerulonephritis and hemoptysis.

Guillain-Barré syndrome—After a viral infection, the patient develops bilateral leg weakness, progressive ascending paralysis, and absent reflexes in the lower extremities.

Hair tourniquet syndrome—A baby who presents with excessive crying and with a purple toe. Hair or thread may be found tightly wound around toes, fingers, or external genitalia.

Hand-foot syndrome—This is seen in patients with sickle cell anemia and presents as a symmetric painful swelling of the hands and feet. It is a pediatric disease, with the patients falling between 6 months and 3 years of age.

Hand foot and mouth syndrome—This is a pediatric viral syndrome presenting with shallow whitish ulcers on the soft palate as well as an erythematous rash on the palms, hands, and feet.

Hemolytic-uremic syndrome (HUS)—These children present with bloody diarrhea, vomiting, abdominal pain, a low hemoglobin, and low platelets.

Hepatorenal syndrome—This is an oliguric renal failure. It complicates severe hepatic cirrhosis and appears to be caused by an altered renal vasoregulation.

Horner's syndrome—Ptosis, miosis, and anhydrosis are the presenting signs of this syndrome, caused by damage to the sympathetic branches of the brachial plexus, often due to an apical pulmonary carcinoma.

Impingement syndrome—There is limitation of active abduction of shoulder with pain on flexion, extension, and internal rotation of the shoulder. It is caused by repeated irritation of the rotator cuff, usually from the repetitive trauma induced by sport activities such as tennis or racquet ball.

Inferior vena cava (IVC) syndrome—This represents a compression of the inferior vena cava, caused by a pancreatic or hepatic tumor, or obstruction caused by vein thrombosis. The patient may present with bilateral lower extremity edema and tachycardia.

Irritable bowel syndrome (IBS)—The patient has acute and chronic abdominal pain, cramps, diarrhea, and no evident pathology. It is a somatizing syndrome thought to be a response to anxiety and life stress.

Leriche's syndrome—The patient presents with bilateral claudication of the hip or thigh with pain on activity, impotence, and hairlessness of the lower extremities. This is caused by arteriosclerotic vascular disease of the aorta and iliac and femoral arteries.

Meigs' syndrome—The patient develops ascites and a hydrothorax. It is associated with pelvic tumors, especially ovarian carcinoma.

Munchausen syndrome—A person intentionally fakes illness, causes self-injury, or undergoes painful procedures for the purpose of being treated as a patient.

Plummer-Vinson syndrome—Esophageal webs with iron deficiency anemia and cancer. This is often seen in the elderly female patient who may present with weakness, fatigue, and breathlessness induced by the anemia.

Ramsey-hunt syndrome—This is seen in patients with herpes zoster of CN VII. The patient often has vesicles on the eardrum.

Red man syndrome—This is caused by histamine release when vancomycin IV is too rapidly infused. It does not represent a drug allergy.

Reiter's syndrome—This is an autoimmune disease that presents with the triad—conjunctivitis, arthritis, and nongonococcal urethritis.

Serotonin syndrome—This toxicologic disease is thought to occur from high levels of serotonin that are induced by drug combinations. For example, combining SSRI (selective serotonin reuptake inhibitor) drugs with tricyclic antidepressants. The patient presents with confusion, increased muscle tone, hyperreflexia, hyperthermia, and "wet dog shakes."

Shaken baby syndrome—This is seen in abused children, and the presentation may be difficult to recognize before the physical examination. The child will have retinal hemorrhages.

Staphylococcal scalded skin syndrome (SSSS)—A child presents with a sandpaper-like rash, facial edema, general malaise, and fever. Flaccid bullae form in which the epidermis separates with minor pressure (positive Nikolsky's sign) from the dermis. The mucous membranes are not involved.

Steven's Johnson syndrome—The patient has multiple lesions with blisters < 10% of the body surface area. The mucous membranes are involved. It can follow infections but is often induced by medications. There is often multisystem involvement.

Sudden infant death syndrome (SIDS)—This is sudden and unexpected death of a healthy infant between one month to one year of age. It often occurs during sleep and is thought to be due to sleeping prone.

Superior vena cava (SVC) syndrome—This results from compression of the SVC. The patient may present with jugular venous distention (JVD), headache, facial plethora, a feeling of fullness in the arms, tachypnea, shortness of breath, periorbital edema, and facial swelling. The cause is usually oncologic compression by a variety of tumors.

Syndrome of inappropriate antidiuretic hormone (SIADH) secretion—The patient will have hyponatremia, a decreased serum osmolality, an increased urine sodium excretion, and an elevated urine osmolality. This often is caused by blunt head trauma.

Thoracic outlet syndrome—This occurs from compression of the brachial plexus, subclavian vein, or subclavian artery between the cervical spine and the scalene muscles of the neck. Symptoms include pain, swelling, and weakness of the arm, following repetitive arm motions with work or sport, especially those that require extension of the shoulder.

Toxic shock syndrome (TSS)—The patient presents with fever, shock, and a diffuse sunburn-like rash with subsequent desquamation within 1 to 2 weeks involving the palms and soles. There is present multisystem organ failure. The syndrome is caused by exotoxins released from certain strains of staphylococcus aureus and can follow insertion of ear tubes, orthopedic instrumentation, or utilization of vaginal tampons.

Tumor lysis syndrome—Hyperkalemia, hyperuricemia, hyperphosphatemia, and hypocalcemia following treatment with chemotherapy, and subsequent necrosis of a large mass of tumor.

Turner's syndrome—This is a congenital anomaly of female patients, XO. The patient presents with a short webbed-neck, absent ovaries, and often has angiomata of the bowel that may cause gastrointestinal bleeding. It may be seen in a female patient with Down's syndrome (see earlier text).

Wolff-Parkinson-White (WPW) syndrome—An accessory pathway causing preexcitation of the ventricles. On the EKG, there will be a delta wave present before the QRS complex. These patients often present with rapid and hard-to-diagnose tachycardias.

Appendix III:
What's in a Name—
Eponyms

Addison's disease (primary aldosterone insufficiency)—Patient presents with weight loss, fatigue, hypotension, and, often, hyperpigmentation. They also have hyponatremia and hyperkalemia. The acute disease is caused by acute adrenal destruction, as after meningococcemia.

Adie's pupil—There is a minimal reaction to light and impaired accommodation as well as slow papillary constriction and relaxation in change from near to distant vision. The affected pupil may be > normal.

Apt test—This is to determine the presence of maternal blood in the child's circulation. Mix a sample of the baby's blood with enough tap water to cause hemolysis. The sample is then centrifuged and the pink supernatant is mixed with NaOH. Fetal hemoglobin is resistant to an alkali denaturation and remains pink. Adult hemoglobin is denatured turning a yellow-brown color.

Argyll-Robertson pupil—The pupil constricts when the unaffected pupil does by accommodation but does not constrict directly in response to light. This is seen in tertiary syphilis.

Austin-Flint murmur—Soft diastolic rumble. This is auscultated with severe aortic regurgitation and is easy to confuse with mitral stenosis, except that there is usually an accompanying systolic murmur and the other signs of aortic regurgitation.

Bankart's deformity—There is a fracture of the glenoid rim. This occurs with anterior shoulder dislocation

Beck's triad—Seen in pericardial tamponade. The triad is: an elevated central venous pressure (CVP), hypotension, and muffled heart tones. It is often not observed in acute tamponade.

Bell's palsy—There is unilateral mouth drooping, facial smoothing, and an inability to close the eye or wrinkle the forehead on the affected side. This is peripheral CN VII involvement.

Bennet's fracture—This is an oblique fracture into the joint space of the thumb metacarpal.

Borchardt's triad—Sudden severe epigastric pain, abdominal distention, and vomiting, which may be seen in gastric volvulus.

Boutonniere deformity—There is a rupture of the central slip of the proximal interphalangeal (PIP) joint. This produces hyperextension of the distal interphalangeal (DIP) joint with flexion at the PIP.

Boxer's fracture—This is a fracture of the metacarpal of the little or ring finger, or both.

"Bucket handle" tear—There is a tear of the medial meniscus. The displaced central fragment resembles a bucket handle on MRI of the knee joint.

Chagas' disease—This is an infection caused by *trypanosoma cruzi*. The patient presents with fever, conjunctivitis, myocarditis, and megacolon.

Chance fracture—This is caused by lap belt only, seat belt injury of the abdomen, with fractures of the pedicles and vertebral body and of the posterior spinous process. It is usually accompanied by paralysis distal to the fracture, and by intraabdominal injury, classically a tear of the small bowel mesentery.

Charcot joint—The ankle joint feels like a "bag of worms." It is boggy and painless. This occurs in a denervated joint, for example, in a patient with diabetes, and is caused by chronic trauma causing multiple small fractures, which are unperceived by the patient because of the denervation.

Charcot's triad in ascending cholangitis—There is high fever with shaking chills, right upper quadrant (RUQ) abdominal pain, and jaundice.

Clay shoveler's fracture—This is a hyperflexion injury to the spinous process of the cervical vertebra, usually C_7; it is stable.

Colles' fracture—This occurs after a fall on an outstretched hand. It produces a fracture of the radius, with dorsal angulation, and usually an avulsion fracture of the distal ulnar styloid. This produces the classic deformity described as a "silver fork."

Corrigan pulse—Also known as waterhammer pulse, this represents an exaggerated peripheral pulse on palpation due to severe aortic regurgitation.

Crohn's disease (regional enteritis)—There are multiple enteropathic "skip lesions" from mouth to anus involving all bowel layers.

Crutch palsy—Compression of radial nerve caused by allowing the crutch to impinge on the axillae during crutch walking rather than using the forearm and hand to brace the crutch.

Curling's ulcers—These are "stress ulcers in stomach or duodenum" that are seen in patients who sustained bad burns.

Cushing's ulcers—These are "stress ulcers in stomach or duodenum" that are seen in patients with severe brain injury.

de Quervain's tenosynovitis—This is a painful mass in the hand that comes from inflammation of the extensor pollicis brevis and abductor pollicis longus.

"Drop arm test"—The patient's arm is passively raised to 90° of abduction and lowered slowly. If the patient is unable to sustain the abducted position of the arm (the arm "drops"), this is a positive test and indicates a rotator cuff tear.

Dupuytren's contracture—There is an inflammatory contracture of the flexor tendons of the hand. This is seen in chronic alcoholism but may also occur from the repeated trauma of construction work.

Eaton-Lambert—This is an autoimmune disorder of neuromuscular transmission. Patient presents with proximal muscle weakness, especially in the lower extremities, that improves with activity. In addition, there may be autonomic, oropharyngeal, or ocular muscle involvement.

Ehlers-Danlos—This is a congenital connective tissue disease that occurs in many forms. It leads to spontaneous internal hemorrhages, joint laxity and hyperextensible skin. The external deformities may be missing, and the patient presents with severe internal hemorrhage after very minor or no trauma. It may be a cause of aortic transaction.

Ellis fractures types I–III—This is a classification of tooth fractures.
- Type I—This involves only the enamel.
- Type II—The enamel is involved along with exposed dentin.
- Type III—In this form, the pulp is exposed.

Fournier's gangrene—Fulminating gangrene of the scrotum, caused by necrotizing fasciitis from a gram-negative anaerobic bacteria.

Galeazzi's fracture—A radial shaft fracture with dislocation of the radial–ulnar joint.

Gamekeeper's thumb—Rupture of the ulnar collateral ligament of the thumb caused by forced hyperabduction. This is also known as skier's thumb.

Gonococcal dermatitis—Multiple tender lesions with gray necrotic or hemorrhagic centers.

Grave's disease—This is the classical patient with hyperactive thyroid disease. The patient presents with goiter, exophthalmos, tachycardia, heat intolerance, hair loss, weakness, and excessive sweating.

Hamman's crunch—A clicking rub heard over the precordium synchronous with the heartbeat in mediastinitis associated with esophageal rupture.

Hampton's hump—There is a wedge-shaped infiltrate (rounded border facing the hilus) seen on the chest x-ray study caused by pulmonary embolism. It is rare, and late finding, because it represents pulmonary infarction.

Henoch-Schönlein purpura (HSP)—This is a vasculitis presenting with a purpuric rash on the buttocks or abdomen and producing diffuse abdominal and joint pain. It may be confused with nonaccidental trauma and meningococcemia.

Heraldic patch—Solitary round erythematous scaly plaque seen 5 to 10 days before the development of the generalized rash seen in pityriasis rosea.

Herpangina—These are painful ulcerations seen on the posterior pharynx.

Hill-Sachs deformity—Posterior lateral defect of the humeral head as it impacts on the anterior rim of the glenoid fossa. It connotes recurrent episodes of dislocation.

Hirschsprung's disease—This is a congenital disease causing a lack of ganglionic nerve cells in the wall of the large bowel. It causes megacolon, constipation, and, in the infant, may present with fulminating colitis.

Hutchinson fracture—There is an isolated avulsion fracture to the radial styloid. Also known as a "Chauffeur fracture."

Janeway lesions—These are nontender plaques on the palms and soles that are sometimes seen in infective endocarditis.

Jarisch-Herxheimer reaction—There is a marked febrile reaction with an erythematous rash that occurs immediately after penicillin administration in a syphilitic patient.

Jefferson's fracture—Vertical compression of C_1 ring. There is widening of the predental space seen on the lateral cervical-spine x-ray study.

Jones criteria—These are used to diagnose rheumatic fever. A positive diagnosis requires two major, or one major and two minor, criteria to be present.
- **Major**—Arthritis, carditis, chorea, erythema marginatum, or subcutaneous nodules.
- **Minor**—Fever, arthralgias, a history of rheumatic heart disease, an elevated erythrocyte sedimentation rate (ESR), an elevated C-reactive protein (CRP) level, an elevated antistreptolysin-*O* (ASO) titer, and an increased PR interval.

Jones fracture—This is a transverse fracture of the metatarsal base of the little toe.

Kaposi's sarcoma—Painless and raised brown-black or purple nodules that do not blanch. They are seen anywhere on the body in AIDS patients.

Kawasaki's disease—Also known as the mucocutaneous lymph node syndrome. The child presents with prolonged fever, a strawberry tongue, conjunctivitis, a desquamating rash, and enlarged lymph nodes.

Kerley B lines—These are horizontal lines at the edge of the pleural border seen in the chest x-ray study in congestive heart failure.

Keyser-Fleisher ring—These are dark rings around the iris of the eye. Seen in Wilson's disease due to abnormal metabolism of copper resulting in excessive copper deposits in body tissue.

Kienböck's disease—There is collapse of the lunate bone of the wrist due to avascular necrosis.

Kleihauer-Betke (KB) test—KB test is a blood test used to measure the amount of fetal hemoglobin transferred to the bloodstream of an Rh-negative mother. An aliquot of the mother's blood is taken to make a blood smear. Acid bath removes all maternal hemoglobin, and, on subsequent staining, the fetal hemoglobin appears a rose-pink color.

Koplik's spots—Bright red spots with bluish white centers seen on the buccal mucosa. These are seen with rubella (measles). They actually occur throughout the gastrointestinal (GI) tract and can cause a picture of acute appendicitis.

Korsakoff's psychosis—The patient presents with chronic organic brain syndrome with confusion, ataxia, and nystagmus associated with anterograde or retrograde amnesia. This is seen in chronic alcoholism and is the end stage of Wernicke's encephalopathy, the acute organic brain syndrome seen from thiamine deficiency in alcoholics.

Kussmaul's breathing—These are involuntary deep rapid respirations that are often painful and fatiguing and often seen in diabetic ketoacidosis.

Lachman's test—This is a test for anterior cruciate ligament (ACL) integrity. With the patient supine, flex the knee in 20 to 30 degrees. Place one hand on the patient's thigh and the other hand behind the tibia. When pulling anteriorly on the tibia, if the ACL is torn, the tibia will move anterior to the femur.

LeFort—Facial fracture classification:
- I—Fracture alveolar ridge below nose—There is mobility of the upper teeth and hard palate.
- II—Pyramidal area—Maxilla, nasal bones, and medial orbits. There is midface mobility due to the fractures of the orbital pillars, and the patient has a deformed "dish face."
- III—There are fractures through the zygomaticofacial sutures yielding complete craniofacial dislocation.
  Levels of Le Fort fractures are often mixed between sides of the face.

Legg-Calve-Perthes—Idiopathic, avascular osteochondrosis of the femoral head with stress fractures of the affected hip and a limited range of motion. The hip x-ray study reveals a smaller-than-normal femoral head with resorption.

Leibman-Sachs lesions—These are vegetative growths on heart valves seen in endocarditis.

Lichtenberg figures—This is the superficial fern pattern from being struck by lightning.

Lisfranc's fracture—This is a fracture between the midfoot and the forefoot.

Little leaguer's elbow—This is a medial epicondyle avulsion from throwing too far, or too hard.

Ludwig's angina—Fever, brawny induration of the anterior neck and trismus are seen in a patient with infection of the floor of the mouth by anaerobic organisms, which may emanate from a molar infection.

Lyme disease—Malaise, headache, and an annular erythematous rash with central clearing caused by an infected wood tick bite.

Maisonneuve fracture—This is a proximal fibular fracture with an associated ankle fracture and a deltoid ligament tear.

Malgaigne's fracture—This is a fracture of the ileum along with a symphyseal dislocation.

Mallampati classification—This is used to determine the difficulty of intubation:

- Grade I—All of the faucial pillars, soft palate, and uvula are visualized.
- Grade II—The faucial pillars and soft palate are visualized.
- Grade III—Only the base of the uvula is visualized.
- Grade IV—Only the tongue can be seen.

Mallory-Weiss tear—These are mucosal tears (partial thickness) at the junction of the esophagus and stomach following repeated vomiting. They may be seen in patients with bulimia.

Maltese cross—A cross with triangular-shaped arms with the points toward the center. Used to describe intraerythrocyte ring formations in the peripheral blood smear in patients infected with baseosis.

Marfan's syndrome—This is a congenital autosomal-dominant disease with variable degrees of expression. The patients have a connective tissue disorder characterized by long extremities, lens subluxation, and cardiovascular abnormalities, typically aortic dissection.

McMurray's test—This is used to examine for a meniscal tear. Flex the knee to 90°. Place one hand on the lateral side of the knee, and with the other hand rotate the foot externally while extending the knee. If pain or a "click" is felt, the test is considered positive.

Meckel's diverticulum—This is a congenital malformation of the GI tract that produces an outpouching diverticulum of the distal ileum. The diverticulum often has ectopic gastric mucosa present, and this can cause the patient to have GI bleeding, perforation, or abdominal pain that appears like acute appendicitis.

"Meckel's rule of twos"—The diverticulum appears: in 2% of population, 2% will have symptoms, the diverticulum is 2 feet proximal to the terminal ileum, and many of the patients are< 2 years old.

Ménière's disease—This disease produces vertigo, hearing loss, and tinnitus resulting from nonsuppurative disease of the labyrinth.

Mittelschmerz—This is the name given young women with abdominal or pelvic pain that is thought to be caused by midcycle ovulation. It often is confused with appendicitis and ectopic pregnancy.

Mondor's disease—This is a superficial phlebitis of the subcutaneous veins of the breast. It is sometimes seen in nursing mothers who have developed a mastitis. It may be confused with inflammatory breast cancer.

Monteggia's fracture—This is a proximal ulnar fracture with dislocation of the radial head.

Myasthenia gravis—This is an autoimmune neuromuscular disease that presents with weakness that is worse after activity. The circulating antibodies block acetylcholine receptors at the postsynaptic neuromuscular junction, thereby preventing the stimulating effect of acetylcholine.

Nightstick fracture—This is an isolated, ulnar, nondisplaced transverse fracture.

Norwalk virus—A common cause of gastroenteritis with nausea, vomiting, diarrhea, and abdominal cramps.

Nursemaid's elbow—This represents a radial head subluxation. It follows a sudden jerking of the child's arm; the child holds the hand in pronation with elbow flexion.

Nylen-Barany (Hallpike) maneuvers—These are used to treat vertigo. Turn the patient's head quickly from side to side after bringing the patient from an upright seated to a supine position. If this relieves the vertigo, the patient has benign positional vertigo.

Ortolani test—Checks for hip dysplasia in infant. With the infant supine, the examiner abducts the child's knees. During abduction, the examiner hears a distinct "clicking" sound.

Osgood-Schlatter disease—This is osteochondrosis of the tibial tuberosity. The child presents with gradual knee pain that worsens with activities.

Osler nodes—These are tender nodules on the tips of the fingers and toes. They are associated with infective endocarditis.

Ottawa ankle rules—Obtain ankle x-ray if there is tenderness on the posterior edge, or the tip of the distal 6 cm of either malleolus. Also, if the patient is unable to bear weight for four steps either immediately after the injury or in ED.

Paget's disease—This is a chronic disorder of breakdown and reformation of bone tissue resulting in fractures, deformed bones, and a characteristic hyperdense appearance on the x-ray study. The bone appears thicker than normal but is very porous and vascular, and even small fractures may lead to extensive bleeding.

Pantaloon hernia—A direct and indirect inguinal hernia on the same side.

Parkinson's disease—A wasting neurologic disease that presents with cogwheel rigidity, resting tremor, and akinesia or bradykinesia. There is an impairment of posture and equilibrium.

Pellagra—This is a nutritional disorder caused by the lack of niacin (vitamin B_3). It presents with four D's: dermatitis, dementia, diarrhea, and death.

Peyronie's disease—There are thickened plaques involving the tunica albuginea resulting in a curvature of the penis and painful erections.

Posterior drawer test—This is a test for posterior collateral ligament injury. With the patient supine, flex the knee 90°. Grasp the anterior tibia and push backwards. If the tibia moves posteriorly more than normal (compared with the uninjured leg), the test is positive.

Potter's faces—The newborn child will have a flattened nose, recessed chin, prominent epicanthal folds, and abnormal low set ears, possibly due to oligohydramnios secondary to renal disease such as bilateral renal agenesis.

"Pott's puffy tumor"—There is obvious and tender nonpitting swelling of the forehead. This is seen with sinusitis and probably represents osteomyelitis of the frontal bones, along with abscess formation.

Pseudo-Jones fracture—This is a longitudinal avulsion fracture at the tuberosity of the base of the 5th metatarsal.

Quinsy—Synonym for a peritonsillar abscess.

Raynaud's disease—A vascular disorder affecting blood flow to fingers, toes, nose, and ears when exposed to cold temperatures.

Rigler's triad—Also known as gallstone ileus. Pneumobilia, dilated small bowel, and an ectopic calcified single large gallstone. The gallbladder ruptures into the small bowel, and distal movement of the large stone causes obstruction of the small bowel, usually at the terminal ileum, because the stone cannot pass the ileocecal valve. Rarely, it does pass but cannot be expelled from the rectum and causes a large bowel obstruction.

Rinne's test—Test of hearing with tuning fork placed first on the mastoid process and when the sound is no longer heard, the fork is placed just outside the ear. If the patient hears the sound better with the mastoid placement, there is a conductive loss of hearing. If the ear hearing is louder than the bone, this is normal and is considered a normal result. If both are equal, there is a sensorineural hearing loss.

Rocky Mountain spotted fever (RMSF)—This is a rickettsial tick-borne disease causing fever, myalgia, headache, abdominal pain, and rash that spreads from the wrists to the palms and the soles. It is more common in the South than in the Rocky Mountain regions.

Rolando fracture—This is a comminuted intraarticular fracture of the thumb metacarpal joint.

Romberg test—The patient stands with feet together and arms at the sides. If the patient sways or is unable to stand when the eyes are closed, the test is positive and indicates a defect in the spinal cord posterior columns. If the patient cannot stand with eyes open, there is a cerebellar hemorrhage.

Roseola—One of the pediatric viral exanthems; there are 4 to 5 days of high fever. When the fever defervesces, the rash appears.

Roth's spots—Retinal hemorrhages with central clearing. They may be seen in infective endocarditis.

Rubella (German measles)—3 days of rash with large postauricular and postcervical lymph nodes; dangerous during pregnancy.

Rubeola (measles)—Fever, conjunctivitis, otitis media, and often pneumonia.

"St. Anthony's fire" (Erysipelas)—This is a rash that exhibits lesions with a bright red, raised, and well-demarcated border. It is caused by a group A streptococcus.

Salter Harris fractures—Classification of growth plate fractures:
- I—Epiphyseal plate disruption; may not be seen in x-ray study
- II—Epiphyseal plate + metaphysic; no growth disturbance
- III—Epiphyseal plate + epiphysis; growth disturbance may occur
- IV—Epiphyseal plate + metaphysis + epiphysis; growth disturbance in high proportion
- V—Crush injury to epiphysis; growth arrest often

Scarlet fever—The patient presents with fever, strawberry tongue, and sandpaper rash. It is caused by group A beta-hemolytic streptococci.

Schatzki's ring—Diaphragm-like stricture near the gastroesophageal junction; it probably relates to scarring from regurgitation.

Schiotz tonometry—Used to detect glaucoma. The instrument measurements are inversely related to the seriousness or presence of the disease, that is, the lower the number on the tonometer, the higher is the intraocular pressure.

School of fish—Based on the appearance of the Gram's stain: gram-negative bacilli in linear or parallel formation. When seen, it diagnoses chancroid.

Seidel's test—Under blue light, there will be a streaming of the fluorescein dye in a patient with a ruptured globe.

Smith's fracture—This is a radial fracture and volar angulation from a fall on a flexed wrist. This is the opposite of a Colles' fracture, a fall on an extended hand with dorsal angulation of the radial fracture.

Somogyi phenomenon—Hyperglycemic rebound from transient hypoglycemia. The patient is often treated with an increased dose of insulin because of the hyperglycemic level.

Stenson's duct—Parotid gland that empties opposite to the maxillary molars.

Strawberry cervix—This is a punctate appearance of the cervix seen in trichomoniasis.

Sudeck's atrophy—Posttraumatic osteoporosis. It is the same as reflex sympathetic dystrophy.

Tarasoff—"Duty to Warn" concept. If a patient is expressing homicidal thoughts, either warn the person he or she wants to kill, or place the patient on a mental health hold.

Tardieu's spots—These are seen following an asphyxial death. They are petechial hemorrhages seen on the conjunctiva, mucous membranes, and skin cephalad to the strangling ligature.

Tetralogy of Fallot (TOF)—This is a congenital heart defect consisting of a ventricular septal defect (VSD), pulmonary stenosis, overriding aorta, and right ventricular hypertrophy. The child may present within the first few months of life with episodic cyanotic events while feeding; the O_2 saturation does not improve with oxygen administration. The older child also has spells in which relief is obtained by kneeling.

Thompson's test—With the patient supine, squeeze the calf. The test is positive if there is no plantar flexion. The positive test indicates a rupture of the achilles tendon.

Todd's paralysis—This is a focal postictal paralysis that can demonstrate any degree or location of focal finding.

Virchow's triad—Venous stasis, hypercoagulability, and endothelial damage; these are the causes of venous thrombosis.

Volkmann's ischemic contracture—This is muscle atrophy with a disabling flexion contracture of the wrist or hand. This is a complication of ischemia from compartment syndrome induced often by a circular cast that has been placed before fracture swelling has subsided.

von Willebrand disease—This is a genetic autosomal dominant disease that presents with epistaxis, menorrhagia, or GI bleed.

Waldenström's macroglobulinemia—This is a non-Hodgkin's lymphoma that causes overproduction of IgM antibody.

Water-hammer pulse—Visible and bounding peripheral pulses. Seen in severe aortic regurgitation.

Waterhouse-Friderichsen syndrome—Shock, petechiae, and adrenal infarction. This is often caused by meningococcemia.

Water's view—This is a facial imaging view obtained by passing the x-ray beam through the chin at an oblique angle in order to demonstrate the maxillary and frontal sinuses.

Weber test—Place the tuning fork in the middle of the patient's forehead; if hearing is greater on one side, that is a positive test, and indicates conductive hearing loss in that ear. If heard louder in the unaffected ear, then there is a sensorineural loss in the affected ear.

"Welder's flash"—This is an ultraviolet keratitis from tanning, eclipse viewing without dark lens protection, or snow blindness.

Wernicke's encephalopathy—This is an acute organic brain syndrome caused by thiamine deficiency, which produces an acute delirium, ataxia, and nystagmus. It is most often seen in alcoholics. It can theoretically be produced if sugar is administered to a hypoglycemic alcoholic patient prior to thiamine.

Wharton's duct—This drains the submandibular or sublingual gland in the floor of the mouth.

Wilms tumor—This is a malignant kidney tumor that may be present as a palpable mass at birth. It may also present with hematuria in an infant or child.

Wilson's disease—Cirrhosis of liver caused by excessive copper retention.

Zenker's diverticulum—This is a pharyngoesophageal pouch presenting in the upper third of the esophagus.

Appendix IV: Mnemonics

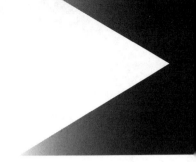

CHAMP—**C**amphor, **H**alogenated, **A**romatic, **M**etals, and **P**esticide.

CHIPS—**C**hloral hydrate, **H**eavy metal, **I**odide, **I**ron, **P**sychotropics, **P**henothiazine, and **S**ustained-release potassium.

DUMBELLS—**D**iaphoresis, **U**rination, **M**iosis, **B**radycardia, **E**mesis, **L**acrimation **L**ethargy, and **S**alivation.

MUDPILES—**M**ethanol, **U**remia, **D**KA, **P**araldehyde, **I**ron, INH, **L**actic acid, **E**thanol, and **S**alicylates.

SALT—**S**alicylates, **A**lcohols, **L**ithium, and **T**heophylline.

SLUDGE—**S**alivation, **L**acrimation, **U**rinary incontinence, **D**iarrhea, **G**I symptoms, and **E**mesis.

Bibliography

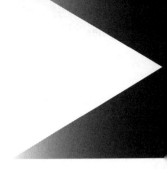

ATLS Advanced Trauma Life Support Program for Doctors. 7th ed. Chicago: American College of Surgeons; 2004.

Brant W, Helms C. *Fundamentals of Diagnostic Imaging.* 2nd ed. Baltimore: Williams and Wilkins; 1999.

Cline DM, Kellen GD. *Just the Facts in Emergency Medicine.* New York: McGraw-Hill; 2004.

Collman D, Plantz S, Adler J. *Emergency Medicine Pearls of Wisdom.* Boston: Boston Medical Publishing; 2000.

Garcia TB, Holtz NE. *Introduction to 12-Lead ECG: The Art of Interpretation.* Sudbury, MA: Jones and Bartlett Publishers; 2003.

Garcia TB, Holtz NE. *12-Lead ECG: The Art of Interpretation.* Sudbury, MA: Jones and Bartlett Publishers; 2001.

Hart RG, Rittenberry TJ, Uehara D. *Handbook of Orthopaedic Emergencies.* Philadelphia: Lippincott-Raven; 1999.

Koenig KL. *Clinical Emergency Medicine Pretest Self-Assess and Review.* New York: McGraw-Hill; 1996.

Koenig KL. *Emergency Medicine Pretest Self-Assessment and Review.* 2nd ed. New York: McGraw-Hill; 2000.

Marx JA, Hockberger RS, Walls RM, eds. *Rosen's Emergency Medicine Concepts and Clinical Practice.* 6th ed. New York: Elsevier Health Sciences; 2006.

Rivers CS, Weber DE. *Preparing for the Written Board Exam in Emergency Medicine.* 3rd ed. Milford, OH: Emergency Medicine Educational Enterprises, Inc.; 2000.

Schaider J, Barkin R, Hayden S, Rosen P, Wolfe R. *5 Minute Emergency Medicine Consult.* Philadelphia: Lippincott William and Wilkins; 2006.

Shah B, Laude T. *Atlas of Pediatric Clinical Diagnosis.* Philadelphia: W.B. Saunders Co.; 2000.

Simon RR, Sherman SC, Koenigsknecht SJ. *Emergency Orthopedics—The Extremities.* 5th ed. Connecticut: Appleton and Lange; 2006.

Thomas J, O'Connor RE, Hoffman GL. *Emergency Medicine Self-Assessment and Review.* St. Louis: Mosby; 1999.

Tintinalli JE, Kelen GD, Stapczynski JS. *Emergency Medicine: A Comprehensive Study Guide.* 6th ed. New York: McGraw-Hill; 2003.

Wagner MJ, ed. *PEER-VII: Physician's Evaluation and Educational Review in Emergency Medicine.* Volume 7. Kansas City, MO: The Covington Group; 2007.

Wiest P, Roth P. *Fundamentals of Emergency Radiology.* Philadelphia: W.B. Saunders Co.; 1996.

Index

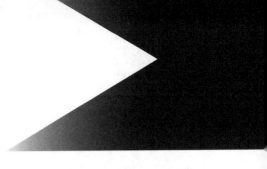